T0141812

Studies in Fuzziness and Soft Computing

Volume 347

Series editor

Janusz Kacprzyk, Polish Academy of Sciences, Warsaw, Poland
e-mail: kacprzyk@ibspan.waw.pl

About this Series

The series "Studies in Fuzziness and Soft Computing" contains publications on various topics in the area of soft computing, which include fuzzy sets, rough sets, neural networks, evolutionary computation, probabilistic and evidential reasoning, multi-valued logic, and related fields. The publications within "Studies in Fuzziness and Soft Computing" are primarily monographs and edited volumes. They cover significant recent developments in the field, both of a foundational and applicable character. An important feature of the series is its short publication time and world-wide distribution. This permits a rapid and broad dissemination of research results.

More information about this series at http://www.springer.com/series/2941

Laécio Carvalho de Barros
Rodney Carlos Bassanezi
Weldon Alexander Lodwick

A First Course in Fuzzy Logic, Fuzzy Dynamical Systems, and Biomathematics

Theory and Applications

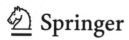 Springer

Laécio Carvalho de Barros
Departamento de Matemática Aplicada
Universidade Estadual de Campinas
São Paulo
Brazil

Rodney Carlos Bassanezi
Centro de Matemática e Computação
Universidade Federal do ABC
Santo André, São Paulo
Brazil

Weldon Alexander Lodwick
Department of Mathematical and Statistical
  Sciences
University of Colorado Denver
Denver, CO
USA

ISSN 1434-9922   ISSN 1860-0808   (electronic)
Studies in Fuzziness and Soft Computing
ISBN 978-3-662-57132-3   ISBN 978-3-662-53324-6   (eBook)
DOI 10.1007/978-3-662-53324-6

This Springer imprint is published by Springer Nature
The registered company is Springer-Verlag GmbH Germany
The registered company address is: Heidelberger Platz 3, 14197 Berlin, Germany

The authors wish to thank all their students who over the years graced our presence and with whom we share a space in time devoted to our mutual love of mathematics and the pursuit of truth. In particular, we would like to thank Estevão Esmi Laurenao for the assistance in reading, editing early versions, and with the layout of the text and figures.

Preface

This book is the result of courses we have given for more than a decade to upper level undergraduate students and to graduate students majoring in mathematics, applied mathematics, statistics, and engineering. In this book the reader will encounter the basic concepts that span the initial notions of fuzzy sets to more advanced notions of fuzzy differential equation and dynamical systems. We follow, in our ordering of topics, a pedagogical unfolding beginning with classical theory such as set theory and probability in such a way that these serve as an opening into the fuzzy case. Moreover, the classical differential and integral calculus is the beginning step from which fuzzy differential and integral analysis are developed.

There are various derivatives and integrals that exist and applied in the context of fuzzy functions. These are clearly delineated and interpreted in our presentation of fuzzy integral and differential equations.

Each of the major topics is accompanied with examples, worked exercises and exercises to be completed. Many applications of our concept to real problems are found throughout the book.

Even though this book may be, and has been, used as a textbook for various courses, in it are sufficient ideas for beginning the research projects in fuzzy mathematics. It is the hope of the authors that our joy, passion, and respect for all who seriously the study of fuzzy mathematics, modeling, and applications, emerges through the written page.

Laécio Carvalho de Barros
Rodney Carlos Bassanezi
Weldon Alexander Lodwick

Acknowledgment

The authors would like to acknowledge and thank the partial support received from CNPq.

Contents

About the Authors

Laécio Carvalho de Barros is Professor of Applied Mathematics at the Institute of Mathematics, Statistics and Computational Sciences, the University of Campinas, and holds a Ph.D. degree in Applied Mathematics from the University of Campinas, São Paulo, Brazil, in 1997. He is the co-author of the book *Fuzzy Logic in Action: Applications in Epidemiology and Beyond*, Studies in Fuzziness and Soft Computing Vol. 232, 2008, Springer-Verlag Berlin Heidelberg, and of the book *Fuzzy Differential Equations in Various Approaches*, SpringerBriefs in Mathematics, Number 1, 2015, Springer International Publishing. His current research interests include modeling of biological phenomena, fuzzy sets theory and fuzzy dynamical systems. Moreover, he has taught fuzzy mathematical modeling and fuzzy set theory classes for over 15 years to both undergraduate and graduate students.

Rodney Carlos Bassanezi is Professor Emeritus of Applied Mathematics at the Institute of Mathematics, Statistics and Computational Sciences at the University of Campinas starting his university teaching career there in 1969. He received a Ph.D. degree in Mathematics from the University of Campinas in 1977. He held post-doctoral and research positions at the Libera Universitad di Trento, Italy 1981, 1985, 1990, and 1993. His research activities cover mathematical analysis (minimal surfaces), biomathematics, and fuzzy dynamical systems. He has published some books in Portuguese, notably one textbook on differential equations (1988), one textbook on mathematical modeling (2002), as well as an introduction to calculus and applications (2015). He has been the president of the Sociedade Latino-Americano de Biomatemática (1999–2001) and the coordinator of the graduate program in mathematics at the Federal University ABC in São Paulo. He has directed 55 Masters and 21 Ph.D. theses and his students have been teaching throughout Latin American.

Weldon Alexander Lodwick is Professor of Mathematics at the University of Colorado Denver. He holds a Ph.D. degree in Mathematics (1980) from Oregon State University, He is the co-editor of the book *Fuzzy Optimization: Recent Developments and Applications*, Studies in Fuzziness and Soft Computing Vol. 254, Springer-Verlag Berlin Heidelberg, 2010, and the author of the monograph *Interval and Fuzzy Analysis: A Unified Approach* in *Advances in Imaging and Electronic Physics,* Vol. 148, pp. 76–192, Elsevier, 2007. His current research interests include interval analysis, distance geometry, as well as flexible and generalized uncertainty optimization. Over the last 30 years he has taught applied mathematical modeling classes to undergraduate and graduate students on topics such as radiation therapy of tumor, fuzzy and possibilistic optimization modeling, molecular distance geometry problems, and neural networks applied to control problems.

Chapter 1
Fuzzy Sets Theory and Uncertainty in Mathematical Modeling

Man is the measure of all things: of things which are, that they are, and of things which are not, that they are not.

(Protagoras – 5th Century BCE)

Abstract This chapter presents a brief discussion about uncertainty based on philosophical principles, mainly from the point of view of the pre-Socratic philosophers. Next, the notions of fuzzy sets and operations on fuzzy sets are presented. Lastly, the concepts of alpha-level and the statement of the well-known Negoita-Ralescu Representation Theorem, the representation of a fuzzy set by its alpha-levels, are discussed.

1.1 Uncertainty in Modeling and Analysis

The fundamental entity of analysis for this book is *set*, a collection of objects. A second fundamental entity for this book is *variable*. The variable represents what one wishes to investigate by a mathematical modeling process that aims to quantify it. In this context, the variable is a symbolic receptacle of what one wishes to know. The quantification process involves a set of values which is ascribed a-priori. Thus, when one talks about a variable being fuzzy, a real-number, a random number, and so on, one is ascribing to the variable its attribution.

A set also has an existence or context. That is, when one is in the process of creating a mathematical model, one ascribes to sets attributions associated with the model or problem at hand. One speaks of a set being a classical set, a fuzzy set, a set of distributions, a random sets, and so on. Given that models of existent problems or conditions are far from ideal deterministic mathematical entities, we are interested in dealing directly with associated inexactitudes and so ascribe to our fundamental objects of modeling and analysis properties of determinism (exactness) and non-determinism (inexactness).

This book is about processes in which uncertainty both in the input or data side and in the relational structure is inherent to the problem at hand. Social and biological

© Springer-Verlag Berlin Heidelberg 2017
L.C. de Barros et al., *A First Course in Fuzzy Logic, Fuzzy Dynamical Systems, and Biomathematics*, Studies in Fuzziness and Soft Computing 347, DOI 10.1007/978-3-662-53324-6_1

the modeling are characterized by such uncertainties. The mathematical theory on which we focus to enable modeling with uncertainty occurring in biological and social systems is fuzzy set theory first developed by L. Zadeh [1].

Uncertainty has long been a concern of researchers and philosophers alike, throughout the ages as it is to us in this present book. The pursuit of the truth, of what is, of what exists, which is one aspect of uncertainty if we characterize truth or existence certainty, has been debated since the dawn of thinking. In ancient Greece individuals and schools explicitly asked the question: "What exists? Is everything in transformation or is there permanence?" These are two dimensions of thought and can be considered completely separate issues and even contradictory issues.

The pre-Socratic philosophers tried to make statements summarizing their thoughts about the Universe in an attempt to explain what is existent in the universe. In the words of Heraclitus of Ephesus (6th to 5th Century BCE), "panta hei", which means "everything flows, everything changes". By way of illustration, consider a situation in which a river is never the same, one cannot bathe in the same river twice. Cratylus, his disciple, took Heraclitus' thoughts to the extreme by saying that we cannot bathe in the river even once, because if we assign an identity to things or give them names, we are also giving stability to these things which, in his view, are undergoing constant change.

The Eleatic school, in contrast to Heraclitus, questions the existence of motion or change itself. According to Parmenides of Elea (6th to 5th Century BCE): "the only thing that exists is the being - which is the same as thinking". Zeno, his main follower, denies that there is motion as this was understood at the time by giving his famous paradox of Achilles and the turtle [2].

The Sophists interpret what Parmenides said as the impossibility of false rhetoric. According to Protagoras (5th Century BCE): "Man is the measure of all things". There is no absolute truth or falsehood. In the Sophists' view, humankind must seek solutions in the practical. The criterion of true or false is related to the theoretical and must therefore be replaced by (more practical) patterns related to the concepts of better or worse. Rhetoric is the way to find such patterns.

Most of the pre-Socratic philosophers with the exception of Heraclitus, believed there was something eternal and unchanging behind the coming-to-be (that which is in the process of being, of becoming), that was the eternal source, the foundation of all beings. According to Thales, it was water; in the opinion of Anaximenes, the air; Pythagoras thought it was numbers; and, Democritus believed that this source lay in the atoms and in the void. This eternal something which was unchangeable and which held all things was called by the Greeks *arche*.

Certainty and uncertainty were widely discussed by Greek philosophers. The Sophists (a term derived from sophistes, sages) were known to teach the art of rhetoric. Protagoras, the most important Sophist along with Górgias, taught students how to turn weaknesses of argument into strengths. Rhetoric, for the Sophists, is a posture or attitude with respect to knowledge that has a total skepticism in relation to any kind of absolute knowledge. This, no matter how things are, is because everything is relative and also depends on who gives judgement about them. Górgias said that rhetoric surpasses all other arts, being the best because it makes all things submit to spontaneity rather than to violence. As is well known, Socrates confronted the Sophists of his day with the question: "What is?" That is, if everything is relative, what exists?

Plato, a disciple of Socrates, initially shared the ideas of Heraclitus that everything is changing, the flow of coming-to-be, everything was in process. However, if everything was in motion then knowledge would not be possible. To avoid falling back into skepticism, Plato thought of a "world of ideas". Around this world, there would be changes, and things would be eternal beyond the space-time dimension. The so-called "sensory world", which is the world as perceived by the five senses, would then come into being. It would be true that the "world of ideas" would be behind the coming-to-be of this "sensory world". For Plato the most important thing was not the final concept, but the path taken to reach it. The "world of ideas" is not accessible by the senses but rather just by intuition, while intellectual dialectics is the movement of asceticism in pursuit of the truth. Therefore, Plato promotes a synthesis between Heraclitus and Parmenides.

On the other hand, for Aristotle, the world of ideas and essences is not contained in things themselves. Universal knowledge is linked to its underlying logic (the Logos, the same reason, the principle of order and study of the consequences) and also the syllogism, which is the formal mechanism for deduction. Based on certain general assumptions, knowledge must strictly follow an order using the concept of the demonstrative syllogism. In short, and perhaps naively, we think that the most important difference between Aristotle and the Sophists is the fact that, for Aristotle, there is an eternal, an immutable, independent of human beings, while the Sophists consider that there is no eternal and absolute truth, but rather just the knowledge obtained from our senses. For Plato and Aristotle, respectively, dialectics and syllogisms are to be used in the quest for the truth. The Sophists consider that rhetoric, the art of persuasion, is convincing in relation to the search for the truth, because truth does not exist as an absolute.

Understanding that subjectivity, imprecision, uncertainty, are inherent to certain terms of language, Górgias denied the existence of absolute truth: even if absolute truth existed, it would be incomprehensible to man, even if it were comprehensible to one man, it would not be communicable to others. In order to stimulate our thought about this aspect of the uncertainty of language, we will try to reach a compromise between the positions of the Sophists, on the one hand, and Plato and Aristotle, on the other, by means of a simple example.

It is common practice to propose a meeting with another person by saying something like "Let's meet at four o'clock". Well, the abstract concept of "four o'clock", indicating a measurement of time, shows a need to establish communication (in the abstract) and also enable the holding of the event, our meeting. If this were not the case, how should we then communicate our meeting? - A point for Plato. On the other hand, if we take this at face value, the meeting would never take place as our respective clocks would never reach four o'clock simultaneously, even if they had been synchronized, as we could not get to the point marked in hours, minutes, seconds, and millionths of seconds. A point for Górgias. Admitting that we often carry out our commitments at the appointed time and place, it looks like we equally need abstract truths and practical standards of a sensible world.

We articulated the thoughts above in order to point out the difficulty of talking about certainty or uncertainty and of fuzzy or determinism. If we look in a dictionary for terms synonymous with uncertainty, we find, for example: subjectivity, inaccuracy, randomness, doubt, ambiguity, and unpredictably, among others. Historically, researchers, from what we have noticed, have, in their quantitative treatment, made distinctions between the different types of uncertainty. The uncertainty arising from the randomness of events has been well documented, and now occupies a prominent position in the gallery of mathematics, in probability theory. Quantum physics has used stochastic theories, and a series of formulae now try to explain the "relationships of uncertainty". One of the most widely known of these is the Uncertainty Principle devised by the physicist W. Heisenberg (1927), which relates the position and the velocity (momentum) of a particle. In a nutshell, Heisenberg's Uncertainty Principle says that one cannot know simultaneous for certain the exact position and speed (momentum) of a subatomic particle. One can know one or the other, but not both.

Unlike randomness, some variables used in our daily lives, and which are perfectly understood when transmitted linguistically between partners, have always remained outside the scope of traditional mathematical treatment. This is the case of some linguistic variables that have arisen from the need to distinguish between qualifications through a grading system. To describe certain phenomena within the sensible world, we have used degrees that represent qualities or partial truths, or "better standards" to use Sophist language. This is the case, for example, with such concepts as tall, heavy smoker, or infections. This kind ambiguity in language which is a type of uncertainty in terms of its precise meaning since these terms are by their very nature, imprecise, is from a linguistic point of view, a *flexibility* regarding what elements belong to the category/set (tall, heavy smoker). Moreover, the main contribution that fuzzy logic made and is making, is to the mathematical analysis of fuzzy sets, these vague, flexible, open concepts. Fuzzy logic gives precision to imprecise (linguistic) terms so that mathematical analysis of these flexible categories is meaningful. In language usage, we could refer to the sets of tall people, smokers or infections. These are typical examples of "sets" whose boundaries can be considered transitional, flexible, vague, since they are defined through subjective or flexible properties or attributes.

Let's consider the example of tall people. To make a formal mathematical representation of this set, we could approach it in at least two different ways. The first is the classical approach, establishing a height above which a person could be considered tall. In this case, the set is well-defined. The second and less conventional approach to this issue would be that of considering all people as being tall with greater or less extent, that is, there are people who are more or less tall or not tall at all. This means that the less tall the individual, the lower the degree of relevance to this class. We can therefore say that all people belong to the set of tall people, with greater or less extent. This latter approach is what we intend to discuss in our book. It was from such notions, where the defining characteristics or properties of the set is flexible, transitional, open, that fuzzy theory appeared. Fuzzy set theory has grown considerably since it was introduced in 1965, both theoretically and in diverse applications especially in the field of technology - microchips.

The word "fuzzy" is of English origin and means (see *Concise Oxford English Dictionary*, 11th edition) indistinct or vague. Other meanings include blurred, having the nature or characteristic of fuzzy. Fuzzy set theory was introduced in 1965 by Lotfi Asker Zadeh [1] (an electrical engineer and researcher in mathematics, computer science, artificial intelligence), who initially intended to impart a mathematical treatment on certain subjective terms of language, such as "about" and "around", among others. This would be the first step in working towards programming and storing concepts that are vague on computers, making it possible to perform calculations on vague or flexible entities, as do human beings. For example, we are all unanimous in agreeing that the doubling of a quantity "around 3" results in another "around 6 ".

The formal mathematical representation of a fuzzy set is based on the fact that any classic subset can be characterized by a function, its characteristic function, as follows.

Definition 1.1 Let U be a non-empty set and A a subset of U. The characteristic function of A is given by:

$$\chi_A(x) = \begin{cases} 1 & \text{if } x \in A \\ 0 & \text{if } x \notin A \end{cases}$$

for all $x \in U$.

In this context, a classical subset A of U can uniquely be associated with its characteristic function. So, in the classical case, we may opt for using the language from either "set theory" or "function theory", depending on the problem at hand.

Note that the characteristic function $\chi_A : U \to \{0, 1\}$ of the subset A shows which elements of the universal set U are also elements of A, where $\chi_A(x) = 1$ meaning that the element $x \in A$, while $\chi_A(x) = 0$ means that x is not element of A. However, there are cases where an element is partially in a set which means we cannot always say that an element completely belongs to a given set or not. For example, consider the subset of real numbers "near 2":

$$A = \{x \in \mathbb{R} : x \text{ is near 2}\}.$$

Question. Does the number 7 and the number 2.001 belong to A? The answer to this question is not no/yes (so is uncertain from this point of view) because we do not know to what extent we can objectively say when a number is near 2. The only reasonable information in this case is that 2.001 is nearer 2 than 7.

We now start the mathematical formalization of fuzzy set theory that shall be addressed in this text, starting with the concept of fuzzy subsets.

1.2 Fuzzy Subset

Allowing leeway in the image or range set of the characteristic function of a set from the Boolean set {0, 1} to the interval [0, 1], Zadeh suggested the formalization of the mathematics behind vague concepts, such as the case of "near 2," using fuzzy subsets.

Definition 1.2 Let U be a (classic universal) set. A fuzzy subset F of U is defined by a function φ_F, called the **membership function** (of F)

$$\varphi_F : U \longrightarrow [0, 1].$$

The subscript F on φ identifies the subset (F in this case) and the function φ_F is the analogue of the characteristic function of the classical subset as defined in Definition 1.1 above. The value of $\varphi_F(x) \in [0, 1]$ indicates the degree to which the element x of U belongs to the fuzzy set F; $\varphi_F(x) = 0$ and $\varphi_F(x) = 1$, respectively, mean x for sure does not belong to fuzzy subset F and x for sure belongs to the fuzzy subset F. From a formal point of view, the definition of a fuzzy subset is obtained simply by increasing the range of the characteristic function from {0, 1} to the whole interval [0, 1]. We can therefore say that a classical set is a special case of a fuzzy set when the range of the membership function φ_F is restricted to $\{0, 1\} \subseteq [0, 1]$, that is, the membership function φ_F retracts to the characteristic function χ_F. In fuzzy language, a subset in the classic sense is usually called a **crisp subset**.

A fuzzy subset F of U can be seen as a standard (classic) subset of the Cartesian product $U \times [0, 1]$. Moreover, we can identify a fuzzy subset F of U with the set of ordered pairs (i.e., the graph of φ_F):

$$\{(x, \varphi_F(x)) : \text{ with } x \in U\}.$$

The classic subset of U defined below

$$\text{supp } F = \{x \in U : \varphi_F(x) > 0\}$$

is called the **support** of F and has a fundamental role in the interrelation between classical and fuzzy set theory. Interestingly, unlike fuzzy subsets, a support is a crisp set. Figure 1.1 illustrates this fact.

It is common to denote a fuzzy subset, say F, in fuzzy set literature, not by its membership function φ_F but simply by the letter F. In this text we have decided to distinguish between F and φ_F. In classical set theory, whenever we refer to a particular set A we are actually considering a subset of a universal set U but for the sake of simplicity or convenience, we say set A even though set A is actually a subset. The fuzzy set literature also uses of these terms. This text will use both terms interchangeably.

We now present some examples of fuzzy subsets.

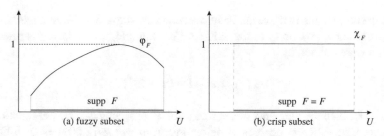

Fig. 1.1 Illustration of subsets fuzzy and crisp

Example 1.1 (Even numbers) Consider the set of natural even numbers:

$$E = \{n \in \mathbb{N} : n \text{ is even}\}.$$

This set E has characteristic function which assigns to any natural number n the value $\chi_E(n) = 1$ if n is even and $\chi_E(n) = 0$ if n odd. This means that the set of even numbers is a particular fuzzy set of the set of natural numbers $\mathbb{N}$, since $\chi_E(n) \in [0, 1]$, in particular

$$\chi_E(n) = \varphi_E(n) = \begin{cases} 1 \text{ if } n \text{ is even} \\ 0 \text{ otherwise.} \end{cases}$$

In this case, it was possible to determine all the elements of E, in the domain of the universal set $\mathbb{N}$ of natural numbers, because every natural number is either even or odd. However, this is not the case for other sets with imprecise boundaries.

Example 1.2 (Numbers near 2) Consider the following subset F of the real numbers near of 2:

$$F = \{x \in \mathbb{R} : x \text{ is near 2}\}.$$

We can define the function $\varphi_F : \mathbb{R} \longrightarrow [0, 1]$, which associates each real value x proximity to point 2 using the expression

$$\varphi_F(x) = \begin{cases} (1 - |x - 2|) & \text{if } 1 \leq x \leq 3 \\ 0 & \text{if } x \notin [1, 3] \end{cases}, \ x \in \mathbb{R}.$$

In this case the fuzzy subset F of points near 2, characterized in φ_F, is such that $\varphi_F(2.001) = 0.999$ and $\varphi_F(7) = 0$. We say that $x = 2.001$ is near to 2 with proximity degree 0.999; $x = 7$ is not near 2.

On the other hand, in the example above, one may suggest a different membership function to show proximity to the value 2. For example, if the closeness proximity function were defined by

$$\nu_F(x) = exp\left[-(x-2)^2\right],$$

with $x \in \mathbb{R}$, then the elements of the fuzzy set F, characterized by the function ν_F, as above, have different degrees of belonging from φ_F: $\nu_F(2.001) = 0.99999$ and $\nu_F(7) = 1.388 \times 10^{-11}$.

We can see that the notion of proximity is subjective and also depends on the membership function which can be expressed in countless different ways, depending on how we wish to evaluate the idea of a "nearness". Note that we could also define the concept "numbers near 2" by a classic set with membership function φ_{F_ϵ}, considering, for example, a sufficiently small value of ϵ and the characteristic function for the interval $(2 - \epsilon, 2 + \epsilon)$, by following expression:

$$\varphi_{\epsilon F}(x) = \begin{cases} 1 & \text{if } |x - 2| < \epsilon \\ 0 & \text{if } |x - 2| \geq \epsilon. \end{cases}$$

Note that being close to 2 means being within a preset neighborhood of 2. The element of subjectivity lies in the choice of the radius of the neighborhood considered.In this specific case, all the values within the neighborhood are close to 2 with the same degree of belonging, which is 1.

Example 1.3 (*Small natural numbers*) Consider the fuzzy subset F containing the small natural numbers,

$$F = \{n \in \mathbb{N} : n \text{ is small}\}.$$

Does the number 0 (zero) belong to this set? What about the number 1.000? In the spirit of fuzzy set theory, it could be said that both do indeed belong to F, but with different degrees depending on the membership function φ_F with respect to the fuzzy set F. The membership function associated with F must be built in a way that is consistent with the term "small", the context of the problem and the application (mathematical model). One possibility for the membership function of F would be

$$\varphi_F(n) = \frac{1}{n+1}, n \in \mathbb{N}.$$

Therefore, we could say that the number 0 (zero) belongs to F with a degree of belonging equal to $\varphi_F(0) = 1$, while 999 also belongs to F, albeit with a degree of belonging equal to $\varphi_F(999) = 0.001$.

It is clear that in this case the choice of the function φ_F was made in a somewhat arbitrary fashion, only taking into account the meaning of "small". To make a mathematical model of the "small natural number" notion, and thus to link F to a membership function, we could, for example, choose any monotonically decreasing sequence, starting at 1 (one) and converging to 0 (zero) as

$$\{\varphi_n\}_{n \in \mathbb{N}}; \text{ with } \varphi_0 = 1.$$

For example,

$$\varphi_F(n) = e^{-n};$$

$$\varphi_F(n) = \frac{1}{n^2 + 1};$$

$$\varphi_F(n) = \frac{1}{\ln(n + e)}.$$

The function to be selected to represent the fuzzy set considered depends on several factors related to the context of the problem under study. From the standpoint of strict fuzzy set theory, any of the previous membership functions can represent the subjective concept in question. However, what should indeed be noted is that each of the above functions produces a different fuzzy set, according to Definition 1.2.

The examples we have presented above possess a universal set U for each fuzzy set that is clearly articulated. However, this is not always the case. In most cases of interest for mathematical modeling, the universal set needs to be delineated and in most instances the support set as well. Let's illustrate this point with a few more examples.

Example 1.4 (*Fuzzy set of young people, Y*) Consider the inhabitants of a specific city. Each individual in this population can be associated to a real number corresponding to their age. Consider the whole universe as the ages within the interval $U = [0, 120]$ where $x \in U$ is interpreted as the age of a given individual. A fuzzy subset Y, of young people of this city, could be characterized by the following two membership functions for young, Y_1, Y_2 according different experts:

$$\varphi_{Y_1}(x) = \begin{cases} 1 & \text{if } x \leq 10 \\ \dfrac{80 - x}{70} & \text{if } 10 < x \leq 80 \ , \\ 0 & \text{if } x > 80 \end{cases}$$

$$\varphi_{Y_2}(x) = \begin{cases} \left(\dfrac{40 - x}{40}\right)^2 & \text{if } 0 \leq x \leq 40 \\ 0 & \text{if } 40 < x \leq 120 \end{cases} .$$

In the first case Y_1, the support is the interval $[0, 80]$ and in the second case Y_2, the support is $[0, 40]$. The choice of which function to be used to represent the concept of young people relies heavily on the context or analysis. Undoubtedly, about to retire professors would choose Y_1. Note that the choice of $U = [0, 120]$ as the interval for the universal set is linked to the fact that we have chosen to show how much an individual is young and our knowledge that statistically in the world, no one has lived beyond 120. If another characteristic were to be adopted, such as the number of grey hairs, to indicate the degree of youth, the universe would be different as well as the support.

The next example shows a bit more about fuzzy set theory in the mathematical modeling of "fuzzy concepts". In this example, we shall present a mathematical modeling treatment that allows the quantification and exploration of a theme of important social concern, poverty. This concept could be modeled based on a variety of appropriate variables, calorie intake, consumption of vitamins, iron intake, the volume of waste produced, or even the income of every individual, among many other features that are possible. However, we have chosen to represent poverty assuming that the only variable is income level. A possible mathematical model for poverty is shown below.

Example 1.5 (*Fuzzy subset of the poor*) Consider that the concept of poor is based on the income level r. Hence, it is reasonable to assume that when you lower the income level, you raise the level of poverty of the individual. This means that the fuzzy subset A_k, of the poor in a given location, can be given by the following membership function:

$$\varphi_{A_k}(r) = \begin{cases} \left\{1 - \left[\left(\frac{r}{r_0}\right)^2\right]\right\}^k & \text{if } r \leq r_0 \\ 0 & \text{if } r > r_0 \end{cases}.$$

The parameter k indicates a characteristic of the group we are considering. This parameter might indicate such things as the environment in which the individual people are situated. The parameter value, r_0, is the minimum income level believed to be required to be out of poverty.

As illustrated in Fig. 1.2 above, we have that if $k_1 \geq k_2$, then $\varphi_{A_{k_1}}(\bar{r}) \leq \varphi_{A_{k_2}}(\bar{r})$ which means that an individual group in k_1, with an income level $\bar{r}$, would be poorer for this income level were the individual in group k_2. We can also say that in terms of income, it is easier to live in the places where k is greatest. So, intuitively, k shows

Fig. 1.2 The membership function of the fuzzy subset of "poor"

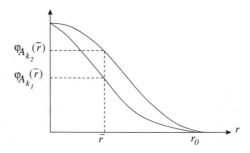

whether the environment where the group lives is less or more favorable to life. The parameter k may give an idea of the degree of saturation that a group has on the environment and, therefore, can be considered as an environmental parameter.

1.3 Operations with Fuzzy Subsets

This section presents the typical operations on fuzzy sets such as union, intersection and complementation. Each one of these operations is obtained from membership functions. Let A and B be two fuzzy subsets of U, with their respective membership functions φ_A and φ_B. We say that A is a fuzzy subset of B, and write $A \subset B$ if $\varphi_A(x) \leq \varphi_B(x)$ for all $x \in U$. Remember that the membership function of the empty set $(\emptyset)$ is given by $\varphi_\emptyset(x) = 0$, while the universal set U has membership function $\varphi_U(x) = 1$ for all $x \in U$. Hence we can say that $\emptyset \subset A$ and $A \subset U$ for all A.

Definition 1.3 (*Union*) The union between A and B is the fuzzy subset of U whose membership function is given by:

$$\varphi_{A \cup B}(x) = max\{\varphi_A(x), \varphi_B(x)\}, x \in U.$$

We note that this definition is an extension of the classic case. In fact, when A and B are classics subsets of U have:

$$max\{\chi_A(x), \chi_B(x)\} = \begin{cases} 1 & \text{if } x \in A \text{ or } x \in B \\ 0 & \text{if } x \notin A \text{ and } x \notin B \end{cases}$$

$$= \begin{cases} 1 & \text{if } x \in A \cup B \\ 0 & \text{if } x \notin A \cup B \end{cases}$$

$$= \chi_{A \cup B}(x), \ x \in U.$$

Definition 1.4 (*Intersection*) The intersection between A and B is the fuzzy subset of U whose membership function is given by the following equation:

$$\varphi_{A \cap B}(x) = min\{\varphi_A(x), \varphi_B(x)\}, x \in U.$$

Definition 1.5 (*Complement*) The complement of A is the fuzzy subset A' in U whose membership function is given by:

$$\varphi_{A'}(x) = 1 - \varphi_A(x), \ x \in U.$$

Exercise 1.1 Suppose that A and B are classic subsets of U.

1. Check that

$$\min\{\chi_A(x), \chi_B(x)\} = \begin{cases} 1 & \text{if } x \in A \cap B \\ 0 & \text{if } x \notin A \cap B. \end{cases}$$

2. Check that $\chi_{A \cap B}(x) = \chi_A(x)\chi_B(x)$. Note that this identity is does not hold in cases where A and B are fuzzy subsets.
3. Check that $\chi_{A \cap A'}(x) = 0 \left(A \cap A' = \emptyset\right)$ and that $\chi_{A \cup A'}(x) = 1 \left(A \cup A' = U\right)$ for all $x \in U$.

Unlike the classical situation, in the fuzzy context (see Fig. 1.3) we can have:

- $\varphi_{A \cap A'}(x) \neq 0 = \varphi_\emptyset(x)$ which means that we may not have $A \cap A' = \emptyset$;
- $\varphi_{A \cup A'}(x) \neq 1 = \varphi_U(x)$ which means that we may not have $A \cup A' = U$.

In the following example, we intend to exploit the special features presented by the concept of the complement of a fuzzy set.

Example 1.6 (*Fuzzy set of the elderly*) The fuzzy set O of the elderly (the old) should reflect a situation opposite of young people given above, when considering the ages that belong to O. While youth membership functions should decrease with age, the elderly should be increase with age. One possibility for the membership function of O is:

$$\varphi_O(x) = 1 - \varphi_Y(x),$$

where φ_Y is the membership function of the fuzzy subset "young". Therefore, the fuzzy set O is the complement of fuzzy Y. In this example, if we take the set of young people Y_1 as having the membership function mentioned in the first part of Example 1.4, then:

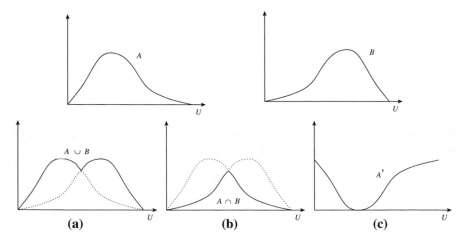

Fig. 1.3 Operations with fuzzy subsets: **a** union, **b** intersection, and **c** complement

Fig. 1.4 Fuzzy subsets of young and elderly

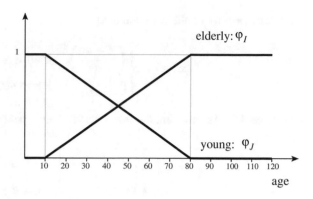

$$\varphi_O(x) = 1 - \varphi_{Y_1}(x) = \begin{cases} 0 & \text{if } x \leq 10 \\ \dfrac{x - 10}{70} & \text{if } 10 < x \leq 80 \\ 1 & \text{if } x > 80 \end{cases}.$$

A graphical representation for O and Y_1 is shown in Fig. 1.4.

Note that this operation, complement, exchanges degrees of belonging for the fuzzy subsets of O and Y_1. This property characterizes the fuzzy complement, which means that while $\varphi_A(x)$ represents the degree of compatibility of x with the linguistic concept in question, $\varphi_{A'}(x)$ shows the incompatibility of x with the same concept.

One consequence of the imprecision of fuzzy sets is that there is a certain overlap of a fuzzy set with its complement. In Example 1.6, an individual who belongs to the of fuzzy set young with grade 0.8, also belongs to its complement O with grade 0.2. Also note that it is quite possible for a member to belong to one set and also its complementary set with the same degree of belonging (in Fig. 1.4 this value is 45), showing that the more doubt we have about an element belonging to the set, the nearer to 0.5 is the degree of belong to this set. That is, the closer to a 0.5 membership value an element is, the greater the doubt of whether or not this element belongs to the set. The degree 0.5 is the maximum doubt (greatest entropy). This is a major difference from classical set theory in which an element either belongs to a set or to its complement, these being mutually exclusive, and there is absolutely no doubt.

Here it must also be noted that we have defined young and elderly (old), which are admittedly linguistic terms of opposite meanings, through the use of fuzzy sets that are not necessarily complementary. For example, we could have used φ_{Y_1}:

$$\varphi_{Y_2}(x) = \begin{cases} \left(\dfrac{40 - x}{40} \right)^2 & \text{if } 0 \leq x \leq 40 \\ 0 & \text{if } 40 < x \leq 120, \end{cases}$$

in which case we could have obtained

$$\varphi_O(x) = \begin{cases} \left(\dfrac{x-40}{80}\right)^2 & \text{if } 40 < x \leq 120 \\ 0 & \text{if } x \leq 40. \end{cases}$$

Exercise 1.2 Assume that the fuzzy set for young people, Y, is given by

$$\varphi_Y(x) = \begin{cases} \left[1 - \left(\dfrac{x}{120}\right)^2\right]^4 & \text{if } x \in [10, 120] \\ 1 & \text{if } x \notin [10, 120] \end{cases}.$$

1. Define a fuzzy set for the elderly.
2. Determine the age of an individual considered of middle age, which means grade 0.5, both in terms of youth and of elderly (old) age, assuming that the fuzzy set of the elderly is the complement to that of the young.
3. Draw the graph of the young and elderly (old) for part 2, and then compare it with Example 1.6.

We will next extend the concept to the complement for $A \subseteq B$ where A is a fuzzy subset of fuzzy set B and both in relation to the universe U. In this case, the complement of A in relation to B is denoted by the fuzzy set A'_B which has the following membership function:

$$\varphi_{A'_B}(x) = \varphi_B(x) - \varphi_A(x), \quad x \in U.$$

Note also that the complement of A in relation to U is a particular case of the complement of A in B since $\varphi_U(x) = 1$.

In the following example, we shall try to further exploit the concept of the ideas of complements with fuzzy subsets as defined in Example 1.5.

Example 1.7 (Fuzzy set of the poor revisited) If the environment in which a group lives suffers any kind of degradation, from what we saw in Example 1.5, this results in a decreased environmental parameter, declining from k_1 to a lower value k_2, so that the individual having income level r in k_1 has degree of poverty $\varphi_{A_{k_1}}(r)$ less than that of another $\varphi_{A_{k_2}}(r)$ with the same income r in k_2. That is,

$$\varphi_{A_{k_1}}(r) < \varphi_{A_{k_2}}(r) \Leftrightarrow A_{k_1} \subset A_{k_2}.$$

Such a change could lead to the poverty level of a pauper, represented by A_{k_2}. The fuzzy complement of A_{k_1} in A_{k_2} is the fuzzy subset given by

$$\left(A'\right)_{A_{k_2}}.$$

This set is not empty, and its membership function is given by

$$\varphi_{(A')_{A_{k_2}}} = \varphi_{A_{k_2}}(r) - \varphi_{A_{k_1}}(r), \ r \in U.$$

A recompense to the group that has suffered such a fall should be that of the same status of poverty as before. That is, given an income of r_1, the group should have an income of r_2 (after the fall) which means that

$$\varphi_{A_{k_2}}(r_2) - \varphi_{A_{k_1}}(r_1) = 0.$$

Therefore $r_2 - r_1 > 0$ and the recompense should be $r_2 - r_1$ (see Fig. 1.5).

We shall now make some brief comments and also look at the consequences of the major operations between fuzzy sets.

If A and B are sets in the classical sense, then the characteristic functions of their operations also satisfy the definitions defined for the fuzzy case, showing coherence between such concepts. For example, if A is a (classic) subset of U, then the characteristic function $\chi_{A'}(x)$ of its complement is such that

$$\begin{cases} \chi_{A'}(x) = 0 & \text{if } \chi_A(x) = 1 \Leftrightarrow x \in A; \\ \chi_{A'}(x) = 1 & \text{if } \chi_A(x) = 0 \Leftrightarrow x \notin A. \end{cases}$$

In this case, either $x \in A$ or $x \notin A$, while the theory of fuzzy sets does not necessarily have this dichotomy. As seen in the Example 1.6, it is not always true that $A \cap A' = \emptyset$ for fuzzy sets, and it may not even true that $A \cup A' = U$. The following example reinforces these facts.

Example 1.8 (Fuzzy sets of fever and/or myalgia, muscular rheumatism) Let's suppose that the universal set U is the set of all patients within a clinic, identified by numbers 1, 2, 3, 4 and 5. Let A and B be fuzzy subsets that represent patients with fever and myalgia, respectively. Table 1.1 shows the operations union, intersection and complement.

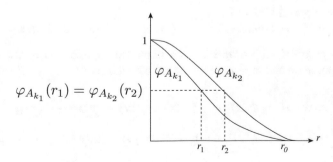

Fig. 1.5 Recompense for changing in environment

Table 1.1 Illustration of operations between fuzzy subsets

Patient	Fever: A	Myalgia: B	$A \cup B$	$A \cap B$	A'	$A \cap A'$	$A \cup A'$
1	0.7	0.6	0.7	0.6	0.3	0.3	0.7
2	1.0	1.0	1.0	1.0	0.0	0.0	1.0
3	0.4	0.2	0.4	0.2	0.6	0.4	0.6
4	0.5	0.5	0.5	0.5	0.5	0.5	0.5
5	1.0	0.2	1.0	0.2	0.0	0.0	1.0

The values in all columns except the first, show the degree to which each patient belongs to the fuzzy sets A, B, $A \cup B$, $A \cap B$, A', $A \cap A'$, $A \cup A'$; respectively, where A and B are hypothetical data. In the column $A \cap A'$, the value of 0.3 shows that patient number 1 is both in the first group of patients with a fever as well as in the group with non-fever. As we have seen, this is a fact that would not be possible in classical set theory in which there is the exclusion law by which any set and its complement are mutually exclusive, $A \cap A' = \emptyset$.

The fuzzy subsets A and B of U are equal if their membership functions are identical, that is, if $\varphi_A (x) = \varphi_B (x)$ for all $x \in U$. Below is listed the main properties of the operations as defined in this section.

Proposition 1.1 *The operations between fuzzy subsets satisfying the following properties:*

- $A \cup B = B \cup A$,
- $A \cap B = B \cap A$,
- $A \cup (B \cup C) = (A \cup B) \cup C$,
- $A \cap (B \cap C) = (A \cap B) \cap C$,
- $A \cup A = A$,
- $A \cap A = A$,
- $A \cup (B \cap C) = (A \cup B) \cap (A \cup C)$,
- $A \cap (B \cup C) = (A \cap B) \cup (A \cap C)$,
- $A \cap \emptyset = \emptyset$ *and* $A \cup \emptyset = A$,
- $A \cap U = A$ *and* $A \cup U = U$,
- $(A \cup B)' = A' \cap B'$ *and* $(A \cap B)' = A' \cup B'$ $\left(DeMorgan's\ Law \right)$.

Proof The proof of each property is an immediate application of the properties between maximum and minimum functions, which means

$$\begin{cases} max\,[\varphi\,(x)\,,\psi\,(x)] = \dfrac{1}{2}\,[\varphi\,(x) + \psi\,(x) + |\varphi\,(x) - \psi\,(x)\,|] \\ min\,[\varphi\,(x)\,,\psi\,(x)] = \dfrac{1}{2}\,[\varphi\,(x) + \psi\,(x) - |\varphi\,(x) - \psi\,(x)\,|]. \end{cases}$$

where φ and ψ are functions with image in $\mathbb{R}$. We will only prove one of De Morgan's laws, because the other properties have similar proofs. If we consider that φ_A is the membership function associated with the subset A, then we have:

$$\varphi_{A' \cup B'}(u) = max \left[1 - \varphi_A(u), 1 - \varphi_B(u) \right]$$

$$= \frac{1}{2} \left[(1 - \varphi_A(u)) + (1 - \varphi_B(u)) + |\varphi_A(u) - \varphi_B(u)| \right]$$

$$= \frac{1}{2} \left[2 - (\varphi_A(u) + \varphi_B(u)) - |\varphi_A(u) - \varphi_B(u)| \right]$$

$$= 1 - \frac{1}{2} \left[\varphi_A(u) + \varphi_B(u) - |\varphi_A(u) - \varphi_B(u)| \right]$$

$$= 1 - min \left[\varphi_A(u), \varphi_B(u) \right] = 1 - \varphi_{A \cap B}(u) = \varphi_{(A \cap B)'}(u),$$

for all $u \in U$.   ■

Exercise 1.3 Consider the fuzzy subset of tall people (in meters) in Brazil as defined by,

$$\varphi_A(x) = \begin{cases} 0 & \text{if } 0 \leq x \leq 1.4 \\ \dfrac{1}{0.4}(x - 1.4) & \text{if } 1.4 < x \leq 1.8 \\ 1 & \text{if } x > 1.8 \end{cases}.$$

And people of average height x (in meters) as follows,

$$\varphi_B(x) = \begin{cases} 0 & \text{if } x \leq 1.4 \\ \dfrac{1}{0.2}(x - 1.4) & \text{if } 1.4 < x \leq 1.6 \\ 1 & \text{if } 1.6 < x \leq 1.7 \\ \dfrac{1}{0.1}(1.8 - x) & \text{if } 1.7 < x \leq 1.8 \\ 0 & \text{if } x > 1.8 \end{cases}.$$

Obtain $(A \cup B)'$ and $A' \cup B'$ and give an interpretation for such operations.

To end this chapter, we look, in the next section, at a special class of crisp sets which are closely related to each fuzzy subset. These crisp sets can be interpreted as representing the level of vagueness represented by each fuzzy set.

1.4   Concept of α-Level

A fuzzy subset A of U is "formed" by elements of U with an order (hierarchy) that is given by the membership degrees. An element x of U will be in an "order class" α if its degree of belonging (its membership value) is at least the threshold level $\alpha \in [0, 1]$ that defines that class. The classic set of such elements is called an α-level of A, denoted $[A]^\alpha$.

Definition 1.6 (α-*level*) Let A be a fuzzy subset of U and $\alpha \in [0, 1]$. The α-level of the subset A is classical set $[A]^\alpha$ of U defined by

$$[A]^\alpha = \{x \in U : \varphi_A(x) \geq \alpha\} \text{ for } 0 < \alpha \leq 1.$$

When U is a topological space, the zero α-level of the fuzzy subset A is defined as the smallest closed subset (in the classic sense) in U containing the support set of A. In mathematical terms, $[A]^0$ is the closure of the support of A and is also denoted by $\overline{\text{supp}A}$. This consideration becomes essential in theoretical situations appearing in this text. Note also that the set $\{x \in U : \varphi_A(x) \geq 0\} = U$ is not necessarily equal to $[A]^0 = \overline{\text{supp}A}$.

Example 1.9 Let $U = \mathbb{R}$ be the set of real numbers and let A be a fuzzy subset of $\mathbb{R}$ with the following function membership function:

$$\varphi_A(x) = \begin{cases} x - 1 & \text{if } 1 \leq x \leq 2 \\ 3 - x & \text{if } 2 < x < 3 \\ 0 & \text{if } x \notin [1, 3) \end{cases}.$$

In this case we have:

$$[A]^\alpha = [\alpha + 1, 3 - \alpha] \text{ for } 0 < \alpha \leq 1 \text{ and } [A]^0 = \overline{]1, 3[} = [1, 3] \text{ (Fig. 1.6)}.$$

Example 1.10 Let $U = [0, 1]$ and A be the fuzzy subset of U whose membership function is given by $\varphi_A(x) = 4(x - x^2)$. Then,

$$[A]^\alpha = \left[\frac{1}{2} \left(1 - \sqrt{1 - \alpha} \right), \frac{1}{2} \left(1 + \sqrt{1 - \alpha} \right) \right]$$

for all $\alpha \in [0, 1]$ (Fig. 1.7).

We observed that if x is an element of $[A]^\alpha$, then x belongs to the fuzzy set A with at least membership function degree α. We have also that if $\alpha \leq \beta$ then $[A]^\beta \subseteq [A]^\alpha$.

The following theorem shows that a fuzzy set is uniquely determined by its α-cuts.

Fig. 1.6 α-level of the fuzzy subset A

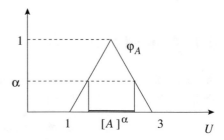

Fig. 1.7 α-level of the fuzzy subset A

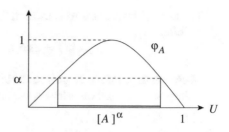

Theorem 1.2 *Let A and B be fuzzy subset of U. A necessary and sufficient condition for $A = B$ to hold is that $[A]^\alpha = [B]^\alpha$, for all $\alpha \in [0, 1]$.*

Proof Of course $A = B \implies [A]^\alpha = [B]^\alpha$ for all $\alpha \in [0, 1]$. Let's now suppose that $[A]^\alpha = [B]^\alpha$ for all $\alpha \in [0, 1]$. If $A \neq B$ then there is an $x \in U$ such that $\varphi_A(x) \neq \varphi_B(x)$. Therefore we have $\varphi_A(x) < \varphi_B(x)$ or that, conversely, $\varphi_A(x) > \varphi_B(x)$. If we imagine that $\varphi_A(x) > \varphi_B(x)$, then we come to the conclusion that $x \in [A]^{\varphi_A(x)}$ and $x \notin [B]^{\varphi_A(x)}$ and therefore $[A]^{\varphi_A(x)} \neq [B]^{\varphi_A(x)}$, which contradicts the hypothesis that $[A]^\alpha = [B]^\alpha$ for all $\alpha \in [0, 1]$. Similar contradiction is reached if we assume that $\varphi_A(x) < \varphi_B(x)$. ∎

One consequence of this theorem is that we now have a relationship between the membership function of a fuzzy subset and the characteristic functions of its α-levels.

Corollary 1.3 *The membership function φ_A of a fuzzy set A can be expressed in terms of the characteristic function of their α-levels, as follows:*

$$\varphi_A(x) = sup\{min\,[\alpha, \chi_{[A]^\alpha}(x)]\}, \text{ where } \chi_{[A]^\alpha}(x) = \begin{cases} 1 & \text{if } x \in [A]^\alpha \\ 0 & \text{if } x \notin [A]^\alpha \end{cases}.$$

The following theorem is of extreme importance in the study of fuzzy set theory and shows a condition which is sufficient for a family of subsets, in the classical sense, of U can be formed by different α-levels of a fuzzy subset.

Theorem 1.4 (Negoita and Ralescu's Theorem of Representation [3]) *Let A_α, $\alpha \in [0, 1]$, be a family of classical subsets of U, such that the following conditions hold:*

1. $\bigcup A_\alpha \subseteq A_0$ *with $\alpha \in [0, 1]$;*
2. $A_\alpha \subseteq A_\beta$ *if $\beta \leq \alpha$;*
3. $A_\alpha = \bigcap_{k \geq 0} A_{\alpha_k}$ *if α_k converges to α with $\alpha_k \leq \alpha$.*

Under these conditions, there is one single fuzzy subset of A in U whose α-levels are exactly the classic subsets A_α, in other words,

$$[A]^\alpha = A_\alpha.$$

The idea of the proof is to construct, for each $x \in U$, the membership function of A, as following,

$$\varphi_A(x) = sup\{\alpha \in [0, 1] : x \in A_\alpha\}.$$

For a complete proof see Negoita and Ralescu [3].

Using the definition of α-levels, we have the following properties:

1. $[A \cup B]^\alpha = [A]^\alpha \cup [B]^\alpha$,
2. $[A \cap B]^\alpha = [A]^\alpha \cap [B]^\alpha$.

On the other hand, since in general $[A]^\alpha \cup [A']^\alpha \neq U$, we have that $[A']^\alpha \neq ([A]^\alpha)'$.

Definition 1.7 A fuzzy set is said to be normal when all its α-levels are not empty or in other words, if $[A]^1 \neq \emptyset$.

Recalling that the support of the fuzzy subset A is the classic set

$$supp A = \{x \in U : \varphi_A(x) > 0\},$$

it is common to describe A using the following notation, when it has a denumerable number of elements in its support, using the following notation,

$$A = \frac{\varphi_A(x_1)}{x_1} + \frac{\varphi_A(x_2)}{x_2} + \dots = \sum_{i=1}^{\infty} \frac{\varphi_A(x_i)}{x_i},$$

and

$$A = \frac{\varphi_A(x_1)}{x_1} + \frac{\varphi_A(x_2)}{x_2} + \dots + \frac{\varphi_A(x_n)}{x_n} = \sum_{i=1}^{n} \frac{\varphi_A(x_i)}{x_i}.$$

when A has finite discrete support. That is, $supp A = \{x_1, x_2, \dots, x_n\}$. It is worth noting that the notation $\dfrac{\varphi_A(x_i)}{x_i}$, does not indicate division. It's just a way to visualize an element x_i and its respective degree of belonging, its membership value, $\varphi_A(x_i)$. Also here the "+" symbol in the notation does not mean addition and $\sum$ does not mean summation. It's just a way to connect the elements of U that are in A with their respective degrees.

Example 1.11 (*Finite fuzzy set*) Let A be the fuzzy set of real numbers represented by

$$A = \sum_{i=1}^{n} \frac{\varphi_A(x_i)}{x_i} = \frac{0.1}{1} + \frac{0.2}{2} + \frac{0.25}{3} + \frac{0.7}{5} + \frac{0.9}{8} + \frac{1.0}{10}.$$

So,

$$A' = \sum_{i=1}^{n} \left[\frac{1 - \varphi_A(x_i)}{x_i} \right] = \frac{0.9}{1} + \frac{0.8}{2} + \frac{0.75}{3} + \frac{0.3}{5} + \frac{0.1}{8} + \frac{0.0}{10}.$$

In this case we have for example, 0.15-level of A and its complement A' are respectively, $[A]^{0.15} = \{2, 3, 5, 8, 10\}$ and $\left[A'\right]^{0.15} = \{1, 2, 3, 5\}$.

Example 1.12 (*Fuzzy set of wolves*) Let A be a pack of n wolves. The degree of predation for each wolf may be associated with their age $x \in]0, 15]$, assuming that the maximum age of a wolf is 15 years. The finite number of wolves means that one has only a finite number of wolves for each wolf ages. We will denote the set of these ages, as $A = \{x_1, x_2, \ldots, x_n\}$ and let us define the degree of predation of a wolf as $\varphi_P(x)$, considering that many young wolves prey less than adults, and that old wolves have reduced their ability for predation. Hence, the fuzzy subset of predators in the pack can be given by the membership function

$$\varphi_P(x) = \begin{cases} 0.5 & \text{if } 0 \leq x \leq 2 \\ 1.0 & \text{if } 2 < x < 10 \\ 0.2\,(15 - x) & \text{if } 10 \leq x \leq 15 \end{cases}.$$

With the above notation, the fuzzy finite subset P is conveniently denoted by

$$P = \frac{\varphi_P(x_1)}{x_1} + \frac{\varphi_P(x_2)}{x_2} + \cdots + \frac{\varphi_P(x_n)}{x_n},$$

meaning that $\varphi_P(x_j)$ is the predation capacity of an individual of age x_j.

1.5   Summary

This chapter has discussed the differences of fuzzy set and uncertainty along with a brief philosophical discussion of the difficulties associated with these concepts. Our main interest is in fuzzy sets and their use in mathematical models of fuzzy logic and fuzzy dynamical systems. Secondly, we defined and illustrated the basic operations of fuzzy sets. More will be introduced in the context of the topics that follow. Lastly, the classical sets, called α-levels, were discussed since they are central to the analysis in the ensuing chapters.

References

1. L.A. Zadeh, Fuzzy sets. Inf. Control **8**, 338–353 (1965)
2. B.J. Caraça, *Conceitos fundamentais da matemática*, 4th edn. (Gradiva Publicações Ltda, Lisboa, 2002)
3. C.V. Negoita, D.A. Ralescu, *Applications of Fuzzy Sets to Systems Analysis* (Wiley, New York, 1975)

Chapter 2
The Extension Principle of Zadeh and Fuzzy Numbers

Everything has numbers and nothing can be understand without numbers.

(Philolaus, Pythagorean-C.470 - C.385 BCE)

Abstract This chapter presents the *Extension Principle of Zadeh*, and as the name suggests, it is a method used to extend to fuzzy set theory the typical operations of classical set theory. It gives the framework to calculate the membership degree of elements of a fuzzy set and functions of fuzzy sets, which are the result of operations. Also, in the context of fuzzy sets, the concepts of fuzzy number and fuzzy number arithmetic are introduced.

2.1 Zadeh's Extension Principle

There is a need to extend concepts from the classical set theory to fuzzy set theory. The extension method proposed by Zadeh, known also as the *Extension Principle*, is one of the basic ideas that induces the extension of nonfuzzy mathematical concepts into fuzzy ones.

The Zadeh's Extension Principle for a function $f : X \longrightarrow Z$ indicates how the image of a fuzzy subset A of X should be computed when the function f is applied. It is expected that this image will be a fuzzy subset of Z.

Definition 2.1 (*Zadeh's Extension Principle*) Let f be a function such that $f : X \longrightarrow Z$ and let A be a fuzzy subset of X. *Zadeh's extension* of f is the function $\widehat{f}$ which applied to A gives us the fuzzy subset $\widehat{f}(A)$ of Z with the membership function given by

$$\varphi_{\widehat{f}(A)}(z) = \begin{cases} \sup\limits_{f^{-1}(z)} \varphi_A(x) & \text{if } f^{-1}(z) \neq \emptyset \\ 0 & \text{if } f^{-1}(z) = \emptyset \end{cases}, \tag{2.1}$$

where $f^{-1}(z) = \{x; \ f(x) = z\}$ is the *preimage* of z.

© Springer-Verlag Berlin Heidelberg 2017
L.C. de Barros et al., *A First Course in Fuzzy Logic, Fuzzy Dynamical Systems, and Biomathematics*, Studies in Fuzziness and Soft Computing 347, DOI 10.1007/978-3-662-53324-6_2

We can observe that if f is a bijective function, then

$$\{x : f(x) = z\} = \left\{ f^{-1}(z) \right\},$$

where f^{-1} means the inverse function of f. Thus, if A is a fuzzy subset of X, with the membership function φ_A, and if f is bijective, then the membership function of $\widehat{f}(A)$ is given as follows

$$\varphi_{\widehat{f}(A)}(z) = \sup_{\{x:\, f(x)=z\}} \varphi_A(x) = \sup_{\{x \in f^{-1}(z)\}} \varphi_A(x) = \varphi_A(f^{-1}(z)). \qquad (2.2)$$

The graph of how to construct the extension $\widehat{f}$ of f is illustrated in Fig. 2.1, where we have used a bijective function f. We observe that if f is injective, then $z = f(x)$ belongs to the fuzzy subset $\widehat{f}(A)$ with the same degree α as x belongs to A. This may not happen if f is not injective.

Let $f : X \to Z$ be an injective function and A a countable (or finite) fuzzy subset of X given by

$$A = \sum_{i=1}^{\infty} \varphi_A(x_i) / x_i.$$

Then the extension principle ensures that $\widehat{f}(A)$ is a fuzzy subset of Z given by

$$\widehat{f}(A) = \widehat{f}\left(\sum_{i=1}^{\infty} \varphi_A(x_i) / x_i \right) = \sum_{i=1}^{\infty} \varphi_A(x_i) / f(x_i).$$

Therefore, the image of A by $\widehat{f}$ can be derived from the knowledge of the images of x_i through f. The membership degree of $z_i = f(x_i)$ in $\widehat{f}(A)$ is the same as x_i in A.

Example 2.1 Let A be a fuzzy set with countable support, $f(x) = x^2$ and $x \geq 0$. Then

$$\widehat{f}(A) = \sum_{i=1}^{\infty} \varphi_A(x_i) / f(x_i) = \sum_{i=1}^{\infty} \varphi_A(x_i) / x_i^2.$$

The extension principle extends the concept to fuzzy sets of a function applied to a classical subset of X. Indeed, let $f : X \longrightarrow Z$ be a function and A a classical subset

Fig. 2.1 Image of a fuzzy subset from the extension principle for a function f

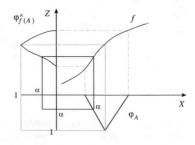

of X. The membership function of A is its characteristic function. The Zadeh's extension of f applied to A is the subset $\widehat{f}(A)$ of Z, which is the characteristic function

$$\varphi_{\widehat{f}(A)}(z) = \sup_{\{x:f(x)=z\}} \chi_A(x) = \begin{cases} 1 & \text{if } z \in f(A) \\ 0 & \text{if } z \notin f(A) \end{cases}$$

$$= \chi_{f(A)}(z)$$

for all z. Clearly, the membership function of the fuzzy set $\widehat{f}(A)$ is just the characteristic function of the crisp set $f(A)$, that is, the fuzzy set $\widehat{f}(A)$ coincides with the classical set $f(A)$:

$$\widehat{f}(A) = f(A) = \{f(a) : a \in A\}.$$

As can be seen in the formula above, when A is a classical set, the image $\widehat{f}(A)$ is clear, i.e., the formula (2.1) is unnecessary since each $f(a)$ belongs to $f(A)$ with membership degree equal to 1. The Zadeh Extension Principle in the context of classical sets is precisely what is called the *united extension* used in set-valued function theory and in interval analysis [1]. The difference between Zadeh's Extension Principle and United Extension is that Zadeh's Extension Principle maps membership functions into membership functions which is equivalent to mapping fuzzy sets to fuzzy sets but does so via a membership functions. Set-valued functions including real-valued intervals, map directly from set to set (without the intermediate membership function).

We can also notice that if A is a classical set, then $[A]^\alpha = A$ for all $\alpha \in\,]0, 1]$. Consequently,

$$[\widehat{f}(A)]^\alpha = [f(A)]^\alpha = f(A) = f([A]^\alpha).$$

Recall that for $\alpha = 0$ we mean that $[A]^0$ is the closure of A, that is, the smallest closed set containing the support of A, if X is a topological space. This result, stated here as Theorem 2.1, can also be applied to a fuzzy subset of X [2–4].

Theorem 2.1 *Let $f : X \longrightarrow Z$ be a continuous function and let A be a fuzzy subset of X. Then, for all $\alpha \in [0, 1]$, the following equality holds*

$$[\widehat{f}(A)]^\alpha = f([A]^\alpha). \tag{2.3}$$

This result indicates that the α-levels of the fuzzy set obtained by the Zadeh's Extension Principle coincides with the images of the α-levels by the crisp function (see Fig. 2.2). The proof of this theorem uses Weierstrass Theorem and it can be seen in [2–4].

Example 2.2 Let A be a fuzzy set of real numbers whose membership function is given by

$$\varphi_A(x) = \begin{cases} 4(x - x^2) & \text{if } x \in [0, 1] \\ 0 & \text{if } x \notin [0, 1] \end{cases}.$$

The α-levels of A are the intervals

$$[A]^\alpha = \left[\frac{1}{2}(1 - \sqrt{1 - \alpha}), \frac{1}{2}(1 + \sqrt{1 - \alpha})\right].$$

Let us now consider the real function $f(x) = x^2$ for $x \geq 0$. Since f is an increasing function, we have

$$f([A]^\alpha) = \left[f(\frac{1}{2}(1 - \sqrt{1 - \alpha})), \ f(\frac{1}{2}(1 + \sqrt{1 - \alpha}))\right]$$

$$= \left[\frac{1}{4}(1 - \sqrt{1 - \alpha})^2, \frac{1}{4}(1 + \sqrt{1 - \alpha})^2\right]$$

$$= [\hat{f}(A)]^\alpha.$$

Figure 2.2 illustrates the fuzzy subset $\widehat{f}(A)$.

Fig. 2.2 Subset $\widehat{f}(A)$ from the Example 2.2

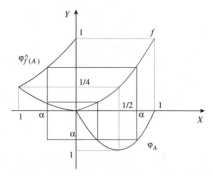

Exercise 2.1 Consider f and A as in Example 2.2. Compute $[\widehat{f}(A)]^\alpha$ for $\alpha = 0$, $\alpha = 3/4$ and $\alpha = 1$.

The relation between classical set functions and fuzzy functions is the following. Let A be a classical set. Its membership function in this context is

$$\chi_A(x) = \mu_A(x) = \begin{cases} 1 & x \in A \\ 0 & \text{otherwise} \end{cases}.$$

Classical set-valued functions compute the range of a classical set A by

$$f(A) = \{y \mid y = f(x), \ x \in A\}.$$

Simply, $f(A)$ is the range set of f over the domain set A. Using Zadeh's Extension Principle, we have for the classical set A,

$$\varphi_{\hat{f}(A)}(z) = \begin{cases} \sup_{x \in f^{-1}(z)} \chi_A(x) & \text{if } f^{-1}(z) \neq \emptyset \\ 0 & \text{if } f^{-1}(z) = \emptyset \end{cases} \tag{2.4}$$

$$= \begin{cases} 1 & z \in f(A) \\ 0 & z \notin f(A) \end{cases}. \tag{2.5}$$

In particular, if $A = [a, b]$, $a \leq b$, $a, b \in \mathbb{R}$,

$$\varphi_{\hat{f}([a,b])}(z) = \begin{cases} \sup_{x \in f^{-1}(z)} \chi_{[a,b]}(x) & \text{if } f^{-1}(z) \neq \emptyset \\ 0 & \text{if } f^{-1}(z) = \emptyset \end{cases} \tag{2.6}$$

$$= \begin{cases} 1 & z \in f([a,b]) \\ 0 & z \notin f([a,b]) \end{cases}. \tag{2.7}$$

This means that Zadeh's Extension Principle is the same as the United Extension on Intervals.

Let us introduce the Extension Principle for functions of two variables looking towards operations between fuzzy numbers that we will present in the next section.

Definition 2.2 Let $f : X \times Y \longrightarrow Z$ be a function and let A and B be fuzzy subsets of X and Y, respectively. The extension $\hat{f}$ of f, applied to A and B is the fuzzy subset $\hat{f}(A, B)$ of Z with membership function given by:

$$\varphi_{\hat{f}(A,B)}(z) = \begin{cases} \sup_{f^{-1}(z)} \min [\varphi_A(x), \varphi_B(y)] & \text{if } f^{-1}(z) \neq \emptyset \\ 0 & \text{if } f^{-1}(z) = \emptyset \end{cases}, \tag{2.8}$$

where $f^{-1}(z) = \{(x, y) : f(x, y) = z\}$.

Example 2.3 Let $f : \mathbb{R} \times \mathbb{R} \to \mathbb{R}$ be a function that satisfies $f(x, y) = x + y$. Consider the finite fuzzy sets of $\mathbb{R}$

$$A = 0.4/3 + 0.5/4 + 1/5 + 0.5/6 + 0.2/7$$
$$B = 0.2/6 + 0.5/7 + 1/8 + 0.5/9 + 0.2/10.$$

Let us compute the membership degree of $z = 10$ in $\hat{f}(A, B)$:

$$\varphi_{\hat{f}(A,B)}(10) = \sup_{\{x+y=10\}} \min[\varphi_A(x), \varphi_B(y)] =$$
$$= \max\{\min[\varphi_A(3), \varphi_B(7)], \min[\varphi_A(4), \varphi_B(6)]\}$$
$$= \max\{0.4; 0.2\} = 0.4.$$

Exercise 2.2 Redo the Example 2.3 for the following two functions:

(a) Defining $f(x, y) = x^2 + y$, determine $\hat{f}(A, B)$ and the membership degrees of $z = 10$ and $z = 25$ in $\hat{f}(A, B)$.

(b) Now, if $f(x, y) = 2x + y$, determine $\widehat{f}(A, B)$ and the membership degree of $z = 18$ in $\widehat{f}(A, B)$.

2.2   Fuzzy Numbers

Concrete problems often involve many quantities that are idealizations of inaccurate information involving numerical values. This is the reason why we use words like "around" in such cases. For example, when we measure the height of a person, what we obtain is a numerical value with a level of imprecision. These imprecisions may be caused by the measuring instrument, by the individuals who took the measurements, by the person who was measured, and for many other reasons. In the end, an "accurate value" (real number) h is chosen to indicate the height of the person. However, it would be more prudent to say that the height is *around* or *approximately* h. Mathematically, we represent the expression *around h* by a fuzzy subset A, whose domain of the membership function φ_A is the set of all real numbers. Also, it is reasonable to expect that $\varphi_A(h) = 1$. The choice of real numbers as the domain is due to the fact that, theoretically, the possible values to the height of a person are real numbers.

Definition 2.3 (*Fuzzy Number*) A fuzzy subset A is called a *fuzzy number* when the universal set on which φ_A is defined is the set of all real numbers $\mathbb{R}$ and satisfies the following conditions:

 (i) all the α-levels of A are not empty for $0 \leq \alpha \leq 1$;
 (ii) all the α-levels of A are closed intervals of $\mathbb{R}$;
(iii) supp $A = \{x \in \mathbb{R} : \varphi_A(x) > 0\}$ is bounded.

Let us represent the α-levels of the fuzzy number A by

$$[A]^\alpha = [a_1^\alpha, a_2^\alpha].$$

We observe that every real number r is a fuzzy number whose membership function is the characteristic function:

$$\chi_r(x) = \begin{cases} 1 & \text{if } x = r \\ 0 & \text{if } x \neq r \end{cases}.$$

We will denote χ_r or just by $\widehat{r}$.

The set of all fuzzy numbers will be denoted by $\mathcal{F}(\mathbb{R})$, and accordingly to what was observed above, the set of the real numbers $\mathbb{R}$ is a subset (classical or crisp) of $\mathcal{F}(\mathbb{R})$. The most common fuzzy numbers are the *triangular, trapezoidal* and the *bell shape* numbers.

Example 2.4 The *fuzzy number* $\widehat{2}$ may be depicted as in Fig. 2.3.

Definition 2.4 A fuzzy number A is said to be *triangular* if its membership function is given by

$$\varphi_A(x) = \begin{cases} 0 & \text{if } x \leq a \\ \frac{x-a}{u-a} & \text{if } a < x \leq u \\ \frac{x-b}{u-b} & \text{if } u < x \leq b \\ 0 & \text{if } x \geq b \end{cases}, \qquad (2.9)$$

where a, u, b are given numbers. The membership function of a triangular fuzzy number has a graphical representation of a triangle with $[a, b]$ being the base of the triangle and the point $(u, 1)$ as the single vertex. Therefore, the real numbers a, u and b define the triangular fuzzy number A which will be denoted by $(a; u; b)$.

The α-levels of triangular fuzzy numbers have the following simplified form

$$[a_1^\alpha, a_2^\alpha] = [(u-a)\alpha + a, (u-b)\alpha + b], \qquad (2.10)$$

for all $\alpha \in [0, 1]$.

Notice that a triangular fuzzy number is not necessarily symmetric, since $b - u$ may be different from $u - a$, however, $\varphi_A(u) = 1$. We can say that a fuzzy number A is a reasonable mathematical model for the linguistic expression "*nearly u*". For the expression "*around u*" we expect symmetry. Imposing symmetry results in a simplification of the definition of a triangular fuzzy number. Indeed, let u be symmetric in relation to a and b, that is, $u - a = b - u = \delta$. In this case,

$$\varphi_A(x) = \begin{cases} 1 - \frac{|x-u|}{\delta} & \text{if } u - \delta \leq x \leq u + \delta \\ 0 & \text{otherwise} \end{cases}.$$

Example 2.5 The expression *around four o'clock* can be mathematically modeled by the symmetric triangular fuzzy number A, whose membership function is given by

$$\varphi_A(x) = \begin{cases} 1 - \frac{|x-4|}{0.2} & \text{if } 3.8 \leq x \leq 4.2 \\ 0 & \text{otherwise} \end{cases},$$

and is represented in Fig. 2.4. From (2.10) we obtain the α-levels of this fuzzy subset, which are the intervals $[a_1^\alpha, a_2^\alpha]$, where

Fig. 2.3 Representation of
the fuzzy number $\widehat{2}$

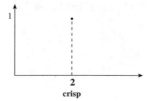

$$a_1^\alpha = 0.2\,\alpha + 3.8 \text{ and } a_2^\alpha = -0.2\,\alpha + 4.2.$$

Definition 2.5 A fuzzy number A is said to be *trapezoidal* if its membership function has the form of a trapezoid and is given by

$$\varphi_A(x) = \begin{cases} \frac{x-a}{b-a} & \text{if } a \leq x < b \\ 1 & \text{if } b \leq x \leq c \\ \frac{d-x}{d-c} & \text{if } c < x \leq d \\ 0 & \text{otherwise} \end{cases},$$

where a, b, c, d are given numbers.

The α-levels of a trapezoidal fuzzy set are the intervals

$$[a_1^\alpha, a_2^\alpha] = [(b-a)\alpha + a, \ (c-d)\alpha + d] \tag{2.11}$$

for all $\alpha \in [0, 1]$.

Example 2.6 The fuzzy set of the *teenagers* can be represented by the trapezoidal fuzzy number with the membership function

$$\varphi_A(x) = \begin{cases} \frac{x-11}{3} & \text{if } 11 \leq x < 14 \\ 1 & \text{if } 14 \leq x \leq 17 \\ \frac{20-x}{3} & \text{if } 17 < x \leq 20 \\ 0 & \text{otherwise} \end{cases},$$

and it is illustrated in Fig. 2.5. Equation (2.11) provides the α-levels for this example

$$[3\,\alpha + 11, \ -3\,\alpha + 20], \text{ with } \alpha \in [0, 1].$$

Definition 2.6 A fuzzy number has the *bell shape* if the membership function is smooth and symmetric in relation to a given real number. The following membership function has those properties for fixed u, a and δ (see Fig. 2.6).

Fig. 2.4 Representation of the fuzzy number "around 4"

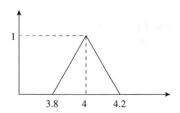

$$\varphi_A(x) = \begin{cases} \exp\left(-\left(\dfrac{x-u}{a}\right)^2\right) & \text{if } u - \delta \le x \le u + \delta \\ 0 & \text{otherwise} \end{cases}.$$

The α-levels of fuzzy numbers in bell shape are the intervals:

$$[a_1^\alpha, a_2^\alpha] = \begin{cases} \left[u - \sqrt{\ln\left(\dfrac{1}{\alpha^{a^2}}\right)}, u + \sqrt{\ln\left(\dfrac{1}{\alpha^{a^2}}\right)}\right] & \text{if } \alpha \ge \overline{\alpha} = e^{-\left(\frac{\delta}{a}\right)^2} \\ [u - \delta, u + \delta] & \text{if } \alpha < \overline{\alpha} = e^{-\left(\frac{\delta}{a}\right)^2} \end{cases}. \quad (2.12)$$

We next present the arithmetic operations for fuzzy numbers, that is, the operations that allow us "to compute" with fuzzy sets.

2.2.1 Arithmetic Operations with Fuzzy Numbers

The arithmetic operations involving fuzzy numbers are closely linked to the interval arithmetic operations. Let us list some of those operations for closed intervals on the real line $\mathbb{R}$.

Interval Arithmetic Operations

Let λ be a real number and, A and B two closed intervals on the real line given by

$$A = [a_1, a_2] \text{ and } B = [b_1, b_2].$$

Definition 2.7 (*Interval Operations*) The arithmetic operations between intervals can be defined as:

(a) The *sum* between A and B is the interval

Fig. 2.5 Trapezoidal fuzzy number

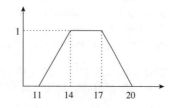

Fig. 2.6 Fuzzy number in the bell shape

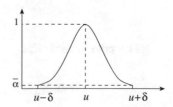

$$A + B = [a_1 + b_1, a_2 + b_2].$$

(b) The *difference* between A and B is the interval

$$A - B = [a_1 - b_2, a_2 - b_1].$$

(c) The *multiplication* of A by a scalar λ is the interval

$$\lambda A = \begin{cases} [\lambda a_1, \lambda a_2] & \text{if } \lambda \geq 0 \\ [\lambda a_2, \lambda a_1] & \text{if } \lambda < 0 \end{cases}.$$

(d) The *multiplication* of A by B is the interval

$$A \cdot B = [\min P, \max P],$$

where $P = \{a_1 b_1, a_1 b_2, a_2 b_1, a_2 b_2\}$.

(e) The *quotient* of A by B, if $0 \notin B$, is the interval

$$A/B = [a_1, a_2] \cdot \left[\frac{1}{b_2}, \frac{1}{b_1} \right].$$

Exercise 2.3 Compute the results of the operations defined above for the intervals

$$A = [-1, 2] \quad \text{and} \quad B = [5, 6].$$

Notice that the arithmetic operations for intervals extend the respective operations for real numbers. To see this, it is sufficient to observe that each real number can be considered as a closed interval with equal endpoints. Also the membership functions obtained by interval arithmetic operations can be derived directly from the respective operations for real numbers. Such a procedure uses the *extension principle*, which will be a tool to obtain the arithmetic operations of fuzzy numbers.

Let us consider an arbitrary binary operation "$\otimes$" between real numbers. Let χ_A and χ_B be the characteristic functions of the intervals A and B, respectively. The theorem that follows gives us the interval arithmetic operations for the respective operations for real numbers via the *extension principle*.

Theorem 2.2 *(Extension Principle for Real Intervals) Let A and B be two closed intervals of $\mathbb{R}$ and $\otimes$ one of the arithmetic operations between real numbers. Then*

$$\chi_{A \otimes B}(z) = \sup_{\{(x,y):x \otimes y = z\}} \min[\chi_A(x), \chi_B(y)]$$

It is simple to verify that

$$\min(\chi_A(x), \chi_B(y)) = \begin{cases} 1 & \text{if } x \in A \text{ and } y \in B \\ 0 & \text{if } x \notin A \text{ or } y \notin B \end{cases}.$$

Thus, for the sum case ($\otimes = +$), we have

$$\sup_{\{(x,y):x+y=z\}} \min[\chi_A(x), \chi_B(y)] = \begin{cases} 1 & \text{if } x \in A + B \\ 0 & \text{if } x \notin A + B \end{cases}.$$

The other cases can be obtained analogously.

An important consequence of the Theorem 2.2 for operations with fuzzy numbers is the corollary that follows.

Corollary 2.3 *The α-levels of the crisp set $A + B$ with the characteristic function $\chi_{(A+B)}$ are given by*

$$[A + B]^\alpha = A + B$$

for all $\alpha \in [0, 1]$.

Remember that the intervals A and B are fuzzy sets of the real line, so that the result of this corollary is an immediate consequence of the characteristic function definition of a classical set. The arithmetic operations for fuzzy numbers may be defined from the extension principle for fuzzy sets in analogous way. Actually, they are particular cases of the extension principle where the functions that must be extended are traditional operations for real numbers.

Arithmetic Operations with Fuzzy Numbers

The definitions that follow can be interpreted as particular cases of the extension principle, both for a function of one and two variables.

Definition 2.8 Let A and B be two fuzzy numbers and λ a real number.

(a) The *sum* of the fuzzy numbers A and B is the fuzzy number $A + B$, whose membership function is

$$\varphi_{(A+B)}(z) = \sup_{\phi(z)} \min[\varphi_A(x), \varphi_B(y)]$$

where $\phi(z) = \{(x, y) : x + y = z\}$.

(b) The *multiplication* of A by a scalar λ is the fuzzy number λA, whose membership function is

$$\varphi_{\lambda A}(z) = \begin{cases} \sup_{\{x:\lambda x=z\}} [\varphi_A(x)] & \text{if } \lambda \neq 0 \\ \chi_{\{0\}}(z) & \text{if } \lambda = 0 \end{cases} = \begin{cases} \varphi_A(\lambda^{-1}z) & \text{if } \lambda \neq 0 \\ \chi_{\{0\}}(z) & \text{if } \lambda = 0 \end{cases},$$

where $\chi_{\{0\}}$ is the characteristic function of $\{0\}$.

(c) The *difference* $A - B$ is the fuzzy number whose membership function is given by:

$$\varphi_{(A-B)}(z) = \sup_{\phi(z)} \min[\varphi_A(x), \varphi_B(y)]$$

where $\phi(z) = \{(x, y) : x - y = z\}$.

(d) The *multiplication* of A by B is the fuzzy number $A.B$, whose membership function is given by:

$$\varphi_{(A.B)}(z) = \sup_{\phi(z)} \min[\varphi_A(x), \varphi_B(y)]$$

where $\phi(z) = \{(x, y) : xy = z\}$.

(e) The *quotient* is the fuzzy number A/B whose membership function is

$$\varphi_{(A/B)}(z) = \sup_{\phi(z)} \min[\varphi_A(x), \varphi_B(y)]$$

where $\phi(z) = \{(x, y) : x/y = z\}$ and $0 \notin supp B$.

Theorem 2.4 below ensures that the result of the arithmetic operations between fuzzy numbers is a fuzzy number. Moreover, it generalizes Corollary 2.3, relating, via α-levels, arithmetic operations for fuzzy numbers with the respective interval arithmetic operations.

Theorem 2.4 *The α-levels of the fuzzy set $A \otimes B$ are given by*

$$[A \otimes B]^\alpha = [A]^\alpha \otimes [B]^\alpha$$

for all $\alpha \in [0, 1]$, where $\otimes$ is any arithmetic operations $\{+, -, \times, \div\}$.

Although the proof of this theorem will be done here, we can say it is a consequence of the Theorem 2.1 applied to the function $\otimes$, since it is continuous as long as we do not divide by zero. The interested reader can find the proof in the classical books of Klir and Yuan [5], Nguyen [6], Pedrycz and Gomide [7] or more generally in Fuller [8].

The combination of the Theorems 2.1 and 2.4 produces "practical methods" to obtain the results of each operation between fuzzy numbers. We observe again that the α-levels of a fuzzy number is always a closed interval of $\mathbb{R}$ given by:

$$[A]^\alpha = \left[a_1^\alpha, a_2^\alpha\right], \text{ with } a_1^\alpha = \min\{\varphi_A^{-1}(\alpha)\} \text{ and } a_2^\alpha = \max\{\varphi_A^{-1}(\alpha)\},$$

where $\varphi_A^{-1}(\alpha) = \{x \in \mathbb{R} : \varphi_A(x) = \alpha\}$ is the preimage of α.

Hereafter we illustrate such "practical methods" through properties given below.

Proposition 2.5 *Let A and B be fuzzy numbers with α-levels respectively given by $[A]^\alpha = \left[a_1^\alpha, a_2^\alpha\right]$ and $[B]^\alpha = \left[b_1^\alpha, b_2^\alpha\right]$. Then the following properties hold:*

(a) The sum of A and B is the fuzzy number $A + B$ whose α-levels are

$$[A + B]^\alpha = [A]^\alpha + [B]^\alpha = \left[a_1^\alpha + b_1^\alpha, a_2^\alpha + b_2^\alpha\right].$$

(b) *The difference of A and B is the fuzzy number* $A - B$ *whose α-levels are*

$$[A - B]^\alpha = [A]^\alpha - [B]^\alpha = \left[a_1^\alpha - b_2^\alpha, a_2^\alpha - b_1^\alpha\right].$$

(c) *The multiplication of A by a scalar λ is the fuzzy number λA whose α-levels are*

$$[\lambda A]^\alpha = \lambda[A]^\alpha = \begin{cases} [\lambda a_1^\alpha, \lambda a_2^\alpha] & if \ \lambda \geq 0 \\ [\lambda a_2^\alpha, \lambda a_1^\alpha] & if \ \lambda < 0 \end{cases}.$$

(d) *The multiplication of A by B is the fuzzy number $A \cdot B$ whose α-levels are*

$$[A \cdot B]^\alpha = [A]^\alpha [B]^\alpha = \left[\min P^\alpha, \max P^\alpha\right],$$

where $P^\alpha = \{a_1^\alpha b_1^\alpha, a_1^\alpha b_2^\alpha, a_2^\alpha b_1^\alpha, a_2^\alpha b_2^\alpha\}$.

(e) *The division of A by B, if $0 \notin$ supp B, is the fuzzy number whose α-levels are*

$$\left[\frac{A}{B}\right]^\alpha = \frac{[A]^\alpha}{[B]^\alpha} = \left[a_1^\alpha, a_2^\alpha\right]\left[\frac{1}{b_2^\alpha}, \frac{1}{b_1^\alpha}\right].$$

Example 2.7 Consider the expressions *nearly* 2 and *nearly* 4 and let A and B be the triangular fuzzy numbers that indicate these expressions. Thus, we define

$$A = (1; 2; 3) \text{ and } B = (3; 4; 5).$$

The results of $A \otimes B$ for each of the arithmetic operations between fuzzy numbers are shown next. First, let us notice that according to formula (2.10)

$$[A]^\alpha = [1 + \alpha, 3 - \alpha] \text{ and } [B]^\alpha = [3 + \alpha, 5 - \alpha].$$

Then by Proposition 2.5 we get

(a) $[A + B]^\alpha = [A]^\alpha + [B]^\alpha = [4 + 2\alpha, 8 - 2\alpha]$. Thus, $A + B = (4; 6; 8)$;
(b) $[A - B]^\alpha = [A]^\alpha - [B]^\alpha = [-4 + 2\alpha, -2\alpha]$. Thus, $A - B = (-4; -2; 0)$;
(c) $[4 \cdot A]^\alpha = 4[A]^\alpha = [4 + 4\alpha, 12 - 4\alpha]$. Thus, $4A = (4; 8; 12)$;
(d) $[A \cdot B]^\alpha = [A]^\alpha [B]^\alpha = [(1 + \alpha)(3 + \alpha), (3 - \alpha)(5 - \alpha)]$;
(e) $\left[\frac{A}{B}\right]^\alpha = \frac{[A]^\alpha}{[B]^\alpha} = [(1 + \alpha)/(5 - \alpha), (3 - \alpha)/(3 + \alpha)]$.

Notice that the fuzzy numbers obtained in (d) and (e) are not triangular. However, it is easy to verify that with triangular fuzzy numbers, the sum, the difference and the multiplication by a scalar results in a triangular fuzzy number. To see this, it suffices to consider the numbers $A = (a_1; u; a_2)$ and $B = (b_1; v; b_3)$. Then, from Eq. (2.10), we have

$$[A]^\alpha = [(u - a_1)\alpha + a_1, (u - a_2)\alpha + a_2]$$
$$[B]^\alpha = [(v - b_1)\alpha + b_1, (v - b_2)\alpha + b_2].$$

Thus

$$[A + B]^\alpha = [A]^\alpha + [B]^\alpha$$

and then

$$[A+B]^\alpha = [\{(u+v)-(a_1+b_1)\}\alpha+(a_1+b_1), \{(u+v)-(a_2+b_2)\}\alpha+(a_2+b_2)].$$

Using Eq. (2.10) again, we see that these intervals are the α-levels of the following triangular fuzzy number:

$$((a_1 + b_1); (u + v); (a_2 + b_2)).$$

Finally, it is possible to conclude that $(A - B) + B \neq A$ so that it follows that $A - A \neq 0$. That is, the space of fuzzy numbers is not a vector space since there are no additive (nor multiplication) inverses. This is a property that hampers many areas of the fuzzy mathematics, for example, the area of fuzzy differential equations (see Chap. 8) and is a challenge to fuzzy linear systems to mention but two areas.

Exercise 2.4 Redo the Example 2.7 from the point of view of the extension principle.

The next example presents an explicit way to obtain the function $\widehat{f}$ in the case that f is linear.

Example 2.8 Let $f : \mathbb{R} \to \mathbb{R}$ be the function $f(x) = \lambda x$, with $\lambda \neq 0$ a scalar. If A is a fuzzy number with membership function φ_A, then according to the Definition 2.1, the membership function of $\widehat{f}(A)$ is given by

$$\varphi_{\widehat{f}(A)}(z) = \sup_{\{x:f(x)=z\}} \varphi_A(x) = \sup_{\{x:\lambda x=z\}}\varphi_A(x)$$
$$= \sup_{\{z/\lambda\}}\varphi_A(x) = \varphi_A(z/\lambda) = \varphi_A(\lambda^{-1}z),$$

which, according to Definition 2.9b, is the membership function of λA. Thus, if $f(x) = \lambda x$, then $\widehat{f} : \mathcal{F}(\mathbb{R}) \to \mathcal{F}(\mathbb{R})$ is given by $\widehat{f}(A) = \lambda A$.

Exercise 2.5 Verify that if $f(x) = \lambda x + b$, with $\lambda \neq 0$, then for any fuzzy number A the fuzzy set $\widehat{f}(A)$ has the following membership function

$$\varphi_{\widehat{f}(A)}(z) \doteq \varphi_A(\lambda^{-1}(z - b)).$$

After, verify that $\widehat{f}(A)$ is a triangular fuzzy number if A is triangular.

Exercise 2.6 From Theorem 2.1 and the proprieties of the arithmetic operations, show that Zadeh's Extension of an affine function $f(x) = ax + b$, is the affine function $\widehat{f}(X) = aX + \widehat{b}$ if $X \in \mathcal{F}(\mathbb{R})$.

Let us use the extension principle to compute the image of a triangular fuzzy number by a known function. Similar to the example of the operations of division and multiplication, the image of a function of triangular numbers may not be triangular even if the function is continuous.

Example 2.9 Consider the function $f(x) = e^x$ and the triangular fuzzy number $A = (0; \ln 2; \ln 3)$.

According to Theorem 1.2, $\widehat{f}(A)$ is determined by its α-levels. From (2.10) it is easy to see that the α-levels of A are the intervals

$$[A]^\alpha = [(\ln 2)\alpha, (\ln 2 - \ln 3)\alpha + \ln 3] = \left[\ln 2^\alpha, \ln\left(3\left(\frac{2}{3}\right)^\alpha\right)\right],$$

with $\alpha \in [0, 1]$.

Now, we obtain the α-levels of $\widehat{f}(A)$ using Theorem 2.1, that is,

$$[\widehat{f}(A)]^\alpha = f([A]^\alpha) = f\left(\left[\ln 2^\alpha, \ln 3\left(\frac{2}{3}\right)^\alpha\right]\right) = \left[2^\alpha, 3\left(\frac{2}{3}\right)^\alpha\right],$$

with $\alpha \in [0, 1]$. Figure 2.7 illustrates $\widehat{f}(A)$ of this example. Therefore,

- if $\alpha = 0$ then $[\widehat{f}(A)]^0 = [1, 3]$;
- if $\alpha = \frac{1}{2}$ then $[\widehat{f}(A)]^{\frac{1}{2}} = [\sqrt{2}, \sqrt{6}]$;
- if $\alpha = 1$ then $[\widehat{f}(A)]^1 = \{2\}$.

Now, it is easy to verify that the points $(1, 0)$; $(\sqrt{2}, \frac{1}{2})$ and $(2, 1)$ are not aligned, that is, not a straight line. So $\widehat{f}(A)$ is not a triangular number.

Example 2.10 Consider that a bus trip from the city of Campinas to São Paulo is subject to the following:

- The distance between the two cities is nearly 100 km;
- The speed can not exceed 120 km/h;
- The traffic is usually intense and the speed also decreases at the toll booths;
- The bus usually leaves Campinas late, but the lateness never exceeds more than 30 min.

Question: What is the total time (T) spent on a trip from Campinas to São Paulo by bus?

The solution to this problem from a classical mathematics point of view with an exact real number answer is impossible, since we just have partial information and ill-defined reports. An intuitive approach to solve this problem as may be answered by a person questioned about the solution of this problem may be something like: "*the total time is just a little bit more than one hour*" or "*between one and one hour and a half*". These answers may be based on personal experience of those who have faced the same or similar situations. The reasoning may be as follows: This bus goes fast on the road but the intense traffic and the toll booths force the bus to slow down, besides,

Fig. 2.7 Zadeh's Extension of the triangular fuzzy number $A = (0; \ln 2; \ln 3)$ for $f(x) = e^x$

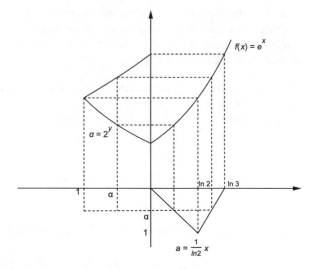

the bus usually leaves the station late. Therefore, if we want a precise value (real number) for the answer, we need to adopt precise values for the data. For example, a mean speed of 90 km/h and a delay of 15 min (T_1) would result in the answer:

$$T = T_1 + T_2 = 15 \, \text{min} \, + (1 \, \text{h and } 6.66 \, \text{min}) = 1.36 \, \text{h}.$$

But the idea here is to propose a mathematical model for this "intuitive arithmetic" that allows people to compute with imprecise data (as the ones in our problem) to obtain a result with information based on fuzzy numbers, even though they might be linguistic answers and at the same time informative and numerically based. Therefore, we want a model that allows this type of reasoning used by people.

Let approach this example from a fuzzy set theoretic point of view.

- Since the distance (D) of the route is approximate, we can consider it a fuzzy number around 100 km. It can be, for example, a triangular number $D = (90; 100; 110)$ whose membership function is

$$\varphi_D(x) = \begin{cases} 0 & \text{if} & x \le 90 \\ \frac{x}{10} - 9 & \text{if} & 90 < x \le 100 \\ 11 - \frac{x}{10} & \text{if} & 100 < x \le 110 \\ 0 & \text{if} & x > 110 \end{cases}$$

and α-levels given by $[D]^\alpha = [10\alpha + 90, -10\alpha + 110]$. Notice that formula (2.6) can be used to get these α-levels.

- The uncertain about the speed of the bus (V) can also be modeled by a triangular fuzzy number. Taking into account that the speed never exceeds 120 km/h and that we have some low speeds in route, we can suppose that $V = (30; 100; 120)$, whose α-levels are $[V]^\alpha = [70\alpha + 30, -20\alpha + 120]$.

- The fact that the bus usually leaves the station late indicates that we should have an extra time (T_1) that does not exceed *half an hour*. This time can be modeled by the triangular fuzzy number $T_1 = (0; 0; 0.5)$, whose α-levels are

$$[T_1]^\alpha = [0, -0.5\alpha + 0.5] = \left[0, \frac{1-\alpha}{2}\right].$$

From physics, the time that is spent on the road (T_2) is obtained by the fuzzy number $T_2 = \frac{D}{V}$. From Proposition 2.5 we have that the α-levels of T_2 are:

$$[T_2]^\alpha = [10\alpha + 90, 110 - 10\alpha]\left[\frac{1}{120 - 20\alpha}, \frac{1}{70\alpha + 30}\right].$$

Therefore, the total time (T) is given by the fuzzy number $T = T_1 + T_2$ whose α-levels are:

$$[T]^\alpha = \left[0, \frac{1-\alpha}{2}\right] + \left[\frac{10\alpha + 90}{120 - 20\alpha}, \frac{110 - 10\alpha}{70\alpha + 30}\right]$$

$$= \left[\frac{10\alpha + 90}{120 - 20\alpha}, \frac{1-\alpha}{2} + \frac{110 - 10\alpha}{70\alpha + 30}\right]$$

$$= [f(\alpha), g(\alpha)].$$

This would be the fuzzy solution of the problem which includes the times between $\frac{3}{4}$ h and $\frac{25}{6}$ h. We can also observe that the time with the highest possibility $(\alpha = 1)$ is $t = 1$ h. The time $t = 1.36$ h given at the beginning of the discussion (with precise data) would have membership degree of $\alpha^* \simeq 0.8$ in the total time set T, since

$$1.36 = \frac{1 - \alpha^*}{2} + \frac{110 - 10\alpha^*}{70\alpha^* + 30}.$$

In the fuzzy context, a real number - obtained a-posteriori by the defuzzification of the fuzzy set T (see Sect. 5.4) or considering the fuzzy expectation of T (Definition 7.10) - could also be used to represent the solution to this problem.

Exercise 2.7 Redo the example, but now, using the arithmetic operations from the extension principle. For that, the reader must consider the membership functions of each fuzzy set. Also, verify that, even though all the sets are triangular, the answer T is not a triangular fuzzy number. Sketch the graphs of $f(\alpha)$ and $g(\alpha)$ to observe that.

Definition 2.9 (*Hukuhara Difference: $A -_H B$*) Let A and B be two fuzzy numbers. If there exists a fuzzy number C such that $A = B + C$, then C is called the Hukuhara Difference of A and B and we denote it by $A -_H B$.

In terms of α-levels this is equivalent to saying that

$$[A -_H B]^\alpha = [a_1^\alpha - b_1^\alpha, a_2^\alpha - b_2^\alpha] \ \forall \ \alpha \in [0, 1].$$

Since

$$[A - B]^\alpha = [a_1^\alpha - b_2^\alpha, a_2^\alpha - b_1^\alpha],$$

it follows that

$$A - B = A -_H B \ \Leftrightarrow \ b_1^\alpha = b_2^\alpha,$$

that is,

$$A - B = A -_H B \ \Leftrightarrow \ B \in \mathbb{R}.$$

Notice that, in general,

$$A - B = A + (-1)B \neq A -_H B.$$

This difference, historically, was first used to study derivatives of fuzzy functions (see Chap. 8).

Let us look at a relationship between the extension principle and the probability theory before we close this chapter. Consider the following Tables 2.1 and 2.2.

The question is: "How can we obtain the uncertain distribution for $Z = X + Y$?". It is clear that the "possible" values for $Z = X + Y$ are the elements of the set $\{5, 6, 7\}$. Table 2.3 shows the values of $\varphi_{X+Y}(z_i)$ and $P_{X+Y}(z_i)$, where P denote the probability and φ the membership function:

According to the formulas

$$\varphi_{X+Y}(z_i) = \sup_{x_j + y_k = z_i} \min(\varphi_A(x_j), \varphi_B(y_k)) \tag{2.13}$$

and

$$P_{X+Y}(z_i) = \sum_{x_j + y_k = z_i} P_{(X,Y)}(X = x_j, Y = y_k), \tag{2.14}$$

where $P_{(X,Y)}(X = x_j, Y = y_k)$ is the joint probability distribution of the random vector (X, Y) (see [9, 10]).

The main observation that we have here is that to obtain the probability of $X + Y$, we need to add the independence hypothesis. However, to compute the membership distribution of $X + Y$ according to the extension principle, the analogous hypothesis is not needed. We stress that if X and Y are independent and we note that the formulas

Table 2.1 Membership and probability distributions of X

$X = x_j$	$\varphi_X(x_j)$	$P_X(x_j)$
2	0.5	0.5
3	0.5	0.5

Table 2.2 Membership and probability distributions of Y

$Y = y_k$	$\varphi_Y(y_k)$	$P_Y(y_k)$
3	0.5	0.5
4	0.5	0.5

Table 2.3 Membership and probability distributions of $X + Y$

$Z = X + Y$	$\varphi_{X+Y}(z_i)$	$P_{X+Y}(z_i)$
5	0.5	0.25
6	0.5	0.50
7	0.5	0.25

(2.13) and (2.14) have some kind of similarity, exchanging **sup** by Σ and **min** by **product**.

Finally, we observe that the last two columns of the Table 2.3 represent, respectively, the "membership" and the "occurrence" of each element of the first column to the sum set. Intuitively, a higher probability for 6 is expected, since its "occurrence" is more than the others. On the other hand, from the fuzzy set theory point of view, which is an extension of the classical set theory, the value 6 belongs to the sum set with the same membership of the others. The number of times that it "occurs" does not matter.

References

1. R.E. Moore, W. Strother, C.T. Yang, *Interval integrals*, Technical Report LMSD-703073, Lockheed Aircraft Corporation: Missiles and Space Division, Sunnyvale, California (1960)
2. L.C. Barros, *Sobre sistemas dinâmicos fuzzy - teoria e aplicação*, Tese de Doutorado, IMECC-UNICAMP, Campinas (1997)
3. M.S. Ceconello, *Sistemas Dinâmicos em Espaços Métricos Fuzzy - Aplicações em Biomatemática*, Tese de Doutorado, IMECC-UNICAMP, Campinas (2010)
4. H. Román-Flores, L.C. Barros, R.C. Bassanezi, A note on zadeh's extensions. Fuzzy Sets Syst. **117**(3), 327–331 (2001)
5. G. Klir, B. Yuan, *Fuzzy Sets and Fuzzy Logic Theory and Applications* (Prentice-Hall, Upper Saddle River, 1995)
6. H.T. Nguyen, E.A. Walker, *A First Course of Fuzzy Logic* (CRC Press, Boca Raton, 1997)
7. W. Pedrycz, F. Gomide, *An Introduction to Fuzzy Sets: Analysis and Design* (The MIT Press, Massachusets, 1998)
8. R. Füller, T. Keresztfalvi, On generalization of Nguyen' theorem. Fuzzy Sets Syst. **41**, 371–374 (1990)
9. W.O. Bussab, P.A. Morettin, *Estatística básica*, 5th edn. (Editora Saraiva, São Paulo, 2002)
10. S.M. Ross, *A First Course in Probability* (Pearson Prentice Hall, Upper Saddle River, 2010)

Chapter 3
Fuzzy Relations

Everything that exists in nature is due to chance and need.
(Democritus, C.460–C.370 BCE)

Abstract This chapter presents a short discussion of mathematical relations, basic concepts of fuzzy relations, and the composition between two fuzzy relations. Lastly, the chapter presents the rule for the composition of inferences, which is relevant to the modus ponens discussed in the next chapter.

Do the individuals of a species agree with Democritus: they relate to one another so as to construct the trajectories in the course of their lives only to survive apparently without any interest of optimizing anything? Or do they seek the maximum return for the minimum of effort, as was advocated by Leibniz when he said "that we live in the best of all worlds?" Maybe the difference between these two poles is just a matter of gradual truth.

Studies dealing with associations, relations or interactions between elements of many classes is of great interest in the analysis and understanding of many phenomena of real world problems and mathematics. Such studies are always concerned with establishing such relations. We will see in this chapter that fuzzy relations are a natural extension of classical mathematical relations and these fuzzy relations have wide applications.

3.1 Fuzzy Relations

The concept of relation in mathematics is formalized from the point of view of set theory. We will follow the same path. Intuitively, we say that the relation is *fuzzy* when we adopt a fuzzy set theory point of view, and is *crisp* when we use classical set theory to conceptualize the relation. The choice of the relation depends on the phenomenon that we are studying. However, fuzzy set theory is always more general

© Springer-Verlag Berlin Heidelberg 2017

L.C. de Barros et al., *A First Course in Fuzzy Logic, Fuzzy Dynamical Systems, and Biomathematics*, Studies in Fuzziness and Soft Computing 347, DOI 10.1007/978-3-662-53324-6_3

than classical set theory, since fuzzy set theory includes classical set theory as a particular case (remember that a classical set—*crisp* set—is a particular fuzzy set). A classical relation indicates if there is or is not some association between two elements, while fuzzy relations indicate, in addition, the degree of this association.

Definition 3.1 A (classical) *relation* $\mathcal{R}$ over $U_1 \times U_2 \times \cdots \times U_n$ is any (classical) subset of the Cartesian product $U_1 \times U_2 \times \cdots \times U_n$. If the Cartesian product is formed by just two sets $U_1 \times U_2$, this relation is called a *binary relation* over $U_1 \times U_2$. If $U_1 = U_2 = \cdots = U_n = U$, we say that $\mathcal{R}$ is a *n-ary relation* over U.

A crisp relation $\mathcal{R}$ is a subset of the Cartesian product and can be represented by its characteristic function

$$\chi_\mathcal{R} : U_1 \times U_2 \times \ldots \times U_n \longrightarrow \{0, 1\} ,$$

with

$$\chi_\mathcal{R}(x_1, x_2, \ldots, x_n) = \begin{cases} 1 & \text{if } (x_1, x_2, \ldots, x_n) \in \mathcal{R} \\ 0 & \text{if } (x_1, x_2, \ldots, x_n) \notin \mathcal{R} \end{cases} . \tag{3.1}$$

The mathematical concept of fuzzy relation is formalized from the usual Cartesian product between sets, extending the characteristic function of a classical relation to a membership function.

Definition 3.2 A *fuzzy relation* $\mathcal{R}$ over $U_1 \times U_2 \times \ldots \times U_n$ is any fuzzy subset of $U_1 \times U_2 \times \ldots \times U_n$. Thus, a fuzzy relation $\mathcal{R}$ is defined by a membership function $\varphi_\mathcal{R} : U_1 \times U_2 \times \ldots \times U_n \longrightarrow [0, 1]$.

If the Cartesian product is formed by just two sets $U_1 \times U_2$, the relation is called a *binary fuzzy* relation over $U_1 \times U_2$. If the sets U_i, $i = 1, 2, \ldots, n$, are all equal to U, then we say that $\mathcal{R}$ is a *n-ary fuzzy relation* over U. For example, a binary fuzzy relation over U is a fuzzy relation $\mathcal{R}$ over $U \times U$. If a membership function of the fuzzy relation $\mathcal{R}$ is indicated by $\varphi_\mathcal{R}$, then the number

$$\varphi_\mathcal{R}(x_1, x_2, \ldots, x_n) \in [0, 1]$$

indicates the degree to which the elements x_i that compose the *n-tuple* $(x_1, x_2, \ldots, x_n)$ are related according to the relation $\mathcal{R}$.

The fuzzy inference relationships which are used in making decisions are of great importance, especially in the theory of the fuzzy controllers, as we shall see in Chap. 5. Technically, in fuzzy set theory this operation is similar to intersection, as seen in Chap. 1, Sect. 1.3. The great difference is in the associated universe from which the set comes. While in the intersection of fuzzy subsets, the same universal sets are the same, in the Cartesian product they can be different, as we shall see in the next definition.

Definition 3.3 The *fuzzy Cartesian product* of the fuzzy subsets $A_1, A_2, ..., A_n$ of U_1, $U_2, ..., U_n$, respectively, is the fuzzy relation $A_1 \times A_2 \times \cdots \times A_n$, whose membership function is given by

$$\varphi_{A_1 \times A_2 \times \cdots \times A_n}(x_1, x_2, \ldots, x_n) = \varphi_{A_1}(x_1) \wedge \varphi_{A_2}(x_2) \wedge \cdots \wedge \varphi_{A_n}(x_n),$$

where $\wedge$ represents the minimum.

Notice that if $A_1, A_2, \ldots, A_n$ are classical sets, then the classical Cartesian product $A_1 \times A_2 \times \cdots \times A_n$ may be obtained by Definition 3.3, substituting the membership functions by the respective characteristic functions of the sets $A_1, A_2, \ldots, A_n$. The next example illustrates the application of the Cartesian product.

Example 3.1 Let us consider again the Table 1.1 of the Example 1.8 which relates the diagnostics of 5 patients with two symptoms: fever and myalgia.

Patient	F: Fever	M: Myalgia	D: Diagnosis
1	0.7	0.6	0.6
2	1.0	1.0	1.0
3	0.4	0.2	0.2
4	0.5	0.5	0.5
5	1.0	0.2	0.2

To diagnose a patient the doctor evaluates the symptoms that are specific to each disease. Many diseases can present symptoms like fever and myalgia with different intensities and measures. For example, for flu, the patient with fever and myalgia with intensities that, if represented by fuzzy subsets, must have distinct universal sets. The universe that indicates the fever can be given by the possible temperatures of a person, while the myalgia can be assessed by the numbers of painful areas.

The indication of how much an individual has flu can be taken as the degree of membership of the set of the fever symptoms and the set of myalgia. For example, the patient 1 in Table 1.1 has temperature x whose membership in the fever set F is $\varphi_F(x) = 0.7$ and the value y to myalgia is $\varphi_M(y) = 0.6$. The diagnosis of the patient 1 for the flu is then given by:

$$\text{Patient 1: } \varphi_{\text{flu}}(x, y) = \varphi_F(x) \wedge \varphi_M(y) = 0.7 \wedge 0.6 = 0.6.$$

Here we have used the fuzzy binary relationship "and" as "min". This means that the patient 1 is in the fuzzy subset of the ones who have fever and myalgia with membership degree 0.6 which coincides with the degree of its diagnosis for flu.

This number obtained can give support to a physician's decision of which adopted treatment is best for the patient. It is clear that from the theoretical point of view, the classical Cartesian product could also be employed for the diagnoses. In this case the information would be flu (degree one) or not flu (degree zero). Consequently, just patient 2 of Table 1.1 would be considered to have flu.

Chapter 6, Sect. 6.2.3, will present a more complete study about medical diagnoses. However, we want to note that in the example above we have used the "min" binary relationship because we have assumed that flu occurs with myalgia. However, if myalgia was not a strong correlated part of the diagnosis, we would use a different fuzzy relationship.

Exercise 3.1 Compare the Example 3.1 with the Example 1.8 and explain the difference between them.

Exercise 3.2 Investigate one more symptom that is typical for flu (coryza, for example) and add it as a fuzzy subset in Table 1.1 (create some values) and diagnose the patients who have flu using the "and" operator.

3.1.1 Forms of Representation and Properties of the Binary Relations

This text will just stress the forms of representation and some properties of the binary relations and fuzzy binary relations, which will be illustrated by some examples. The interested reader can consult other texts for more detailed discussion of relationships. The following example will help to illustrate the main representations that we will be using in this text.

Example 3.2 Let U be an ecosystem with the following populations: *eagles* (e), *snakes* (s), *insects* (i), *hare* (h) and *frogs* (f). A possible study between the individuals of these populations might be the predation process, that is, the relation *prey-predator*. To study the relation between two individuals from this ecosystem, this relation can be mathematically modeled by a *binary relation* $\mathcal{R}$ with $\varphi_{\mathcal{R}}(x, y) = 0$ if y is not a predator of x and $\varphi_R (x, y) \neq 0$ if y is a predator of x, where x and y are individuals from the set U.

Next, we will discuss two possible cases of the use of the classical relation and of the fuzzy relation for this example.

- If the interest regarding the relation is just to indicate who is the predator and who is the prey in U, then we can choose the classical theory and $\mathcal{R}$ will be a classical binary relation. In this case,

$$\varphi_{\mathcal{R}}(x, y) = \chi_{\mathcal{R}}(x, y) = \begin{cases} 1 & \text{if } y \text{ is a predator of } x \\ 0 & \text{if } y \text{ is not a predator of } x \end{cases}.$$

A graphic representation for this relation is in Fig. 3.1, where we put the animals in alphabetical order on a pair of axes.

The points that are highlighted in Fig. 3.1 indicate the pairs that belong to the relation $\mathcal{R}$, that is, the relation $\mathcal{R}$ reveals who is the predator of whom accordingly to some specialist.

Fig. 3.1 Representation of
the classical relation between
the predators and their prey

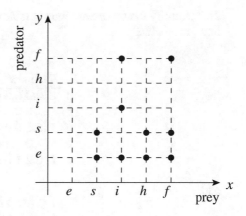

Fig. 3.2 Fuzzy relation and
the many degrees of
preference

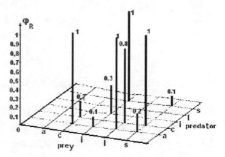

- If there is interest in knowing, for example, the gradual preference of a predator for
  some prey in U, then a good option is to choose $\mathcal{R}$ as a fuzzy relation. In that case,
  $\varphi_{\mathcal{R}}(x, y)$ indicates the preference degree of y for prey x. Supposing that there is no
  difference in the predation degree in each species, one possibility for $\varphi_{\mathcal{R}}(x, y)$ for
  this example, might be measured according to a specialist as illustrated in Fig. 3.2,
  where in the third axis (vertical axis) this (fuzzy) measure is represented as degree
  $\varphi_{\mathcal{R}}(x, y)$.

When X and Y are finite, the most common forms to represent a binary fuzzy
relation in $X \times Y$ are the tabular and the matrix forms. Let us define $X =
\{x_1, x_2, \ldots, x_m\}$, $Y = \{y_1, y_2, \ldots, y_n\}$ and the fuzzy relation $\mathcal{R}$ over $X \times Y$ with
membership function given by $\varphi_{\mathcal{R}}(x_i, y_j) = r_{ij}$, for $1 \leq i \leq n$ and $1 \leq j \leq m$.
The representations of $\mathcal{R}$ can be in table or in matrix form as it follows below.

$$
\begin{array}{c|cccc}
\mathcal{R} & y_1 & y_2 & \cdots & y_n \\
\hline
x_1 & r_{11} & r_{12} & \cdots & r_{1n} \\
x_2 & r_{21} & r_{22} & \cdots & r_{2n} \\
\vdots & \vdots & \vdots & \ddots & \vdots \\
x_m & r_{m1} & r_{m2} & \cdots & r_{mn}
\end{array}
\quad \text{or} \quad
\mathcal{R} =
\begin{bmatrix}
r_{11} & r_{12} & \cdots & r_{1n} \\
r_{21} & r_{22} & \cdots & r_{2n} \\
\vdots & \vdots & \ddots & \vdots \\
r_{m1} & r_{m2} & \cdots & r_{mn}
\end{bmatrix}.
$$

To exemplify the representations in table and in matrix form for Example 3.2 we have, respectively,

		p	r	e	d	a	t	o	r
	$\mathcal{R}$	**e**	**s**	**i**	**h**	**f**			
p	**e**	0.0	0.0	0.0	0.0	0.0			
r	**s**	1.0	0.2	0.0	0.0	0.0			
e	**i**	0.1	0.0	0.3	0.0	1.0			
y	**h**	1.0	0.8	0.0	0.0	0.0			
s	**f**	0.2	1.0	0.0	0.0	0.1			

and

$$\mathcal{R} = \begin{bmatrix} 0.0 & 0.0 & 0.0 & 0.0 & 0.0 \\ 1.0 & 0.2 & 0.0 & 0.0 & 0.0 \\ 0.1 & 0.0 & 0.3 & 0.0 & 1.0 \\ 1.0 & 0.8 & 0.0 & 0.0 & 0.0 \\ 0.2 & 1.0 & 0.0 & 0.0 & 0.1 \end{bmatrix}.$$

The following definition will be used in subsequent analyses.

Definition 3.4 Let $\mathcal{R}$ be a binary fuzzy relation defined over $X \times Y$. The *inverse binary fuzzy relation*, $\mathcal{R}^{-1}$, defined over $Y \times X$, has the following membership function $\varphi_{\mathcal{R}^{-1}} : Y \times X \longrightarrow [0, 1]$, with $\varphi_{\mathcal{R}^{-1}}(y, x) = \varphi_{\mathcal{R}}(x, y)$.

Notice that the matrix of $\mathcal{R}^{-1}$ coincides with the transpose of $\mathcal{R}$, since $\varphi_{\mathcal{R}^{-1}}(y, x) = \varphi_{\mathcal{R}}(x, y)$. For this reason many texts of fuzzy logic adopt the term transpose relation instead of inverse (see Pedrycz and Gomide [1]). Thus, if $\mathcal{R}$ is the fuzzy relation of the Example 3.2, then the matrix representation of its inverse $\mathcal{R}^{-1}$ is given by its transpose

$$\mathcal{R}^{\mathsf{T}} = \begin{bmatrix} 0.0 & 1.0 & 0.1 & 1.0 & 0.2 \\ 0.0 & 0.2 & 0.0 & 0.8 & 1.0 \\ 0.0 & 0.0 & 0.3 & 0.0 & 0.0 \\ 0.0 & 0.0 & 0.0 & 0.0 & 0.0 \\ 0.0 & 0.0 & 1.0 & 0.0 & 0.1 \end{bmatrix}.$$

The transpose, $\mathcal{R}^{-1}$, for our prey-predator example, indicates that x is a prey of y, while by $\mathcal{R}$ we have that y is a predator of x.

3.2 Composition Between Binary Fuzzy Relations

The composition between relations is of great importance in many applications. This operation will be explored extensively in Chap. 6, where the main applications in medical diagnoses are developed. Also in Chap. 6 we will study many types of compositions between fuzzy relations. Here, in this section, we will present only the more traditional compositions of fuzzy logic.

Definition 3.5 Let $\mathcal{R}$ and $\mathcal{S}$ be two binary fuzzy relations in $U \times V$ and $V \times W$, respectively. The *composition* $\mathcal{R} \circ \mathcal{S}$ is a binary fuzzy relation in $U \times W$ whose membership function is given by

$$\varphi_{\mathcal{R} \circ \mathcal{S}}(x, z) = \sup_{y \in V} [\min(\varphi_{\mathcal{R}}(x, y), \varphi_{\mathcal{S}}(y, z))]. \qquad (3.2)$$

Let the sets U, V and W be finite. Then the matrix form of the relation $\mathcal{R} \circ \mathcal{S}$, given by the composition [max–min], is obtained by a matrix multiplication, substituting the product by the minimum and the sum by the maximum. Indeed, suppose that

$$U = \{u_1, u_2, \ldots, u_m\}; V = \{v_1, v_2, \ldots, v_n\} \quad \text{and} \quad W = \{w_1, w_2, \ldots, w_p\}$$

and that

$$\mathcal{R} = \begin{bmatrix} r_{11} & r_{12} & \cdots & r_{1n} \\ r_{21} & r_{22} & \cdots & r_{2n} \\ \vdots & \vdots & \ddots & \vdots \\ r_{m1} & r_{m2} & \cdots & r_{mn} \end{bmatrix}_{m \times n} \quad \text{and} \quad \mathcal{S} = \begin{bmatrix} s_{11} & s_{12} & \cdots & s_{1p} \\ s_{21} & s_{22} & \cdots & s_{2p} \\ \vdots & \vdots & \ddots & \vdots \\ s_{n1} & s_{n2} & \cdots & s_{np} \end{bmatrix}_{n \times p}.$$

According to Definition 3.5, the binary fuzzy relation given by the composition [max–min] has the following matrix form

$$\mathcal{T} = \mathcal{R} \circ \mathcal{S} = \begin{bmatrix} t_{11} & t_{12} & \cdots & t_{1p} \\ t_{21} & t_{22} & \cdots & t_{2p} \\ \vdots & \vdots & \ddots & \vdots \\ t_{m1} & t_{m2} & \cdots & t_{mp} \end{bmatrix}_{m \times p},$$

where

$$t_{ij} = \sup_{1 \leq k \leq n} [\min(\varphi_R(u_i, v_k), \varphi_S(v_k, w_j))] = \sup_{1 \leq k \leq n} [\min(r_{ik}, s_{kj})]. \qquad (3.3)$$

The special case of the composition [max–min], which will be presented next, will be used in a more general way in Chap. 6.

Definition 3.6 (*Rule of inference composition*) Let U and V be two sets with the respective classes of the fuzzy subsets $\mathcal{F}(U)$ and $\mathcal{F}(V)$ and $\mathcal{R}$ a binary relation over $U \times V$.

(i) The relation $\mathcal{R}$ defines a function of $\mathcal{F}(U)$ into $\mathcal{F}(V)$ such that for each $A \in \mathcal{F}(U)$ there is a corresponding element $B \in \mathcal{F}(V)$ whose membership function is given by

$$\varphi_B(y) = \varphi_{\mathcal{R}(A)}(y) = \sup_{x \in U} [\min(\varphi_{\mathcal{R}}(x, y), \varphi_A(x))]. \tag{3.4}$$

This composition is known as the *rule of inference composition* which will produce other rules as we shall see in Chaps. 4 and 5.

(ii) The relation $\mathcal{R}$ also defines a function of $\mathcal{F}(V)$ into $\mathcal{F}(U)$: for each $B \in \mathcal{F}(V)$ there is a corresponding element $A \in \mathcal{F}(U)$ whose membership function is given by

$$\varphi_A(x) = \varphi_{\mathcal{R}^{-1}(B)}(x) = \sup_{y \in V} [\min(\varphi_{\mathcal{R}^{-1}}(y, x), \varphi_B(y))]. \tag{3.5}$$

A is called the *inverse image* of B by $\mathcal{R}$.

Notice that formula (3.4) can be rewritten as

$$\varphi_B(y) = \varphi_{\mathcal{R}(A)}(y) = \sup_{x \in U} [\min(\varphi_A(x), \varphi_{\mathcal{R}}(x, y))].$$

Thus, according to (3.2),

$$B = \mathcal{R}(A) = A \circ \mathcal{R}.$$

In a similar way the inverse image is given by

$$A = B \circ \mathcal{R}^{-1}.$$

Exercise 3.3 Suppose that the universal sets U and V are finite so that A, B and $\mathcal{R}$ can be represented in matrix form. From the observation above verify that

$$B = A \circ \mathcal{R} \quad \text{and} \quad A = B \circ \mathcal{R}^{\mathsf{T}}$$

where A and B are the matrix forms of the respective fuzzy sets whose elements are obtained from (3.3).

We will present some important definitions to deepen our understanding of binary relations which will be made first for classical binary relations and next for the binary fuzzy relations. The definitions for the classical binary relations $\mathcal{R}$ will be made by the use of their characteristic functions $\chi_{\mathcal{R}} : U \times U \longrightarrow \{0, 1\}$, for a better understanding of the fuzzy case.

Definition 3.7 Let $\mathcal{R}$ be a (classical) binary relation over U. Then, for any x, y and z of U, the relation $\mathcal{R}$ is

  (i) *reflexive* if $\chi_{\mathcal{R}}(x, x) = 1$;
 (ii) *symmetric* if $\chi_{\mathcal{R}}(x, y) = 1$ implies $\chi_{\mathcal{R}}(y, x) = 1$;
(iii) *transitive* if $\chi_{\mathcal{R}}(x, y) = \chi_{\mathcal{R}}(y, z) = 1$ implies $\chi_{\mathcal{R}}(x, z) = 1$;
(iv) *anti-symmetric* if $\chi_{\mathcal{R}}(x, y) = \chi_{\mathcal{R}}(y, x) = 1$ implies $x = y$.

Observe that the definitions above represent exactly each one of the traditional definitions used in classical set theory. The use of the characteristic function was just an "artifice" to facilitate the understanding of those concepts in the fuzzy case. There are some little differences in the extensions of the concepts given in the Definition 3.7, when adapted to the fuzzy case, mainly the concept of transitivity (see [2, 3]).

Definition 3.8 Let $\mathcal{R}$ be a binary fuzzy relation over U, whose membership function is $\varphi_{\mathcal{R}}$. Then, for any x, y and z of U, the fuzzy relation $\mathcal{R}$ is

 (i) *reflexive* if $\varphi_{\mathcal{R}}(x, x) = 1$;
 (ii) *symmetric* if $\varphi_{\mathcal{R}}(x, y) = \varphi_{\mathcal{R}}(y, x)$;
(iii) *transitive* if $\varphi_{\mathcal{R}}(x, z) \geq \varphi_{\mathcal{R}}(x, y) \wedge \varphi_{\mathcal{R}}(y, z)$, where $\wedge = \text{minimum}$.
(iv) *anti-symmetric* if $\varphi_{\mathcal{R}}(x, y) > 0$ and $\varphi_{\mathcal{R}}(y, x) > 0$ implies $x = y$.

The reflexive relation is the relation in which all element have the maximum relation to themselves; the symmetric relation is characterized by the reciprocity between their elements; the transitive indicates that the relation between any two individuals can not be simultaneously less than the relation of each of them with the rest; and the last, the anti-symmetric, is the relation that does not admit any reciprocity between distinct elements. Relations that satisfy simultaneously the four properties above are, generally, very artificial. Typically when they are required to fulfill (ii) and (iv) the relation tends to be artificial. For example, if U has just one element x, the Cartesian product $U \times U = \{(x, x)\}$ satisfies the properties (i)–(iv) from the Definition 3.8. Relations that satisfy just the first three conditions are called *equivalence relations*. Concepts (i)–(iv) can be seen in the following example:

Example 3.3 Intuitively, the relation of the military hierarchy ($\mathcal{M}$): "is a higher rank than" is based on the rank of the individual, that is, x is related to y if the rank of x is higher than y. So, $\mathcal{M}$ is reflexive, transitive and anti-symmetric but not symmetric. On the other hand, the relation ($\mathcal{A}$): "*is friend of*" is reflexive, symmetric but not transitive.

The relations $\mathcal{M}$ and $\mathcal{A}$ are not necessarily fuzzy relations. However, if we want to indicate the degree that x *is higher than* y, based not on rank but in subjective factors, say status, then $\mathcal{M}$ can be considered a fuzzy relation. The same can be said about the relation $\mathcal{A}$.

References

1. W. Pedrycz, F. Gomide, *An Introduction to Fuzzy Sets: Analysis and Design* (The MIT Press, Massachusets, 1998)
2. G. Klir, B. Yuan, *Fuzzy Sets and Fuzzy Logic Theory and Applications* (Prentice-Hall, Upper Saddle River, 1995)
3. H.T. Nguyen, E.A. Walker, *A First Course of Fuzzy Logic* (CRC Press, Boca Raton, 1997)

Chapter 4
Notions of Fuzzy Logic

The purpose of theoretical science is the truth.
(Aristotle – C.384 – 322 BCE)

Abstract This chapter presents the basic notions of classical and fuzzy logic followed by the concepts of t-norms, t-conorms, fuzzy negation, and fuzzy implication, which are the key ideas of propositional calculus of fuzzy logic. Next the chapter discusses modus ponens and generalized modus ponens together with the concepts of linguistic variables that are used in logical reasoning. The chapter closes with linguistic modifiers and the concept of interactivity between fuzzy sets.

The task of knowledge, according to Aristotle, is the truth, without practical concerns. On the other hand, for sophist philosophers, knowledge must be concerned with practical things and, for this reason, the search for "true" or "false" must be replaced by measurements of "better" or "worse". In this and the next two chapters these "measurements" will be elaborated, mainly through study of *generalized modus ponens*.

The literature uses the term "fuzzy logic" in at least two ways: the first one is to represent and manipulate inexact information with the purpose of making decisions through use of the fuzzy set theory, its membership functions and algebras. The second one refers to the extension of the classical logic which is the main goal of this chapter.

From an historical point of view, logic was developed from studies of Aristotelian syllogisms whose purpose was to better understand "truth". Building on the work of Plato, who was a disciple of Socrates; Aristotle developed laws governing thought whose aim was to deduce knowledge from hypotheses. In this case, there is no possible interpretations from the method of deduction in the sense it is either true or false (but not both). Thus, the motto of Sophists "man is the measure of all things", seems to be mistaken. An example truth in sense of Aristotle is given by statement about Socrates:

© Springer-Verlag Berlin Heidelberg 2017
L.C. de Barros et al., *A First Course in Fuzzy Logic, Fuzzy Dynamical Systems, and Biomathematics*, Studies in Fuzziness and Soft Computing 347, DOI 10.1007/978-3-662-53324-6_4

"Every human is mortal
Socrates is human
Then, Socrates is mortal"

The syllogism above is typical of the structure of *logic* which illustrates "true knowledge" as developed by Aristotle.

The study of Aristotelian logic was restarted only in seventeenth century when Leibniz created symbolic logic. In the nineteenth century, Boole created an algebra for this symbolic logic. This tool started to be widely used in the first half of the twentieth century for computer circuits and in the computer language. In the same century, logic was studied by great mathematicians like Peano, Frege, Whitehead, Russel and Gödel, among others. During the first half of the twentieth century, there arose many scholars who extended the *logic of two values* to logics with many values known as *multi-valued logic*. Among them we stress the Lukasiewicz's logic which in a way is considered the precursor of the fuzzy logic [1, 2]. However, it was only in 1960 that there arises the first study that is the originator of fuzzy logic [3].

Chapter 1 already commented that it is important to understand that fuzzy logic is "subjective". However, this does mean that fuzzy logic is not part of logic. Logic is a discipline that studies implications. Indeed, fuzzy logic is a logic with methodology of its own [1]. On the other hand, fuzzy logic does not deal with ambiguity. The uncertainties of fuzzy logic are monotonic, in the sense that the less the premises are uncertain, the less the conclusions will be uncertain as well. Ambiguity is not monotonic in this sense. Intuitively, we can say that the fuzzy logic tends to classical logic when the uncertainties go to zero.

The main success of the fuzzy logic is due to its practical approach, since it can handle uncertain propositions to obtain conclusions. The field that deals with the formalization of these propositions is known as **approximate reasoning** whose structure has the same structure as the method proposed by Socrates. For example,

Intense flu causes high fever;
High fever frequently causes headache;
Conclusion: Intense flu frequently causes headache.

The conclusion above is a deduction obtained from the assumptions. However, some of these predicates are not precise terms (for example: *intense*, *high* and *frequently*) and for this reason classical logic can not handle these sentences. The next section delineates some concepts of traditional logic that will be a foundation for our fuzzy logic development.

4.1 Basic Connectives of Classical Logic

The first steps in mathematical logic begin with the study of connectives: *"and"*, *"or"*, *"not"* and *"implication"*. These connectives are typically used in the mathematical modeling in sentences like:

"If a is in A **and** b is in B,

then c is in C **or** d is **not** in D" (4.1)

The logical values for each connective are studied using truth tables. Thus, the logical value of a sentence, formed from two or more propositions, is obtained by the composition of the truth tables for the connectives in this sentence. If we suppose that A and B are sets, the proposition

"a is in A **and** b is in B"

is true only if a belongs to A is true **and** also that b belongs to B. The logical value of this sentence is a consequence of the classical truth table to the connective **and**.

True sentences have a logical value **1**, while false sentences have a logical value **0** in classical logic. In the extension to the fuzzy case, truth values range between 0 and 1. Regardless, for either the classical or the fuzzy case we are going to use the notation $\wedge$ (minimum) for the conjunction **and**, $\vee$ (maximum) for **or**, $\neg$ for the **negation**, and $\Longrightarrow$ for the **implication** (Tables 4.1, 4.2 and 4.3).

Let p and q be two propositions. The classical truth tables for the connectives presented above are given in Table 4.4. We can notice that in each truth table, p and q just have the values 0 and 1. For that reason, the classical logic is sometimes called "two-valued logic".

Each one of the logical connectives above can be seen as a mathematical operator whose values match with the respective truth tables, and it is this fact that justifies the notation $\wedge$ for **and** and $\vee$ for **or**. With the exception of the negation, the other connectives are binary operations.

Table 4.1 Truth table of $\wedge$

p	q	$p \wedge q$
1	1	1
1	0	0
0	1	0
0	0	0

Table 4.2 Truth table of $\vee$

p	q	$p \vee q$
1	1	1
1	0	1
0	1	1
0	0	0

Table 4.3 Truth table of $\neg$

p	$\neg p$
1	0
0	1

Table 4.4 Truth table of $\Longrightarrow$

p	q	$p \Longrightarrow q$
1	1	1
1	0	0
0	1	1
0	0	1

• Connective **and**: $\wedge$

$$\wedge : \{0, 1\} \times \{0, 1\} \longrightarrow \{0, 1\}$$
$$(p, q) \longmapsto \wedge (p, q) = p \wedge q = \min \{p, q\} \,.$$

Thus,

$$\wedge(1, 1) = 1 \wedge 1 = 1;$$
$$\wedge(1, 0) = 1 \wedge 0 = 0;$$
$$\wedge(0, 1) = 0 \wedge 1 = 0;$$
$$\wedge(0, 0) = 0 \wedge 0 = 0.$$

• Connective **or**: $\vee$

$$\vee : \{0, 1\} \times \{0, 1\} \longrightarrow \{0, 1\}$$
$$(p, q) \longmapsto \vee (p, q) = p \vee q = \max \{p, q\} \,.$$

Therefore,

$$\vee(1, 1) = 1 \vee 1 = 1;$$
$$\vee(1, 0) = 1 \vee 0 = 1;$$
$$\vee(0, 1) = 0 \vee 1 = 1;$$
$$\vee(0, 0) = 0 \vee 0 = 0.$$

• The negation is an unary operation: $\neg$

$$\neg : \{0, 1\} \longrightarrow \{0, 1\}$$
$$p \longmapsto \neg p,$$

where, $\neg 1 = 0$ and $\neg 0 = 1$. It is interesting to notice that $\neg p = 1 - p$.
• Implication: $\Longrightarrow$

$$\Longrightarrow : \{0, 1\} \times \{0, 1\} \longrightarrow \{0, 1\}$$
$$(p, q) \longmapsto \Longrightarrow (p, q) = (p \Longrightarrow q).$$

We can observe that

$$(p \Longrightarrow q) = \begin{cases} 1 \text{ if } p \le q \\ 0 \text{ if } p > q \end{cases}$$

that is, $(p \Longrightarrow q)$ is true if q is at least p.

The previous connectives generate at least three formulas that reproduce the truth table associated with implication:

(1) $(p \Longrightarrow q) = (\neg p) \vee q$;
(2) $(p \Longrightarrow q) = (\neg p) \vee (p \wedge q)$;
(3) $(p \Longrightarrow q) = \max\{x \in \{0, 1\} : p \wedge x \le q\}$.

Let us verify that "not p or q" is the implication "p implies q", that is, $(\neg p) \vee q = (p \Longrightarrow q)$ is in fact an implication:

$$\Longrightarrow (1, 1) = (1 \Longrightarrow 1) = (\neg 1) \vee 1 = 1;$$
$$\Longrightarrow (1, 0) = (1 \Longrightarrow 0) = (\neg 1) \vee 0 = 0;$$
$$\Longrightarrow (0, 1) = (0 \Longrightarrow 1) = (\neg 0) \vee 1 = 1;$$
$$\Longrightarrow (0, 0) = (0 \Longrightarrow 0) = (\neg 0) \vee 0 = 1.$$

We leave as exercise for the reader to verify the other two cases.

Although each one of the operators (1), (2) and (3), define the same classical implications, this does not occur when we extend each one of these formulas to the fuzzy case. In general, case (2) does not define a fuzzy implication as we are going to see later.

Let us go back to sentence (4.1). This sentence can have a logical evaluation using logical values of the connectives. Since we are dealing with classical sets, this evaluation can only take the values 0 or 1. Let us consider

$$\overbrace{\text{If } a \text{ belongs to } A \;\mathbf{and}\; b \text{ belongs to } B,}^{P} \;\mathbf{then}\; \overbrace{c \text{ belongs to } C \;\mathbf{or}\; d \text{ is } \mathbf{not} \text{ in } D}^{Q}.$$

The values of each expressions p, q, r and s can only be 0 or 1, depending if each element belongs or not to the indicated set. For example, $p = 1$ if $a \in A$ while $p = 0$ if $a \notin A$. Analogously, the same is true for q, r and s. Thus, it is easy to evaluate sentence (4.1) for each situation. For example, if

$$a \in A (p = 1); \; b \notin B (q = 0); \; c \in C (r = 1) \text{ and } d \notin D (s = 1),$$

then the logical value of sentence (4.1) is

$$(1 \wedge 0) \Longrightarrow (1 \vee 1) = (0 \Longrightarrow 1) = 1.$$

Note that the logical value of the sentence p : "a belongs to A" coincides with that value obtained from the membership function of the set A evaluated at a, that is, the value of p is given by $\chi_A(a)$. In the same way, χ_B gives the logical value of q; χ_C, of r and the value of s is given by $1 - \chi_D$.

The next section is dedicated to the mathematical formulation of (4.1), keeping in mind that now the sets are fuzzy.

4.2 Basic Connectives of Fuzzy Logic

We observe that, to logically evaluate the expression (4.1) defined by connectives in the classical case, it can only assume the values 0 or 1. This assumption is consistent with the fact that the related sets are classical. Now, if we allow the sets in (4.1) to be fuzzy sets, how can we logically evaluate this expression? Initially, we need to give a value that indicates how much the proposition "*a belongs to A*" is true, where A is a fuzzy set and knowing that an element a can belong to A with values in the set $[0, 1]$. To do the logical evaluation of the connectives in the fuzzy case, we need to extend the classical ones. These extensions are obtained by triangular norms and conorms. These operators were originally developed for the study of metric spaces associated with statistical analysis (Menger, 1942 [4]). The name, triangular norm (conorm), comes from the generalization of the triangular property for these spaces [5].

4.2.1 Operations T-Norm and T-Conorm

Definition 4.1 (*t-norm*) The operator $\triangle : [0, 1] \times [0, 1] \longrightarrow [0, 1]$, $\triangle(x, y) = x \triangle y$, is a *t-norm*, if it satisfies the following conditions:

(t_1) *Neutral element*: $\triangle(1, x) = 1 \triangle x = x$;
(t_2) *Commutative*: $\triangle(x, y) = x \triangle y = y \triangle x = \triangle(y, x)$;
(t_3) *Associative*: $x \triangle (y \triangle z) = (x \triangle y) \triangle z$;
(t_4) *Monotonicity*: if $x \leq u$ and $y \leq v$, then $x \triangle y \leq u \triangle v$.

The operator *t-norm* extends the operator $\wedge$ that models the connective "**and**".

Example 4.1 Let us consider the operator

$$\triangle_1(x, y) = \min\{x, y\} = x \wedge y.$$

It is easy to see that this operator reproduces the truth table of the connective $\wedge$. The proof is left to the reader. Other examples of t-norms are:

$$\triangle_2(x, y) = xy;$$
$$\triangle_3(x, y) = \max\{0, x + y - 1\};$$
$$\triangle_4(x, y) = \begin{cases} x \text{ if } y = 1 \\ y \text{ if } x = 1 \\ 0 \text{ otherwise} \end{cases}.$$

Exercise 4.1 Verify that $\triangle_1$, $\triangle_2$, $\triangle_3$ are t-norm and $\triangle_3 \leq \triangle_2 \leq \triangle_1$.

Definition 4.2 (*t-conorm*) The operator $\triangledown(x, y) = x \triangledown y$ is a *t-conorm* if it satisfies the following conditions

(c_1) *Neutral element*: $\triangledown(0, x) = 0 \triangledown x = x$;
(c_2) *Commutative*: $\triangledown(x, y) = x \triangledown y = y \triangledown x = \triangledown(y, x)$;
(c_3) *Associative*: $x \triangledown (y \triangledown z) = (x \triangledown y) \triangledown z$;
(c_4) *Monotonicity*: if $x \leq u$ and $y \leq v$, then $x \triangledown y \leq u \triangledown v$.

The operator *t-conorm* $\triangledown : [0, 1] \times [0, 1] \longrightarrow [0, 1]$ extends the operator $\vee$ of the connective "**or**".

Example 4.2 The operator

$$\triangledown_1(x, y) = \max\{x, y\} = x \vee y.$$

is a *t-conorm* that reproduces the truth table of the connective $\vee$. Other examples of t-conorm are (verify!):

$$\triangledown_2(x, y) = \min\{1, x + y\};$$
$$\triangledown_3(x, y) = x + y - xy.$$

The following operation extends the truth table for the negation:

Definition 4.3 (*negation*) A map $\eta : [0, 1] \longrightarrow [0, 1]$ is a negation if it satisfies the following conditions:

(n_1) *Boundary conditions*: $\eta(0) = 1$ and $\eta(1) = 0$;
(n_2) *Monotonicity*: η is decreasing.

Moreover if η is strictly decreasing, (n_1) holds and

(n_3) *Involution*: $\eta(\eta(x)) = x$,

then η is called **strong negation**.

The maps

$$\eta_1(x) = 1 - x \quad \text{and} \quad \eta_2(x) = \frac{1 - x}{1 + x}$$

reproduce the negation truth table $\neg$. In reality, they are strong negations. However,

$$\eta_3(x) = \begin{cases} 0 \text{ if } x = 1 \\ 1 \text{ if } x \in [0, 1[\end{cases}$$

is a negation but not a strong one. Moreover, we observe that the operations $\triangle = \wedge$, $\triangledown = \vee$, and $\eta = 1 - x$, satisfy the De Morgan's laws, that is, for all pairs (x, y) of $[0, 1] \times [0, 1]$ we have

$$\eta (x \wedge y) = \eta(x) \vee \eta (y)$$
$$\eta (x \vee y) = \eta(x) \wedge \eta (y).$$

Exercise 4.2 Prove that for any t-norm $\triangle$, t-conorm $\triangledown$ and strong negation η, De Morgan's laws are satisfied. That is, in the formulas above, change $\wedge$ to $\triangle$ and $\vee$ to $\triangledown$.

We say that the t-norm $\triangle$ and the t-conorm $\triangledown$ are **dual** with respect to a negation η if they satisfy the two laws of De Morgan.

Exercise 4.3 Verify that

$$\eta_\lambda(x) = \frac{1 - x}{1 + \lambda x}, \quad \lambda > -1$$

is a strong negation.

Exercise 4.4 Verify which of the systems given below are dual t-norms and t-conorms with respect to the negation $\eta(x) = 1 - x$:

(1) $\begin{cases} x \triangle y = \max \{x + y - 1, 0\} \\ x \triangledown y = \min \{x + y, 1\} \end{cases}$;

(2) $\begin{cases} x \triangle y = xy \\ x \triangledown y = x + y - xy \end{cases}$;

(3) $\begin{cases} x \triangle y = \max \{x + y - 1, 0\} \\ x \triangledown y = x + y - xy \end{cases}$;

(4) $\begin{cases} x \triangle_H y = \dfrac{xy}{a + (1 - a)(x + y - xy)} \\ \\ x \triangledown_H y = \dfrac{(a - 2)xy + x + y}{1 + (a - 1)xy} \end{cases}$, $a \geq 0$;

$\triangle_H$ and $\triangledown_H$ are known as t-norm and t-conorm of Hamacher [5].

(5) $\begin{cases} x \triangle_F y = \log_a \left[1 + \dfrac{(a^x - 1)(a^y - 1)}{a - 1} \right] \\ \\ x \triangledown_F y = 1 - \log_a \left[1 + \dfrac{(a^{1-x} - 1)(a^{1-y} - 1)}{a - 1} \right] \end{cases}$, $0 < a \neq 1$;

$\triangle_F$ and $\triangledown_F$ are the denominated t-norm and t-conorm of Frank [5].

A complete study about t-norms and t-conorms can be found in [5].

Definition 4.4 (*Fuzzy implication*) An operator $\Rightarrow: [0, 1] \times [0, 1] \rightarrow [0, 1]$ is a fuzzy implication if it satisfies the following conditions:

1. Reproduces the classical implication table;
2. Is decreasing in the first variable, that is, for each $x \in [0, 1]$ we have

$$(a \Rightarrow x) \leq (b \Rightarrow x) \text{ if } a \geq b;$$

3. Is increasing in the second variable, that is, for each $x \in [0, 1]$ we have

$$(x \Rightarrow a) \geq (x \Rightarrow b) \text{ if } a \geq b.$$

Thus, the class of fuzzy implications consists of all the maps from the square $[0, 1] \times [0, 1]$ to $[0, 1]$, whose restrictions on the vertices coincide with the values of the classical implication and are decreasing with respect to the abscissas, and increasing with respect to the ordinates. As we have already mentioned in the exposition of the classical implication, it can be represented by one of the formulas:

(1) $(p \Longrightarrow q) = (\neg p) \vee q$;
(2) $(p \Longrightarrow q) = (\neg p) \vee (p \wedge q)$;
(3) $(p \Longrightarrow q) = \max\{x \in \{0, 1\} : p \wedge x \leq q\}$.

For the fuzzy case, these formulas do not produce the same fuzzy implications (verify this fact!). Moreover, due to the second condition in Definition 4.4, formula (2) above does not always reproduce a fuzzy implication. Thus, we distinguish formulas (1) and (3):

(4) A S-implication has the form $(x \Longrightarrow y) = \eta(x) \triangledown y$;

S-implications are build from the conorms, which are frequently called s-norms [5].

(5) A R-implication has the form

$$(x \Longrightarrow y) = \sup\{z \in [0, 1] : x \triangle z \leq y\}.$$

The R-implication name comes from the residual operation [5] and can be interpreted as $(x \Longrightarrow y)$ is the greatest value for which y overcomes x according to $\triangle$. In other words, it is the residue of x with respect to y, according to $\triangle$.

Notice that for the classical case, $(p \Longrightarrow q)$ is what is "lacking" in order that p is q according to $\wedge$. For a more complete study about the extension of formula (2) $((\neg p) \vee (p \wedge q))$ to the fuzzy case, the reader might consult [6].

Exercise 4.5 Verify that each of the operators S and R, of Definition 4.4 are in fact fuzzy implications for any *t-norms*, *t-conorms* and *negation*. Next, verify (using examples) that (2) does not always reproduces a fuzzy implication, except when the negation is given by

$$\eta(x) = \begin{cases} 0 \text{ if } x = 1 \\ 1 \text{ if } x \in [0, 1[\end{cases}.$$

Example 4.3 (Fuzzy implications) The following operators are fuzzy implications:

(a) Gödel's implication:

$$(x \implies y) = g(x, y) = \begin{cases} 1 & \text{if } x \leq y \\ y & \text{if } x > y \end{cases}.$$

(b) Goguen's implication:

$$(x \implies y) = g_n(x, y) = \begin{cases} 1 & \text{if } x \leq y \\ \dfrac{y}{x} & \text{if } x > y \end{cases}.$$

(c) Lukasiewicz's implication:

$$(x \implies y) = \ell(x, y) = \min\{(1 - x + y), 1\}.$$

(d) Kleene-Dienes' implication:

$$(x \implies y) = k_d(x, y) = \max\{(1 - x), y\}.$$

(e) Reichenbach's implication:

$$(x \implies y) = r(x, y) = (1 - x + xy).$$

(f) Gaines–Rescher's implication:

$$(x \implies y) = g_r(x, y) = \begin{cases} 1 & \text{if } x \leq y \\ 0 & \text{if } x > y \end{cases}.$$

(f) Wu's implication:

$$(x \implies y) = w(x, y) = \begin{cases} 1 & \text{if } x \leq y \\ \min\{1 - x, y\} & \text{if } x > y \end{cases}.$$

Exercise 4.6 Solve the items below.

(a) Verify that the Gödel's and Goguen's implications are R-implications, supposing that $\triangle = \min$ for Gödel's and $\triangle = \text{product}$ for Goguen's.
(b) Among the fuzzy implications above, give examples of S-implications and of R-implications, supposing $\eta(x) = 1 - x$.
(c) Verify that $g(x, y) \leq g_n(x, y)$ for x and y in the interval $[0, 1]$.

Exercise 4.7 Graphically depict of the implications from Example 4.3.

The reader who wants to know more about logical operators and fuzzy propositional calculus can consult Baczynski and Jayaram [6], Hajék [1], Nguyen [2],

Klir and Yuan [7], Pedrycz and Gomide [8], Wangning [9] and their references. Our interest here is focused on calculations and interpretations of formulas in which these basic connectives appear.

Example 4.4 Let us return to expression (4.1) and obtain its logical value when we consider $\triangle = \wedge$, $\triangledown = \vee$, $\eta(x) = 1 - x$ and the Gödel's implication. Initially, for each cell p, q, r and s of expression (4.1), we take its logical value as a membership degree of each element from the related set. For example, let us consider that those values are: $\varphi_A(a) = 0.6$; $\varphi_B(b) = 0.7$; $\varphi_C(c) = 0.4$ and $\varphi_D(d) = 0.7$. Then, we have:

$$
\begin{aligned}
p \triangle q &= \min(0.6; 0.7) = 0.6; \\
s &= 1 - \varphi_D(d) \quad = 1 - 0.7 = 0.3; \\
r \triangledown s &= \max(0.4; 0.3) = 0.4.
\end{aligned}
$$

Therefore, the logical value of (4.1) is the result of

$$(p \triangle q) \Longrightarrow (r \triangledown s).$$

Assuming that the implication is the Gödel implication, then

$$(p \triangle q) \Longrightarrow (r \triangledown s) = \begin{cases} 1 & \text{if } (p \triangle q) \le (r \triangledown s) \\ (r \triangledown s) & \text{if } (p \triangle q) > (r \triangledown s) \end{cases} = 0.4;$$

since $(p \triangle q) = 0.6$ and $(r \triangledown s) = 0.4$. Thus, for the memberships above, expression (4.1) is true with degree 0.4.

Exercise 4.8 Redo the Example 4.4 for other implications given by Example 4.3.

Many of the implications in Example 4.3 are obtained from the combination of t-norms and t-conorms and they are used to model *fuzzy propositions* in *approximate reasoning*. This topic is of great interest in the resolution methods of the *relational equations* and of the *systems based on fuzzy rules*, such as Mamdani's controllers. These topics will be studied in Chaps. 5 and 6. The reader who wants greater details about fuzzy implications for process modeling in engineering should consult [2, 7–9]. In biomathematics, we have expanded some classical models and changed the product operation to t-norms in mathematical models of epidemics [10].

4.3 Approximate Reasoning and Linguistic Variables

Approximate reasoning refers to the process where we can make conclusions from uncertain premises. When this uncertainty involves fuzzy sets, it is common to use the term fuzzy reasoning.

The following form of reasoning is very common in life:

$$\text{"If the banana is yellow then the banana is ripe"} \qquad (4.2)$$

that is,

"If we have a yellow banana, it is automatic classified as ripe".

In a general form we obtain something like:

$$\text{"If } X \text{ is } \Diamond \text{ then } Y \text{ is } \Box.\text{"} \qquad (4.3)$$

In this case, if we know that X is $\Diamond$, we conclude that Y is $\Box$.

This is a generalization of the well known deductive method **modus ponens**. The difference between the classical modus ponens and fuzzy modus ponens is the subjectivity of the predicates involved. The general sentences (4.3) above are expressed in a "natural" language without the formalism of the mathematical language. Our interest here is in a mathematical model for some sentences using fuzzy logic.

Sentence (4.1) is substantially different from sentence (4.3). In (4.3) there is no set (classical or fuzzy) involved, only qualifications about the variables X and Y. To formally express sentences with variables like (4.3) we relate fuzzy set theory to fuzzy logic. To obtain a logical evaluation of (4.3) the idea is to rewrite it in the way that the sentence (4.1) appears, and for that, it is necessary to define the concept of *linguistic variable*.

Definition 4.5 (*Linguistic Variable*) A *linguistic variable* X in the universe U is a variable whose values are fuzzy subsets of U.

Intuitively, a linguistic variable is a noun, while its values are adjectives represented by fuzzy sets. For example, "flu" is a linguistic variable that can assume the attributes "intense" or "weak".

Sentences where linguistic variables appear with its subjective values (attributes) are commonly called as fuzzy propositions. However, the interest here are those variables whose assumed values are **fuzzy numbers** where the universe of discourse is the set of real numbers. In this case, we say that the support of variable is the set of real numbers and X is a real linguistic variable.

The logical value of "$X = x$ is A" is given by number $\varphi_A(x)$ that indicates how much $X = x$ is in agreement with the linguistic term modeled by the fuzzy set A. For this reason, and to have an easier notation when there is no doubt about the variables, we will use just the values of interest assumed by them in each fuzzy proposition, that is, we are going to use "x is A", instead of "$X = x$ is A".

Next, we are going to use the notion of linguistic variables to formulate the deductive method of **modus ponens** for the fuzzy case.

4.4 Modus Ponens and Generalized Modus Ponens

Our initial interest is to model mathematically the **fuzzy modus ponens**:

$$p \Longrightarrow q: \quad \text{If } x \text{ is } A \text{ then } y \text{ is } B$$
$$\text{Fact:} \qquad x \text{ is } A$$
$$\text{Conclusion:} \qquad y \text{ is } B$$

Notice that $(p \Longrightarrow q)$ is a conditional fuzzy proposition that is modeled by a fuzzy relation $\mathcal{R}$ of $U \times V$, whose membership function is

$$\varphi_{\mathcal{R}}(x, y) = [\varphi_A(x) \Longrightarrow \varphi_B(y)],$$

where x and y are values of linguistic variables in U and V, respectively. Thus, the sentence value "If x is A then y is B" depends on the chosen implication.

The classical implication, that is, $\varphi_A(x) \in \{0, 1\}$ and $\varphi_B(y) \in \{0, 1\}$, produces a fuzzy relation whose membership function is given by:

$$\varphi_{\mathcal{R}}(x, y) = \chi_{\mathcal{R}}(x, y) = (\chi_A(x) \Longrightarrow \chi_B(y))$$
$$= \begin{cases} 1 & \text{if } (x \notin A \text{ and } y \text{ is arbitrary}) \text{ or } (x \in A \text{ and } y \in B) \\ 0 & \text{if } x \in A \text{ and } y \notin B \end{cases}$$

so that

$$\sup_{x \in U} [\chi_{\mathcal{R}}(x, y) \wedge \chi_A(x)] = \begin{cases} 1 & \text{if } y \in B \\ 0 & \text{if } y \notin B \end{cases} = \chi_B(y).$$

That is, for the classical case, the modus ponens can be mathematically written by the formula:

$$\chi_B(y) = \sup_{x \in U} [\chi_{\mathcal{R}}(x, y) \wedge \chi_A(x)].$$

According to the notation that was seen in Chap. 3, the classical modus ponens can be given by the $max - min$ inference composition rule $B = A \circ \mathcal{R}$, where the relation $\mathcal{R}$ is obtained by a fuzzy implication that models the conditional sentence

$$\text{"If } x \in A \text{ then } y \in B\text{"}.$$

Our aim is to inference with fuzzy sets, so this formula will be extended to fuzzy situations which we will call the **fuzzy modus ponens** and the **generalized fuzzy modus ponens**. The fuzzy modus ponens models the following syllogism:

Rule: *"If the banana is yellow, then it is ripe"*
Fact: *"The banana is yellow"*
Conclusion: *"The banana is ripe"*

Fuzzy logic reveals its great potential when modeling each of the sentences above. The nouns and its attributes are modeled by the fuzzy sets (by membership functions), while the connectives are modeled by operators like t-norms and t-conorms, implications and/or negations. The conclusion, which must be a fuzzy set, is obtained by the extension of the inference composition rule

$$\chi_B(y) = \sup_{x \in U} [\chi_{\mathcal{R}}(x, y) \wedge \chi_A(x)], \tag{4.4}$$

replacing the characteristic functions by membership functions and the operator $\wedge$ by some t-norm, that is,

$$\varphi_B(y) = \sup_{x \in U} [\varphi_{\mathcal{R}}(x, y) \, \triangle \, \varphi_A(x)]. \tag{4.5}$$

In short, the formula (4.5) is the inference rule that models the **modus ponens fuzzy**

Rule:	"if x is A, then y is B"
Fact:	"x is A"
Conclusion:	" is B"

The right side of the Eq. (4.5) demands that the t-norm and the fuzzy implication that is adopted are chosen in a way that the output coincides with $\varphi_B(y)$ for all y.

This is a problem of relational equations and can engender some difficulties. Our focus here is in approximate reasoning so we only study these issues by mentioning that they may arise and leave their more detailed discussion to Chap. 6. For this reason, we extend Eq. (4.5) by admitting an input A^* instead of A and we will make it more flexible by not demanding that the output B^* be B for the input $A = A^*$. In this case we will call the syllogism a **generalized fuzzy modus ponens**, which has the general form:

Rule:	"If x is A, then y is B"
Fact:	"x is A^*"
Conclusion:	"y is B^*"

The output from the **generalized fuzzy modus ponens** is a fuzzy set B^*, whose membership function is

$$\varphi_{B^*}(y) = \sup_{x \in U} [\varphi_{\mathcal{R}}(x, y) \, \triangle \, \varphi_{A^*}(x)], \tag{4.6}$$

which, by analogy to the inference composition rule seen in Chap. 3, has the form

$$\mathcal{R}(A^*) = A^* \otimes^t \mathcal{R} = B^*,$$

where $\otimes^t$ is a similar operation to the composition " $\circ$ ", that replaces the minimum t-norm by $\triangle$. In Chap. 6 we will see this operation in more details.

It is worth stressing that: in the classical case, we always have $\mathcal{R}(A) = B$. Although, in fuzzy case, depending on the t-norm and the implication, we will not ever have $\mathcal{R}(A) = B$. This fact does not belie the use of formulas (4.5) or (4.6).

It is very common to obtain a theoretical functional that does not reproduce the data that generated it. This is the case of the well known least-squares method, whose main property is to obtain the functional with the lowest possible quadratic error of the data set. Methods to obtain functionals that reproduce exactly the data that generated it are called interpolation methods. This subject will appear again in subsequent chapters where we will make further observations.

Example 4.5 Suppose we have the product t-norm $x \triangle y = xy$, and the implication

$$(x \Longrightarrow y) = \begin{cases} 1 & \text{if } x = 0 \\ 1 \wedge \dfrac{y}{x} & \text{if } x \neq 0 \end{cases}.$$

Given the fuzzy numbers A and B, we have

$$(\varphi_A(x) \Longrightarrow \varphi_B(y)) \cdot \varphi_A(x) = \varphi_A(x) \wedge \varphi_B(y).$$

Thus,

$$\begin{aligned} \sup_{x \in U}[\varphi_R(x, y) \triangle \varphi_A(x)] &= \sup_{x \in U}[(\varphi_A(x) \Longrightarrow \varphi_B(y)) \cdot \varphi_A(x)] \\ &= \sup_{x \in U}[\varphi_A(x) \wedge \varphi_B(y)] = \varphi_B(y). \end{aligned}$$

that is, $\mathcal{R}(A) = B$.

Exercise 4.9 Verify whether or not $R(A) = B$ with the minimum t-norm, $x \triangle y = x \wedge y$, for:

(a) Reichenbach's implication;
(b) Wu's implication.

Let us analyze a case where the sets are finite.

Example 4.6 Consider the fuzzy subsets:

$$A = 0.4/x_1 + 1.0/x_2 + 0.6/x_3 \quad \text{and} \quad B = 0.8/y_1 + 0.4/y_2$$

the Lukasiewicz's implication,

$$(x \Longrightarrow y) = \min\{(1 - x + y), 1\}$$

and the t-norm $\triangle_1 = \wedge$.

Let us obtain the outputs from the formula (4.5) for each input. Recall that the relation is given by

$$\varphi_{\mathcal{R}}(x, y) = (\varphi_A(x) \Longrightarrow \varphi_B(y))$$

and for the Lukasiewicz, implication, we have

$$\mathcal{R} = 1.0/(x_1, y_1) + 1.0/(x_1, y_2) + 0.8/(x_2, y_1) +$$
$$+ 0.4/(x_2, y_2) + 1.0/(x_3, y_1) + 0.8/(x_3, y_2).$$

So, for the input
$$A = 0.4/x_1 + 1.0/x_2 + 0.6/x_3,$$

we have the output $\widetilde{B}$ with the membership function

$$\varphi_{\widetilde{B}}(y_1) = \max_{x_i} [\varphi_{\mathcal{R}}(x_i, y_1) \wedge \varphi_A(x_i)] =$$
$$= \max[\min(1.0; 0.4); \min(0.8; 1.0); \min(1.0; 0.6)] = 0.8;$$
$$\varphi_{\widetilde{B}}(y_2) = \max_{x_i} [\varphi_{\mathcal{R}}(x_i, y_2) \wedge \varphi_A(x_i)] =$$
$$= \max[\min(1.0; 0.4); \min(0.4; 1.0); \min(0.8; 0.6)] = 0.6.$$

and for the input
$$A^* = 0.6/x_1 + 0.9/x_2 + 0.7/x_3,$$

we have the output of B^* with membership function

$$\varphi_{B^*}(y_1) = \max_{x_i} [\varphi_{\mathcal{R}}(x_i, y_1) \wedge \varphi_A(x_i)]$$
$$= \max[\min(1.0; 0.6); \min(0.8; 0.9); \min(1.0; 0.7)] = 0.8;$$
$$\varphi_{B^*}(y_2) = \max_{x_i} [\varphi_{\mathcal{R}}(x_i, y_2) \wedge \varphi_A(x_i)]$$
$$= \max[\min(1.0; 0.6); \min(0.4; 0.9); \min(0.8; 0.7)] = 0.7.$$

So, for this example, the outputs obtained from generalized fuzzy modus ponens are

$$\mathcal{R}(A) = \widetilde{B} = 0.8/y_1 + 0.6/y_2 \text{ and } \mathcal{R}(A^*) = B^* = 0.8/y_1 + 0.7/y_2.$$

It is interesting to notice that $B \subset \widetilde{B}$. This fact is of interest for approximate reasoning, because it indicates that B could be an optimal output in some sense. Studies that investigate properties like this one and/or that $\widetilde{B} = B$ will be seen in a little different context in Chap. 6. The reader who wants to know more about this topic may consult [9, 11–13] and many other articles about approximate reasoning.

Practical Method

The observation presented after formula (4.6) means we have

$$B^* = A^* \otimes^t \mathcal{R},$$

where for the finite domain case, A^* and B^* are written as row vectors and

$$[\mathcal{R}] = [\varphi_{\mathcal{R}}(x_i, y_j)]_{i \times j}$$

where "$\otimes^t$" is the composition sup–t (see Chap. 6).

The previous example has

$$\mathcal{R} = [\varphi_{\mathcal{R}}(x_i, y_j)]_{3 \times 2} = \begin{bmatrix} 1.0 \ 1.0 \\ 0.8 \ 0.4 \\ 1.0 \ 0.8 \end{bmatrix}_{3 \times 2},$$

$$A = \begin{bmatrix} 0.4 \ 1.0 \ 0.6 \end{bmatrix}$$

and the composition is the max-min once we have $\triangle = \wedge$.

So,

$$\tilde{B} = A \circ \mathcal{R} = \begin{bmatrix} 0.4 \ 1.0 \ 0.6 \end{bmatrix} \circ \begin{bmatrix} 1.0 \ 1.0 \\ 0.8 \ 0.4 \\ 1.0 \ 0.8 \end{bmatrix} = \begin{bmatrix} 0.8 \ 0.6 \end{bmatrix},$$

that is,

$$\tilde{B} = \frac{0.8}{y_1} + \frac{0.6}{y_2}.$$

Our objective now is to use the generalized modus ponens to model situations where the attributes may be modified. For example, in the case "banana", if it is observed that its color is *almost yellow*, this color may be considered *yellow slightly modified*. In cases like this we use the operators called modifiers.

4.5 Linguistic Modifiers

As its name suggests, linguistic modifiers, are frequently used to change attributes, that is, modeling adverbs. Fuzzy set theory, when combined with the generalized fuzzy modus ponens, helps in the production of fuzzy sets that represent attributes of linguistic variables. In this case, the linguistic modifiers are called fuzzy modifiers.

Definition 4.6 (*Fuzzy modifier*) A *fuzzy modifier* m over U is a map defined on $\mathcal{F}(U)$ with values on $\mathcal{F}(U)$:

$$m : \mathcal{F}(U) \longrightarrow \mathcal{F}(U). \tag{4.7}$$

The main fuzzy modifiers are:

(i) *Expansive* if, for all $A \in \mathcal{F}(U)$, $A \subseteq m(A)$, that is, $\varphi_A(x) \le \varphi_{m(A)}(x)$;
(ii) *Restrictive* if, for all $A \in \mathcal{F}(U)$, $A \supseteq m(A)$, that is, $\varphi_A(x) \ge \varphi_{m(A)}(x)$.

The most commonly used fuzzy modifiers are of power type. A modifier is a *power* type if for each $A \in \mathcal{F}(U)$ we have

$$m_s(A) := (A)^s,$$

that is,

$$\varphi_{m(A)}(x) = (\varphi_A(x))^s,$$

for some $s \in [0, \infty)$.

We can observe that if $s < 1$ then m_s is expansive and if $s > 1$ then m_s is restrictive, since $\varphi_A(x) \in [0, 1]$.

Example 4.7 Consider the fuzzy set of young individuals defined by the membership function

$$\varphi_Y(x) = \begin{cases} 1 & \text{if } x \leq 25 \\ \left(1 + \dfrac{x-25}{5}\right)^{-2} & \text{if } x > 25 \end{cases}.$$

When we apply fuzzy modifiers on primary terms like the adjective "young", we define new fuzzy terms like "very young". Thus, if we define for "very young" the fuzzy subset VY, whose membership function is given by

$$\varphi_{VY}(x) = \varphi_{m(Y)}(x) = (\varphi_Y(x))^2,$$

we have the modifier $m(A) = (A)^2$ and, for an individual whose age is $x = 30$, his/her membership degree to the "young" set is $\varphi_Y(30) = 0.25$ while for the "very young" set we have $\varphi_{VY}(30) = 0.25^2 = 0.0625 < \varphi_Y(30)$.

For a more complete study, the reader may consult [7, 14].

Example 4.8 Let us return to the "banana" example, which motivated the study of this section.

Rule:	*"If the banana is yellow, then it is ripe"*
Fact:	*"The banana is yellow"*
Conclusion:	*"The banana is ripe"*

Now the idea is to rewrite the conditional

"If the banana is yellow then it is ripe"

in the form

"If X is A then Y is B",

and then obtain the relation $\mathcal{R}$, given by an implication function, whose membership function is

$$\varphi_{\mathcal{R}}(x, y) = (\varphi_A(x) \Longrightarrow \varphi_B(y)).$$

The concept "yellow" is represented here by a fuzzy set that is obtained from a set of coloration which shows different types of yellow. That is, various yellow colors are not equal. We can describe the concept of yellow by a membership function obtained by the color spectrum that goes from green to yellow, whose wave-length λ varies between 530 and 597 nm. We use for the shade associated with the yellowness of a banana the difference between its wave-length and the green one 530 nm. So, the membership function that defines "yellow banana" can be given by:

$$\varphi_A(x) = \begin{cases} \dfrac{x}{60} & \text{if} \quad 0 \le x \le 60 \\ 1 & \text{if} \quad 60 < x \le 67 \end{cases}.$$

This memberships supposes that for x between 60 and 67 nm, the yellow shades are indistinguishable and therefore in this interval the membership degree to the fuzzy set "yellow" will be 1 (see Fig. 4.1).

Modeling of the term "ripe banana" is related to the percentage of sugar in the fruit. Experts say that a banana is ripe for sure when the sugar concentration is between 19 and 25 %. A way to detect the sugar level is the human palate. For our purposes, the membership function of the fuzzy set "ripe banana" can be given by (see Fig. 4.2).

$$\varphi_B(y) = \begin{cases} \dfrac{y}{19} & \text{if } 0 \le y \le 19 \\ 1 & \text{if } 19 < y \le 25 \end{cases}.$$

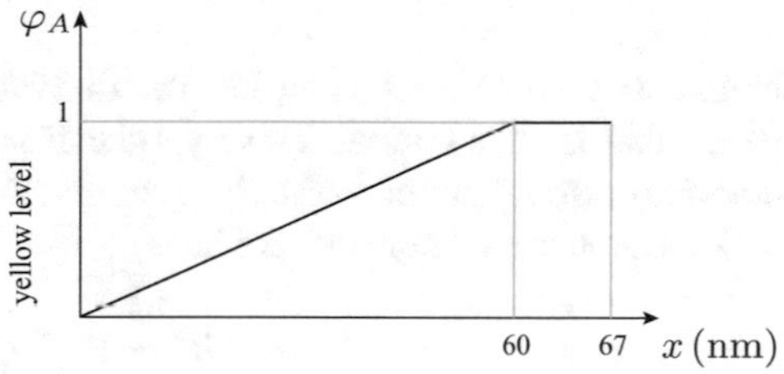

Fig. 4.1 Membership function of the fuzzy set "*yellow*" in nanometers

Fig. 4.2 Membership function of the fuzzy set "ripe banana"

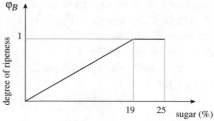

Now let us suppose that the term "almost yellow" is modeled by a fuzzy set A^*, that is obtained by a map of an expansive fuzzy modifier to the fuzzy subset A:

$$\varphi_{A^*}(x) = \varphi_{m(A)}(x) = (\varphi_A(x))^s \text{ with } s \leq 1.$$

Lastly, to obtain the output B^* that indicates the term "almost ripe", we will adopt a generalized modus pones with the Wu's implication and the minimum t-norm: $x \triangle y = x \wedge y$.

So, $B^* = \mathcal{R}(A^*)$, whose membership function is given by

$$\varphi_{B^*}(y) = \varphi_{\mathcal{R}(A^*)}(y) = \varphi_{\mathcal{R}m(A)}(y) = \sup_x \left[\varphi_\mathcal{R}(x, y) \wedge \varphi_{m(A)}(x)\right]$$

$$= \sup_x \left[(\varphi_A(x) \Longrightarrow \varphi_B(y)) \wedge \varphi_{m(A)}(x)\right]$$

$$= \max \left\{\sup_{\varphi_A(x) \leq \varphi_B(y)} \left[\varphi_{m(A)}(x) \wedge 1\right], \sup_{\varphi_A(x) > \varphi_B(y)} \left[(1 - \varphi_A(x)) \wedge \varphi_B(y) \wedge \varphi_{m(A)}(x)\right]\right\}$$

$$= \max \left\{\sup_{\varphi_A(x) \leq \varphi_B(y)} (\varphi_A(x))^s, \sup_{\varphi_A(x) > \varphi_B(y)} \left[(1 - \varphi_A(x)) \wedge \varphi_B(y) \wedge (\varphi_A(x))^s\right]\right\}$$

$$= \max \left\{\sup_{\varphi_A(x) \leq \varphi_B(y)} (\varphi_A(x))^s, \sup_{\varphi_A(x) > \varphi_B(y)} (1 - \varphi_A(x)) \wedge \varphi_B(y)\right\}$$

$$= \max \left\{(\varphi_B(y))^s, (1 - \varphi_B(y)) \wedge \varphi_B(y)\right\} = (\varphi_B(y))^s.$$

Therefore,
$$\varphi_{B^*}(y) = (\varphi_B(y))^s \geq \varphi_B(y), \text{ for } s \in (0, 1].$$

Notice that $\mathcal{R}(A) = B$ ($s = 1$). The derivation above is valid because $Im(\varphi_A) = [0, 1]$, that is, A is normal. This hypothesis is necessary [7], because otherwise, the derivation would not be valid. See Exercise 4.8 (b) with data from Example 4.6.

In set-theoretic language, we have

$$B^* = m(B) \supset B.$$

The fact that B is contained in $m(B)$ means that a banana that is almost ripe will always be less than ripe (Fig. 4.3). If a yellow banana is ripe, then a less yellow banana will be less ripe. The conclusion given by the set B^* "almost ripe" or "less ripe" can be seen in Fig. 4.3b.

To conclude this example, let us explore a little more the condition $B^* = m(B)$. Notice that
$$\mathcal{R}(m(A)) = \mathcal{R}(A^*) = B^* = m(B) = m(\mathcal{R}(A)),$$

or in diagram form this can be seen in Fig. 4.4. The fact that $\mathcal{R}(m(A)) = m(\mathcal{R}(A))$ indicates that the diagram commutes and means that *the modified output of A is the*

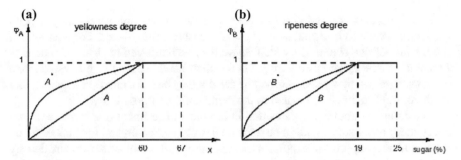

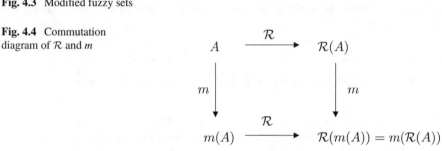

Fig. 4.3 Modified fuzzy sets

Fig. 4.4 Commutation
diagram of $\mathcal{R}$ and m

same as the output modification of A. For our example, the commutativity of the
above diagram means that the modification degree undergone by banana maturation
is the same modification degree of its shade. In fuzzy logic, the commutativity of the
diagram is still not explored very much and the reader is invited to investigate such
property both from a theoretical standpoint as well as in applications.

Exercise 4.10 Redo the Example 4.8 considering the power modifier with $s > 1$
and verify for this case whether $\mathcal{R}(m(A)) = m(\mathcal{R}(A))$ holds. Next, use other implications and t-norms to obtain new output fuzzy sets B^*.

4.6 Independence and Non-interactivity

This section briefly introduces the concept of possibilistic non-interactivity introduced by Zadeh [15], which is closely related to probabilistic independence. The
term "possibilistic" is used here as a reference to "membership degree". This concept will be formalized in the next chapter in Sect. 7.1.3.

There are currently a large number of researchers interested in interactivity and
non-interactivity, with applications in many fields (see [16–19]). Our main goal
here is in how this concept is linked to modus ponens. Intuitively, independence is
associated to the idea of "noninterference" while interactivity is linked to "mutual
action" between two or more things. For example, two chemical substances are non-
interactive if their particles can be identified when we look at them separately and
then jointly. For example, consider water and oil.

Both independence and non-interactivity between two objects strongly depend on what we want to measure, as well as the measurement adopted. For example, in the mixture of two chemical substances we may be interested in changes in density first seen separately and then jointly. On the other hand, we may be interested in the color change, separately and jointly. The density may be associated to the probability while the color may be associated to the membership, or possibility.

The comment above illustrates that in the same experiment (the mixture of two substances) many studies might be done on density and color, and for each of them, we should adopt appropriate tools. In this case, probability is used to measure density and possibility is used to measure color. In order to draw a parallel with the theme that we will study, we next present the concept of probabilistic independence and non-interactivity.

4.6.1 Probabilistic Independence and Non-interactivity

We will limit ourselves to just the discrete case. The continuous case is analogous by replacing the probability distribution with the probability density function. Let X and Y be two discrete random variables. Suppose that $P_{(X,Y)}$ is the joint probability distribution of the random vector (X, Y), we know that [7, 20]:

(p_1) The *marginal distributions* of X and Y are given, respectively, by

$$P_X(x) = \sum_y P_{(X,Y)}(x, y) \quad \text{and} \quad P_Y(y) = \sum_x P_{(X,Y)}(x, y);$$

(p_2) X and Y are *non-interactive*, probabilistically, if

$$P_{(X,Y)}(x, y) = P_X(x)P_Y(y)$$

for all pairs (x, y). Otherwise, they are called *interactive* [7];

(p_3) The *conditional distributions* of X and Y are given, respectively, by

$$P_{X|Y}(x|y) = \frac{P_{(X,Y)}(x, y)}{P_Y(y)} \Leftrightarrow P_{(X,Y)}(x, y) = P_{X|Y}(x|y)P_Y(y)$$

if $P_Y(y) \neq 0$ and

$$P_{Y|X}(y|x) = \frac{P_{(X,Y)}(x, y)}{P_X(x)} \Leftrightarrow P_{(X,Y)}(x, y) = P_{Y|X}(y|x)P_X(x)$$

if $P_X(x) \neq 0$;

(p_4) X and Y are *independent*, probabilistically, if

$$P_{(X|Y)}(x|y) = P_X(x) \quad \text{and} \quad P_{(Y|X)}(y|x) = P_Y(y)$$

for all pairs (x, y). Otherwise, they are called *dependent*.

Of course the concepts of independence (p_4) and probabilistic non-interactivity (p_2) are equivalent if the marginal do not cancel themselves. This fact is the consequence of the mathematical operation "multiplication" used to model such concepts.

However, there are authors who do not agree that we have an equivalence between (p_2) and (p_4) and instead use more general mathematical operations to represent these concepts. These operations are known as copula and have close relations to t-norms. As we already know, the operation "multiplication" used in (p_2) and (p_4) is a particular t-norm. A general result that relates the joint probability distribution with the marginal via copulas is due to Sklar [5].

4.6.2 *Possibilistic Independence and Non-interactivity*

Here the mathematical objects are fuzzy sets instead of random variables. Consequently, possibility distributions as used here are synonymous to membership function. Unlike the probabilistic case, where the most common copula is the product, in the fuzzy case the most common operator to deal with the non-interactivity is the minimum. However, in this text we will use a general t-norm to mathematically deal with the involved concepts.

Suppose that $\varphi_{(A,B)}$ is a possibility distribution (see Definition 7.5) of the universal set $U \times V$ of the fuzzy sets A and B. That is, $\varphi_{(A,B)}(x, y) \in [0, 1]$, for $x \in U$ and $y \in V$.

(f_1) Reference [19] The *marginal distributions of possibilities* of A and B are respectively given by

$$\varphi_A(x) = \sup_{y} \varphi_{(A,B)}(x, y) \quad \text{and} \quad \varphi_B(y) = \sup_{x} \varphi_{(A,B)}(x, y).$$

(f_2) A and B are possibilistically *non-interactive*, according to the $\triangle$ t-norm, if

$$\varphi_{(A,B)}(x, y) = \varphi_A(x)\triangle\varphi_B(y),$$

for all pair (x, y). In particular, A and B are called *non-interactive* if $\triangle$ is the minimum t-norm, that is

$$\varphi_{(A,B)}(x, y) = \varphi_A(x) \wedge \varphi_B(y),$$

or equivalently $[(A, B)]^\alpha = [A]^\alpha \times [B]^\alpha$.

(f_3) The *distributions conditional possibilities* of A and B, according to the $\triangle$ t-norm are respectively, given by the formulas

$$\varphi_{(A,B)}(x, y) = \varphi_{(A|B)}(x|y)\triangle\varphi_B(y)$$

and

$$\varphi_{(A,B)}(x, y) = \varphi_{(B|A)}(y|x) \triangle \varphi_A(x)$$

for all (x, y).

(f_4) A and B are possibilistically *independent* if

$$\varphi_{(A|B)}(x|y) = \varphi_A(x) \quad \text{and} \quad \varphi_{(B|A)}(y|x) = \varphi_B(y).$$

for all (x, y). Otherwise, they are possibilistically *dependent*.

Unlike the probabilistic case, non-interactivity is not equivalent to independence. Independence implies non-interactivity. However, the converse is not generally true. It is interesting to notice that in both cases - probabilistic and possibilities - the marginals are related to the joint distribution by similar formulas except that in the probabilistic case we use the sum, while for the possibilistic case we use **sup** instead of sum.

4.6.3 The Conditional Distributions and Modus Ponens

The conditional rule

$$R : \text{If } x \text{ is } A \text{ then } y \text{ is } B$$

in the modus ponens may be interpreted as "y is B with degree $\varphi_B(y)$, given that x is A with degree $\varphi_A(x)$". From this point of view, the membership function φ_R that represents the rule R is a typical distribution of conditional membership, that is,

$$\varphi_R(x, y) = (\varphi_A(x) \Rightarrow \varphi_B(y)) = \varphi_{B|A}(y|x). \tag{4.8}$$

With this interpretation, we have a formula to obtain conditional distribution, that is, for a causality logical rule, we have a way to obtain its membership conditional distribution. For that, we just have to know the fuzzy implication to be adopted and from this, use formula (4.8). So, from the modus ponens, formula (4.5) becomes

$$\varphi_{R(A)}(y) = \sup_x (\varphi_{B|A}(y|x) \triangle \varphi_A(x)). \tag{4.9}$$

Extrapolating this idea for the generalized modus ponens, we can say that $\varphi_{B^*}(y) = \varphi_{R(A^*)}(y)$ is the possibility distribution of B when we observe A^* and (4.6) becomes

$$\varphi_{R(A^*)}(y) = \sup_x (\varphi_{B|A}(y|x) \triangle \varphi_{A^*}(x)). \tag{4.10}$$

The interested reader might want to consult [21–23].

Thus, we have a way to obtain the conditional distribution $\varphi_{B|A}(y|x)$ using (4.8). However, in general, we do not have a formula that give us the conditional distributions from the marginals. Moreover, it is worth noticing that the conditional rule

$$R : \text{``if } x \text{ is } A \text{ then } y \text{ is } B\text{''} \tag{4.11}$$

is not always causal as is the case of fuzzy controllers (see Chap. 5). The relation R associated with fuzzy controllers represents the Cartesian product, that is, each pair (x, y) is an element of the Cartesian product. The relation R above is usually modeled by the minimum t-norm. In this case φ_R may be interpreted as the joint distribution. This was initially suggested by Zadeh [15].

Thus, we have that (4.11) is given by

$$\varphi_R(x, y) = \varphi_{(A,B)}(x, y) = \varphi_A(x) \triangle \varphi_B(y), \tag{4.12}$$

suggesting non-interactivity between the fuzzy sets A and B, according to the $\triangle$ t-norm. Specifically in Mamdani's method (Chap. 5), we have an assumption in (4.12) of non-interactivity where $\triangle = \wedge$. That is Mamdani uses (4.12) for fuzzy controllers with $\triangle = \wedge$ which means that it is assuming non-interactivity.

Exercise 4.11 Verify that if A and B are crisp, then they are non-interactivity if and only if they are possibilistically independent.

Exercise 4.12 Check that possibilistic independence is equivalent to the non-interactive if the adopted t-norm is the product.

Exercise 4.13 Verify that if A and B are non-interactive and $\triangle = \wedge$ in (4.9), then

$$\varphi_{B|A}(y|x) = \begin{cases} \varphi_B(y) & \text{if } \varphi_B(y) < \varphi_A(x) \\ \alpha \in [\varphi_A(x), 1] & \text{if } \varphi_B(y) \geq \varphi_A(x) \end{cases}.$$

Exercise 4.14 Give examples, if possible, of fuzzy sets A and B with:

(a) Discrete and continuous fuzzy numbers such that B is possibilistically independent of A, when $\varphi_{B|A}(y|x)$ is given by the modus ponens, that is, when

$$\varphi_{B|A}(y|x) = (\varphi_A(x) \Rightarrow \varphi_B(y)).$$

(b) Noninteractivity where B depends possibilistically on A.

Exercise 4.15 Consider the fuzzy sets from Example 4.6.

(a) If the implication is the Gödel implication and $\triangle = \wedge$, check to see if the distributions of $\mathcal{R}(A)$ and B match;
(b) Do the same as in (a) for Lukasiewicz's implication and $\triangle = \wedge$;
(c) Do the same an in (a) for Goguen's implication and the *product* t-norm.

References

1. P. Hájek, *Metamathematics of Fuzzy Logic* (Kluwer Academic Publisher, Dordrecht, 1997)
2. H.T. Nguyen, E.A. Walker, *A First Course of Fuzzy Logic* (CRC Press, Boca Raton, 1997)
3. L.A. Zadeh, Fuzzy sets. Inf. Control **8**, 338–353 (1965)
4. K. Menger, Statistical metrics. Proc. Natl. Acad. Sci. **28**(12), 535–537 (1942)
5. E.P. Klement, R. Mesiar, E. Pap, *Triangular Norms* (Kluwer Academic Publishers, Netherlands, 2000)
6. M. Baczyński, B. Jayaram, *Fuzzy Implications* (Springer, Berlin, Heidelberg, 2008)
7. G. Klir, B. Yuan, *Fuzzy Sets and Fuzzy Logic Theory and Applications* (Prentice-Hall, Upper Saddle River, 1995)
8. W. Pedrycz, F. Gomide, *An Introduction to Fuzzy Sets: Analysis and Design* (The MIT Press, Massachusets, 1998)
9. W. Wangning, Fuzzy reasoning and fuzzy relational equations. Fuzzy Sets Syst. **20**, 67–78 (1986)
10. F.S. Pedro, L.C. Barros, The use of t-norms in mathematical models of epidemics, in, *2013 IEEE International Conference on Fuzzy Systems (FUZZ)*, pp. 1–4 (2013)
11. M. Mizumoto, S. Fukani, and K. Tanaka, *Some methods of fuzzy reasoning*, Advances in Fuzzy Sets Theory and Applications (Amsterdan) (M. M. Gupta et al, ed.), North-Holland, 1979
12. M. Mizumoto, H.J. Zimermann, Comparison of fuzzy reasoning methods. Fuzzy Sets Syst. **8**, 253–283 (1986)
13. M. Ying, Reasonableness of compositional rule of fuzzy inference. Fuzzy Sets Syst. **36**, 305–310 (1990)
14. M. De Cock, E.E. Kerre, Fuzzy modifiers based on fuzzy relations. Inf. Sci. **160**, 173–199 (2004)
15. L.A. Zadeh, Fuzzy sets as a basis for a theory of possibility. Fuzzy Sets Syst. **1**, 3–28 (1978)
16. M.Z. Ahmad, B.D. Baets, A predator-prey model with fuzzy initial populations, Cd-rom, in *Proceeding of IFSA-EUSFLAT Conference*. Lisbon (2009)
17. J.M. Baetens, B.D. Baets, Incorporating fuzziness in spatial susceptible-infected epidemic models, Cd-rom, in *Proceding of IFSA-EUSFLAT Conference*. Lisbon (2009)
18. V.M. Cabral, L.C. Barros, Fuzzy differential equation with completely correlated parameters. Fuzzy Sets Syst. **265**, 86–98 (2015)
19. R. Füller, P. Majlender, On interactive fuzzy numbers. Fuzzy Sets Syst. **143**, 355–369 (2004)
20. W.O. Bussab, P.A. Morettin, *Estatística básica*, 5th edn. (Editora Saraiva, São Paulo, 2002)
21. E. Hisdal, Conditional possibilities independence and noninteraction. Fuzzy Sets Syst. **1**(4), 283–297 (1978)
22. H.T. Nguyen, On conditional possibility distributions. Fuzzy Sets Syst. **1**(4), 299–309 (1978)
23. L. Stephane, B. Bobée, Revision of possibility distributions: a bayesian inference pattern. Fuzzy Sets Syst. **116**(2), 119–140 (2000)

Chapter 5
Fuzzy Rule-Based Systems

There are and there will be many tasks that men can do easily, which that is beyond any machine and any logical system that we can conceive of today.

(Lotfi A. Zadeh)

Abstract This chapter explores fuzzy logic controllers from the point of view of its applications. The chapter covers the fuzzy logic controllers of Mamdani and Takagi-Sugeno-Kang. These are illustrated with applications in biology, ecology, HIV dynamics, and pharmacological decay.

All of us agree intuitively with Zadeh's thought as stated above. However, as it is well known, it was his first studies about fuzzy set theory that originated what nowadays is called fuzzy logic, a subject with many applications in execution and control of tasks that in many domains is challenging human abilities to perform tasks.

Human actions control many systems in the world using inaccurate information. Each individual works as a "black box"; receives information that is interpreted according to her or his parameters and then decides which action should be taken. For a computer procedure, the control and the execution of tasks must follow a sequence of linguistic "instructions" translated by a set of rules that can be decoded by the controller. The following example illustrates the above remark.

Example 5.1 An expert is able to wash clothes until they are clean (according to her or his concept of clean). The following scheme (Fig. 5.1) represents, in a simple way, the actions of the expert (human controller) in the execution of the laundry task. In this example, we can observe a possible way to automate this task. The rules and the orders in which they must be followed can be given by Frame 5.1.

An attempt to reproduce the strategy of a human controller in his or her task execution is made by a **Fuzzy Controller** which is a typical case of a **Fuzzy Rule-Based Sytem (FRBS)**, that is, a system that makes use of the fuzzy logic to produce outputs for each fuzzy input. Many examples of this process can be found in various texts [1–4].

© Springer-Verlag Berlin Heidelberg 2017
L.C. de Barros et al., *A First Course in Fuzzy Logic, Fuzzy Dynamical Systems, and Biomathematics*, Studies in Fuzziness and Soft Computing 347, DOI 10.1007/978-3-662-53324-6_5

Fig. 5.1 A scheme for a human control system to do laundry

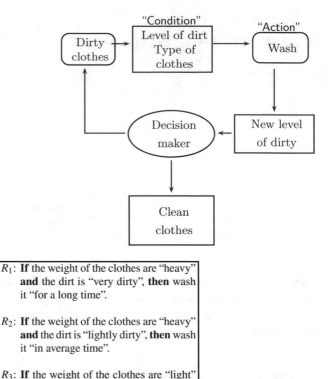

R_1: **If** the weight of the clothes are "heavy" **and** the dirt is "very dirty", **then** wash it "for a long time".

or

R_2: **If** the weight of the clothes are "heavy" **and** the dirt is "lightly dirty", **then** wash it "in average time".

or

R_3: **If** the weight of the clothes are "light" **and** the dirt is "lightly dirty", **then** wash it "very briefly".

or

R_4: **If** the weight of the clothes are "light" **and** the dirt is "very dirty", **then** wash it "briefly".

Frame 5.1: Rules for an automation system to wash clothes

The *modus ponens* seen in Chap. 4 is an example of fuzzy rule-based system. The particularity of the various fuzzy controllers is in their interpretation. In the first FRBS applications that arose, each output represented the "action" relative to the "condition" or to the FRBS input. When the inputs and outputs have this connotation the FRBS are called *Fuzzy Controllers*. With the aid of the methods that we saw in approximate reasoning, in Chap. 4, it becomes possible to translate linguistic terms that are regularly used by experts, whose goal is to control some tasks, into mathematical formulas, enabling the automation of some tasks. This is one fundamental distinction between fuzzy control theory and classical control theory. Classical control has the aim of developing strategies for a dynamical system to optimize a given criterion, or in a more technical language, a cost functional. In fuzzy controllers the tasks are controlled using terms of common language, related to some variable of interest. It is in this context that linguistic variables play an important role in this methodology. The linguistic terms translated by fuzzy sets are used to translate the knowledge base into a collection of fuzzy rules bases, called **Fuzzy Rule Bases**. From this rule base we can obtain a fuzzy relation, which will produce the output from input.

5.1 Fuzzy Rule Bases

A fuzzy rule base has the form

R_1: "**Fuzzy proposition** 1"
or
$\quad R_2$: "**Fuzzy proposition** 2"
....
or
$\quad R_r$: "**Fuzzy proposition** r"

Frame 5.2: General form of a fuzzy rule base

In systems based on fuzzy rules each fuzzy proposition has the form

If "*state*" **then** "*answer*"

where each "*state*" and each "*answer*" is a fuzzy value taken on by linguistic variables. The fuzzy sets that compose the "*state*" are called *antecedents*. On the other hand, the fuzzy sets that compose the "*answer*" are called *consequents*. The characteristic of fuzzy controllers, as we have already observed, is that each rule has the form

If "*condition*" **then** "*action*".

Example 5.1 above supposes that each task is executed by a human being, which requires no mathematical tool. This is not the case with fuzzy controllers. The variables of interest are: clothes (**r**) to be washed; its level of dirt (**s**) and the adopted control (**e**), having classifications "*heavy load*" or "*light load*" for the clothes, and "*lighty dirty*" or "*very dirty*" for the dirt, "*for a long time*", "*very briefly*" or "*average time*" for the action of washing process that must be modeled by fuzzy sets. In a similar way to that of Chap. 4, each one of the classifications of the variables that are in the rule base are modeled by a fuzzy set. Fuzzy logic is the other part used to obtain the fuzzy relation that synthesizes the mathematical informations in the base rule.

The rule base fulfills the role of "translate" mathematically the informations that form the knowledge base of the fuzzy system. In a certain way, we can say that the more accurate such results are, the less fuzzy (more crisp) will be the fuzzy relations that represents the knowledge base. In an ideal situation such relations are functions in the classical way.

The following section deals with the methodology of the fuzzy controllers and their associated basic modules.

5.2 Fuzzy Controller

Fuzzy Controllers consists of a fuzzy system, where the inputs represent "conditions" while the outputs are "actions". However, if the input is crisp (an element of $\mathbb{R}^n$), we expect that the output is also crisp (an element of $\mathbb{R}^m$). In that case, a fuzzy system is a function of $\mathbb{R}^n$ into $\mathbb{R}^m$ built in an specific way. The following modules indicate a process for the construction of this function.

5.2.1 Fuzzification Module

Fuzzification is the step where the inputs of the system are modeled by fuzzy sets with their respective domains. It is this step that great importance is given to experts in the domain of the modeled phenomenon. Together with the experts, the membership functions are formulated for each fuzzy set involved in the process. If the input is crisp, it will be fuzzyfied by its characteristic function.

5.2.2 Base-Rule Module

The Rule-Base Module may be considered as a module forming part of the "kernel" of the fuzzy controller. It consists of the fuzzy propositions and each one of these propositions is described by the linguistic form

$$
\begin{aligned}
&\textbf{If} \quad && x_1 \text{ is } A_1 \quad &&\text{and} \quad && x_2 \text{ is } A_2 \quad &&\text{and} \quad &&\dots \quad &&\text{and} \quad && x_n \text{ is } A_n \\
&\textbf{Then} \quad && u_1 \text{ is } B_1 \quad &&\text{and} \quad && u_2 \text{ is } B_2 \quad &&\text{and} \quad &&\dots \quad &&\text{and} \quad && u_m \text{ is } B_m
\end{aligned}
$$

according to information gathered from the expert. It is at this point that the variables and its linguistic classifications are delineated and subsequently modeled by fuzzy sets, that is, its membership functions. Methods to obtain those membership functions are many: intuitive appeal, curve fitting, interpolation and even neural networks [1, 4, 5].

5.2.3 Fuzzy Inference Module

The Fuzzy Inference Module, using fuzzy logic techniques, translates fuzzy proposition into fuzzy relations. It is this module where we define which t-norms, t-conorms and inference rules, including fuzzy implications are used to obtain the fuzzy relation that models the rule base. This module is as important as the rule base module.

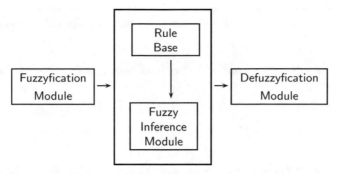

Fig. 5.2 General sketch of a fuzzy controller

Basically, it is from this that the success of the fuzzy controller depends since it will give the fuzzy output (control) to be utilized by the controller from each fuzzy input.

5.2.4 Defuzzification Module

The last module is Defuzzification. In stochastic theory is common to indicate the *mathematical expectation* (or mean) as the number that best represents a random variable (or distribution of data). Other values such as *mode* and the *median* are also used to represent the centralization of such distributions. In the fuzzy set theory, it is the defuzzification process that allows us to represent a fuzzy set by a crisp value (real number).

Figure 5.2 represents a general sketch of a fuzzy controller. The rule base is mathematically modeled by a fuzzy relation $\mathcal{R}$. The membership function of $\mathcal{R}$ is given by

$$\varphi_{\mathcal{R}}(x, u) = \bigtriangledown(\varphi_{R_i}(x, u)), \;\; \text{with } 1 \leq i \leq r, \tag{5.1}$$

where $\bigtriangledown$ is a t-conorm and R_i is a fuzzy relation obtained from rule i, whose membership function φ_{R_i} is obtained by various means – for example, by the generalized *modus ponens*. The values x and u represent the state and the control, respectively.

The inference that represents the control B for a state A is given by an inference composition rule

$$\varphi_B(u) = \sup_x(\varphi_{\mathcal{R}}(x, u) \bigtriangleup \varphi_A(x)), \tag{5.2}$$

where $\bigtriangleup$ is a t-norm. We illustrate how to obtain the relation $\mathcal{R}$ in a similar way as was done for the generalized modus ponens, as we can see in Frame 5.3.

The first published article in automation having to do with control tasks that was based in fuzzy logic was proposed by Mamdani and Assilian [6]. Their experiments dealt with the control of a steam engine. They based their controls on the fact that

R_1: "If x_1 is A_{11} and $\cdots$ and x_n is A_{1n} then u_1 is B_{11} and $\cdots$ and u_m is B_{1m}"

or

R_2: "If x_1 is A_{21} and $\cdots$ and x_n is A_{2n} then u_1 is B_{21} and $\cdots$ and u_m is B_{2m}"

or

$\vdots$ $\vdots$

or

R_r: "If x_1 is A_{r1} and $\cdots$ and x_n is A_{rn} then u_1 is B_{r1} and $\cdots$ and u_m is B_{rm}"

Fact: $A = x_1$ is A_1 and x_2 is A_2 and $\cdots$ and x_n is A_n

Conclusion: u is $B = \mathcal{R}(A)$

Frame 5.3: Illustration of the relation $\mathcal{R}$

human operators express control strategies in linguistic form and not in a mathematical way. This research influenced others to use fuzzy controllers in the control theory. Nowadays, fuzzy controllers are used in electrical appliances, Japan was the first country to invest extensively in the "fuzzy industry". The next section will illustrate Mamdani inference method.

5.3 Mamdani Inference Method

Mamdani proposed, from the theoretical point of view, a binary fuzzy relation $\mathcal{M}$ between x and u to mathematically model the rule base. The Mamdani method is based on the inference composition rule max–min according to the following procedure.

- Each rule R_j from the fuzzy rule base, the conditional "**if** x **is** A_j **then** u **is** B_j" is modeled by the operation $\wedge$ (minimum). This has been wrongly called Mamdani's implication. We say "wrongly called Mamdani's implication" because $\wedge$ is not a fuzzy implication since it does not preserve the classical implication table.
- It uses the t-norm $\wedge$ (minimum) for the logical conective "**and**";
- For the logical connective "**or**" the t-conorm $\vee$ (maximum) is adopted that connects the fuzzy rules of the rule base.

Formally, the fuzzy relation $\mathcal{M}$ is the fuzzy subset of $X \times U$ whose membership function is given by

$$\varphi_{\mathcal{M}}(x, u) = \max_{1 \leq j \leq r}(\varphi_{R_j}(x, u)) = \max_{1 \leq j \leq r}[\varphi_{A_j}(x) \wedge \varphi_{B_j}(u)], \tag{5.3}$$

where r is the number of rules that compose the rule base and, A_j and B_j are the fuzzy subsets of the rule j. Each one of the values $\varphi_{A_j}(x)$ and $\varphi_{B_j}(u)$ is interpreted as the degree that x and u are in the fuzzy subsets A_j and B_j, respectively. Thus, $\mathcal{M}$ is nothing more than the union of the fuzzy Cartesian products between the antecedents and the consequents of each rule.

There are various types of fuzzy controllers, Mamdani–Assilian being one of the most important. Another important fuzzy controller is the Takagi–Sugeno [7] controller which will be discussed after we present the Mamdani–Assilan controller.

Observations:

(1) It is common to find in the literature the initials **MISO** (multiple inputs and single output) and **MIMO** (multiple inputs and multiple outputs).
(2) The fuzzy subsets A_j and B_j that appears in the formula (5.3) can represent the fuzzy Cartesian product of the fuzzy subsets A_{ji} and B_{jk}. For example, it might occur that

$$\varphi_{A_j}(x) = \varphi_{A_{j1}}(x_1) \wedge \varphi_{A_{j2}}(x_2) \text{ and } \varphi_{B_j}(u) = \varphi_{B_{j1}}(u_1) \wedge \varphi_{B_{j2}}(u_2),$$

so it is a **MIMO** fuzzy controller with two inputs and two outputs.

The next example illustrates the Mamdani inference method for the case of a fuzzy system with two inputs and a single output.

Example 5.2 Consider a fuzzy controller with two inputs and a single output, whose rule base is given in Frame 5.4.

R_1: If x_1 is A_{11} and x_2 is A_{12} then u is B_1
or
R_2: If x_1 is A_{21} and x_2 is A_{22} then u is B_2

Frame 5.4: Rule base for a controller with two inputs and a single output

For each $t = (x_1, x_2, u)$, we have

$$\varphi_{\mathcal{M}}(t) = \{\varphi_{A_{11}}(x_1) \wedge \varphi_{A_{12}}(x_2) \wedge \varphi_{B_1}(u)\} \vee \{\varphi_{A_{21}}(x_1) \wedge \varphi_{A_{22}}(x_2) \wedge \varphi_{B_2}(u)\}$$
$$= \max\{\varphi_{A_{11}}(x_1) \wedge \varphi_{A_{12}}(x_2) \wedge \varphi_{B_1}(u), \varphi_{A_{21}}(x_1) \wedge \varphi_{A_{22}}(x_2) \wedge \varphi_{B_2}(u)\}$$

representing the fuzzy relation obtained from the rule base by the Mamdani method.

Now, for a given fuzzy set with input $A = A_1 \times A_2$, where A_1 and A_2 are two fuzzy numbers, the output fuzzy set, which represents the control to be adopted for A by the Mamdani method, is given by $B = \mathcal{M} \circ A$, whose membership function is

$$\varphi_B(u) = (\varphi_{\mathcal{M} \circ A})(u) = \sup_x \{\varphi_{\mathcal{M}}(x, u) \wedge \varphi_A(x)\}.$$

Since
$$A = A_1 \times A_2,$$

then
$$\varphi_A(x_1, x_2) = \varphi_{A_1}(x_1) \wedge \varphi_{A_2}(x_2).$$

Therefore,

$$
\begin{aligned}
\varphi_B(u) &= \sup_x \{\varphi_{\mathcal{M}}(x, u) \wedge \varphi_A(x)\} \\
&= \sup_{(x_1, x_2)} \{\varphi_{\mathcal{M}}(x_1, x_2, u) \wedge [\varphi_{A_1}(x_1) \wedge \varphi_{A_2}(x_2)]\} \\
&= \sup_{(x_1, x_2)} \{[(\varphi_{A_{11}}(x_1) \wedge \varphi_{A_{12}}(x_2) \wedge \varphi_{B_1}(u)) \vee \\
&\qquad (\varphi_{A_{21}}(x_1) \wedge \varphi_{A_{22}}(x_2) \wedge \varphi_{B_2}(u))] \wedge [\varphi_{A_1}(x_1) \wedge \varphi_{A_2}(x_2)]\} \\
&= \sup_{(x_1, x_2)} \{[\varphi_{A_1}(x_1) \wedge \varphi_{A_{11}}(x_1)] \wedge [\varphi_{A_2}(x_2) \wedge \varphi_{A_{12}}(x_2)] \wedge \varphi_{B_1}(u)\} \vee \\
&\qquad \sup_{(x_1, x_2)} \{[\varphi_{A_1}(x_1) \wedge \varphi_{A_{21}}(x_1)] \wedge [\varphi_{A_2}(x_2) \wedge \varphi_{A_{22}}(x_2)] \wedge \varphi_{B_2}(u)\} \\
&= \varphi_{B_{R_1}}(u) \vee \varphi_{B_{R_2}}(u).
\end{aligned}
$$

where B_{R_1} and B_{R_2} are the partial outputs due to the rules R_1 and R_2, respectively. We can observe, from the formula above, that the output from the Mamdani method results from the union between the partial outputs of each rule. To obtain each partial output, we proceed in the following manner. Perform an intersection of each input with each antecedent of the rule and next, calculate the Cartesian product (distinct universes) of these intersections with the rule consequents. The projection of this Cartesian product onto the space U is the partial output for the fuzzy set of input A.

Graphically we have Fig. 5.3.

The general output is given by the union of the partial outputs according to Fig. 5.4.

Notice that the last graphic of Fig. 5.4 represents the membership function φ_B of the control B that was obtained by the conective $\vee$, which is the maximum t-conorm.

The following example is a particular case of the last one in the sense that now the input A is crisp.

Example 5.3 For the last example consider the case where the input fuzzy set A is crisp and whose membership function is concentrated at a point $(x_0, y_0) \in \mathbb{R} \times \mathbb{R}$. Thus,

$$\varphi_A(x, y) = \begin{cases} 1 \text{ if } (x, y) = (x_0, y_0) \\ 0 \text{ if } (x, y) \neq (x_0, y_0) \end{cases},$$

that is,

$$A = A_1 \times A_2$$

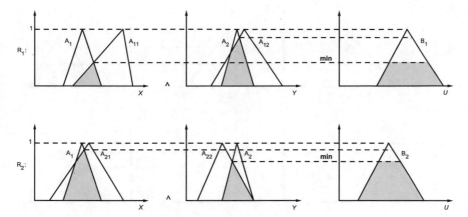

Fig. 5.3 Partial outputs in the Mamdani method

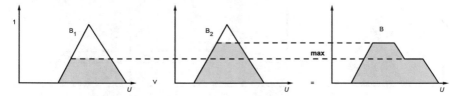

Fig. 5.4 Final output of the Mamdani fuzzy controller

where

$$\varphi_{A_1}(x) = \begin{cases} 1 \text{ if } x = x_0 \\ 0 \text{ if } x \neq x_0 \end{cases} \text{ and } \varphi_{A_2}(y) = \begin{cases} 1 \text{ if } y = y_0 \\ 0 \text{ if } y \neq y_0 \end{cases}.$$

In this case, the fuzzy control B is obtained according to the graphic given by Fig. 5.5.

The final output B is represented in Fig. 5.6.

Example 5.3 shows that the output from the fuzzy controller given by the Mamdani inference method, is a fuzzy subset even for the case with a crisp input. Thus, when it is necessary to have a real number final output we need to defuzzify the output fuzzy subset to obtain a crisp value that represents it.

5.4 Defuzzification Methods

A fuzzy controller produces fuzzy output that indicates the control to be adopted. However, if the input is a real number, it is expected that the related output is also a real number. But, in general, it does not occur in fuzzy controllers, because even for a crisp input, the output is fuzzy. Thus, we must indicate a method to defuzzificate the

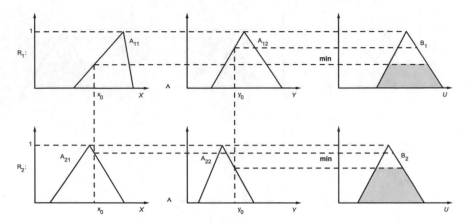

Fig. 5.5 Partial outputs of the Mamdani's fuzzy controller for Example 5.3

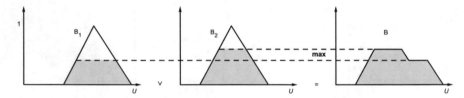

Fig. 5.6 Final output of the Mandani's fuzzy controller for the Example 5.3

output and obtain a real number that will finally indicate the control to be adopted. There are many methods of defuzzification that can be adopted. Any real number that somehow can reasonably represent the fuzzy set B can be called a defuzzification of B. Here, we will present the most common ones.

5.4.1   Centroid or Center of Mass or Center of Gravity (G(B))

This defuzzification method is similar to the arithmetic mean for frequency distributions of a given variable, with the difference that here the weights are the values $\varphi_B(u_i)$, which indicates the degree of compatibility of the value u_i with the concept modeled by the fuzzy set B. Among all the methods of defuzzification, this one is preferred, even though it might be the most complicated one. Equations (5.4) and (5.5) refer to the discrete domain and continuous domain, respectively. The Fig. 5.7 shows the graphic of the defuzzificator $G(B)$.

$$G(B) = \frac{\sum\limits_{i=0}^{n} u_i \varphi_B(u_i)}{\sum\limits_{i=0}^{n} \varphi_B(u_i)}. \tag{5.4}$$

Fig. 5.7 Defuzzificator
center of gravity $G(B)$

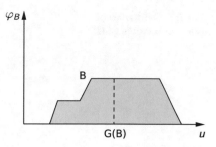

$$G(B) = \frac{\displaystyle\int_{\mathbb{R}} u\varphi_B(u)\mathrm{d}u}{\displaystyle\int_{\mathbb{R}} \varphi_B(u)\mathrm{d}u}. \tag{5.5}$$

5.4.2 Center of Maximum (C(B))

This is a radical procedure, in the sense that it takes into account just the regions of major possibility among the possible values of the variable that models the fuzzy concept involved. In that case, we have:

$$C(B) = \frac{i+s}{2}, \tag{5.6}$$

where

$$i = \inf\{u \in \mathbb{R} : \varphi_B(u) = \max_u \varphi_B(u)\}$$

and

$$s = \sup\{u \in \mathbb{R} : \varphi_B(u) = \max_u \varphi_B(u)\}. \tag{5.7}$$

Figure 5.8 illustrates this defuzzificator

5.4.3 Mean of Maximum (M(B))

For discrete domains it is common to use as defuzzificator the mean of maximum whose definition is given by

$$M(B) = \frac{\sum u_i}{n}, \tag{5.8}$$

Fig. 5.8 Defuzzificator
center of maximum $C(B)$

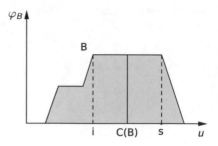

where n is given and u_i, with $1 \le i \le n$, are the values with highest membership to
the fuzzy set B.

Fuzzy controllers, as we have mentioned, are composed of four modules: fuzzification, rule base, inference and defuzzification. The method of Mamdani is a typical
case. However, for some situations, the module of defuzzification might be sup-
pressed. This is the case of Takagi–Sugeno–Kang's inference method that we will
describe next.

5.5 Takagi–Sugeno–Kang Inference Method (TSK)

The basic differences between the Takagi–Sugeno–Kang inference method (now
called TSK) and of Mamdani is in the way we write the consequent of each rule and
in the procedure of defuzzification to obtain the general output of the system. With
the TSK method, the consequent of each rule is explicitly given by a function of the
input values of this rule.

As an illustration of this method we can imagine a rule base with r fuzzy rules,
where each one of them has n inputs $(x_1, x_2, \ldots, x_n) \in \mathbb{R}^n$, and an output $u \in \mathbb{R}$,
according to Frame 5.5, which A_{ij} are fuzzy subsets of $\mathbb{R}$.

The general output of the method is given by

$$u = f_r(x_1, x_2, \ldots, x_n)$$

$$= \frac{\displaystyle\sum_{j=1}^{r} \omega_j g_j(x_1, x_2, \ldots, x_n)}{\displaystyle\sum_{j=1}^{r} \omega_j} = \frac{\displaystyle\sum_{j=1}^{r} \omega_j u_j}{\displaystyle\sum_{j=1}^{r} \omega_j}, \tag{5.9}$$

where the weights ω_j are given by

$$\omega_j = \varphi_{A_{j1}}(x_1) \, \triangle \, \varphi_{A_{j2}}(x_2) \cdots \triangle \, \varphi_{A_{jn}}(x_n),$$

R_1: If x_1 is A_{11} and x_2 is A_{12} and $\cdots$ and x_n is A_{1n} then u is $u_1 = g_1(x_1, x_2, \ldots, x_n)$

or

R_2: If x_1 is A_{21} and x_2 is A_{22} and $\cdots$ and x_n is A_{2n} then u is $u_2 = g_2(x_1, x_2, \ldots, x_n)$

or

$\vdots$

or

R_r: If x_1 is A_{r1} and x_2 is A_{r2} and $\cdots$ and x_n is A_{rn} then u is $u_r = g_r(x_1, x_2, \ldots, x_n)$

Frame 5.5: Rule base to illustrating the TSK method

and $\triangle$ is a t-norm. The weight ω_j corresponds to the contribution of R_j to the general output. The most common cases of t-norms are the product and the minimum.

For the case of two rules, each one with two input variables and one output, the TSK method is illustrated in Frame 5.6. Supposing that $\triangle$ is the minimum t-norm, we have as general output, representing the control for the actions x_1 and x_2, the value of u given by the equation:

R_1: If x_1 is A_{11} and x_2 is A_{12} then u is $u_1 = g_1(x_1, x_2)$

or

R_2: If x_1 is A_{21} and x_2 is A_{22} then u is $u_2 = g_2(x_1, x_2)$

Frame 5.6: Rule base of two rules for the TSK method

$$u = \frac{\omega_1 u_1 + \omega_2 u_2}{\omega_1 + \omega_2} = \frac{\omega_1 g_1(x_1, x_2) + \omega_2 g_2(x_1, x_2)}{\omega_1 + \omega_2} = f_r(x_1, x_2), \qquad (5.10)$$

where $\omega_i = \min[\varphi_{A_{i1}}(x_1), \varphi_{A_{i2}}(x_2)]$ corresponds to the weight of rule R_i in the general output of the process. In the literature, the case that appears most frequently, due to its efficiency and applicability, is the one which the consequents of each rule are affine linear functions, that is, each one of the functions g_i has the form

$$g_i(x_1, x_2) = a_i x_1 + b_i x_2 + c_i.$$

This case is commonly called Takagi–Sugeno method (TS).

Example 5.4 Consider a fuzzy controller with two inputs and one output, where the fuzzy sets involved, A_{ij}, are triangular fuzzy numbers and the outputs of each rule are

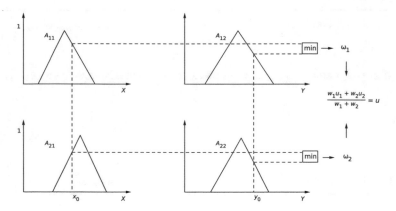

Fig. 5.9 Output of the TSK fuzzy controller for the Example 5.4

given by affine linear functions g_i. For each pair of input x_0 and y_0 Fig. 5.9 depicts how the output is obtained where the output represents the control to be adopted for those inputs. For this example, we have the rule base given in Frame 5.7 In this case the fuzzy control is illustrated in Fig. 5.9 and is given by

---

R_1: If x is A_{11} and y is A_{12} then u is $u_1 = g_1(x, y) = a_1 x + b_1 y + c_1$

or

R_2: If x is A_{21} and y is A_{22} then u is $u_2 = g_2(x, y) = a_2 x + b_2 y + c_2$

Frame 5.7: Rule base for the Example 5.4

$$u = \frac{\omega_1 u_1 + \omega_2 u_2}{\omega_1 + \omega_2} = \frac{\omega_1 g_1(x_0, y_0) + \omega_2 g_2(x_0, y_0)}{\omega_1 + \omega_2}.$$

Example 5.5 Consider the rules in Frame 5.8

R_1: If x is *low* (A_1) then $y_1 = x + 2$

or

R_2: If x is *tall* (A_2) then $y_2 = 2x$

Frame 5.8: Rule base for the Example 5.5

Fig. 5.10 Output y and the rule base of Example 5.5. The lines "under" the abscissa axis represents the membership functions of the antecedents A_1 and A_2. Notice that for "x *low*" the general output y is closer to the line $x + 2$. On the other hand, for "x *tall*" the output y is closer to $2x$

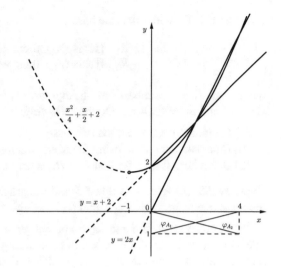

Suppose that the domain is $x \in [0, 4]$,

$$\varphi_{A_1}(x) = 1 - \frac{x}{4} \quad \text{and} \quad \varphi_{A_2}(x) = \frac{x}{4}.$$

The, the output of the system, using the TS method, is

$$y = \frac{\varphi_{A_1}(x)y_1 + \varphi_{A_2}(x)y_2}{\varphi_{A_1}(x) + \varphi_{A_2}(x)} = \varphi_{A_1}(x)y_1 + \varphi_{A_2}(x)y_2$$
$$= \frac{x^2}{4} + \frac{x}{2} + 2$$

which is a concave up parable, whose vertex is $\left(-1, \frac{7}{4}\right)$. Figure 5.10 illustrates the output (y) and the rule base with the membership functions φ_{A_1} and φ_{A_2}. Observe that those functions are represented under the $x - axis$.

Exercise 5.1 Consider the rule base

> R_1 : If x is *short* (A_{11}) *and* y is *short* (A_{12}) then z is *tall* (B_1)
> R_2 : If x is *tall* (A_{21}) *and* y is *tall* (A_{22}) then z is *short* (B_2),

where the fuzzy sets are triangular: $A_{11} = (1; 2; 3)$, $A_{12} = (5; 6; 7)$, $B_1 = (4; 5; 6)$, $A_{21} = (2; 3; 4)$, $A_{22} = (6; 7; 8)$ and $B_2 = (3; 4; 5)$.

(a) Supposing that the inputs are $x = 2.3$ and $y = 6.8$, draw a figure representing the output obtained by the Mamdani inference method for this given rule base.

(b) Is the output of item (a) a real number or a fuzzy set? If it is a fuzzy set, defuzzify it. The fuzzy controller simulates a function f whose domain has what dimension? What is the range?

Exercise 5.2 Consider the rule base

$$R_1 : \text{If } x \text{ is } (A_1) \text{ then } y \text{ is } (B_1)$$
$$R_2 : \text{If } x \text{ is } (A_2) \text{ then } y \text{ is } (B_2),$$

where the fuzzy numbers are triangular: $A_1 = (0; 1; 2)$, $A_2 = (1; 3; 5)$, $B_1 = (2; 3; 4)$ and $B_2 = (3; 4; 5)$. Do the following:

(a) Graphically represent the rule base.
(b) Calculate the output using the Mamdani method if the input is $A = A_1$.
(c) Using item (b), verify that $B = B_1$, where B_1 is the consequent of the rule R_1.

Exercise 5.3 (a) Redo Example 5.5 and the graphical representations by changing the consequents to $y_1 = x + 2$ and $y_2 = 4 - x$.

(b) Redo Example 5.5 and the graphical representations by changing the consequents to $y_1 = 2 - x$ and $y_2 = x$ and considering that the membership function of A_1 is the line that goes through the points $(0, 1)$ and $(10, 0)$ while the membership function of A_2 is the line that goes through the points $(0, 0)$ and $(10, 1)$.

Exercise 5.4 Redo the last exercise changing the membership functions to trapezoids. In particular let fuzzy set A_1 be given by the trapezoid with major base $[0, 3]$ and minor base $[0, 1]$ and the fuzzy set A_2 is a trapezoid whose major base is $[1, 4]$ and minor base $[3, 4]$. Is the output a continuous function? Why or why not?

We have mentioned that fuzzy controllers have the ability to model phenomenon (process) by using linguistic variables. Suppose that a certain phenomenon of interest is modeled by a function. If the output of each rule is given by an affine linear function, we can consider that the function is locally approximated by a line. For example, if we know that the function is smooth, we can use tangent lines to the function to be the consequent function of each rule.

It is interesting to observe that if the functions g_i of the consequents are constants, then the two methods (Mamdani and Takagi–Sugeno) produce the same output if the defuzzification used in the Mamdani's method is the center of gravity. This is particularly easy to see in Example 5.4 where the general output is

$$u = \frac{\omega_1 c_1 + \omega_2 c_2}{\omega_1 + \omega_2}$$

since in this case we have that $a_1 = b_1 = a_2 = b_2 = 0$. This is also the output in the Mamdani's method for this particular case because the membership functions of the consequents are the characteristic functions of the constants c_1 and c_2 (verify this!).

We want to stress that the fuzzy controllers have important mathematical properties such as, for example, the capacity to approximate continuous functions. In Chap. 6 we will show this fact in greater detail for the Takagi–Sugeno–Kang controllers. We note that TSK controllers might be much more general in the sense that the functions of each consequent can have fuzzy arguments and the input values might be fuzzy subsets.

Next we present some comparisons between the two methods presented:

(i) The Mamdani method is simpler and more intuitive than the TSK;
(ii) The Mamdani method is less efficient than the TSK if we speak in terms of speed of computation;
(iii) The Mamdani method has fewer mathematical properties than the TSK;
(iv) Both methods coincides when the consequents are constants and the defuzzification method is the centroid.

Nowadays, the theory of fuzzy controllers is quite advanced and there are specific texts about this subject [2, 4, 8, 9]. We have used fuzzy controllers to compute coefficients of partial differential equations that represents the temporal and spatial evolution of some epidemics [10]. From the initial studies of Castanho [11], who uses fuzzy controllers to classify prostate cancer, Silveira et al [12] developed a computer program with the objective of helping urologists decide the cancer stage of a patient. Using the Gleason Scale, clinical status, and the level of PSA, the software gives the risk (factor) that the tumor might be in some of the following linguistic classes: locally contained initial stage, locally advanced, and metastatic.

The following section will be dedicated to the applications, some which were developed by our students, illustrating the potential that the fuzzy controllers have when used in biomathematics.

5.6 Applications

The following models use the Mamdani and TSK method for the particular case that the initial conditions (inputs) are crisp, with the goal of showing the power of the fuzzy controller methodology. The efficiency, efficacy, and accuracy of the applications fundamentally depends on the information provided by experts for the construction of the fuzzy rule base.

5.6.1 Model 1 – Forecasting the Salinity of an Estuary in Cananeia and Ilha Comprida

This model was developed by Sobrinho [13] together with the town hall of Ilha Comprida, using fuzzy controllers. His goal was to forecast the variation of surface salinity at a given location in Ilha de Cananeia. The input variables were rainfall and the flow rate from Rio Ribeira de Iguape.

The proposed model estimates the surface salinity variation for up to two days and over an area of 80 km in radius. This prediction allows the city to inform the aquaculture employers of the estuary with some antecedence to take appropriate action. Figure 5.11 illustrates the area of the study on the southern coast of the state of São Paulo.

Fig. 5.11 Area of study in
the southern coast of the
state of São Paulo, Brazil

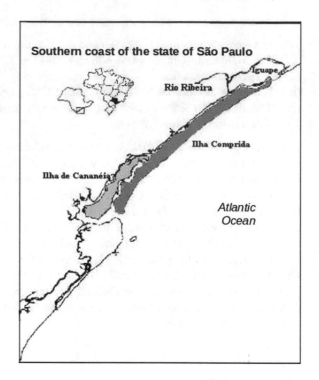

The Problem

The estuary is a lagoon ecosystem that covers three towns located along the southern
coast of state of São Paulo in a region of significant ecological importance due to its
natural state and size. It was classified by IUCN (International Union for the Nature
Conservation) as the third largest estuary in the world with primary productivity
(see in Sobrinho [13]). This estuary is bounded on the north side by the Icapara
sandbar and on the south side by the Cananeia sandbar, both on the Atlantic Ocean.
The supply of fresh water to the estuary is provided by several rivers, the largest
volume coming from the Ribeira river. Its waters enter the estuary on the north side,
through a town by way of a man-made the canal built in the late nineteenth century.
The contribution from the waters of the Ribeira river region was changed in 1978
when a dam was constructed 2 km from the city of Iguape. As a consequence of this
action, the pattern of some environmental variables, such as the surface salinity was
changed.

The Model

The model is based on a system of fuzzy controls using the Mamdani inference
method. The input variables are: *rainfall*, *initial salinity* and *flow of the Ribeira
river*. The output variable is the *final salinity*. The struture of the model is given in
Fig. 5.12.

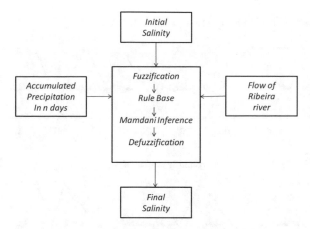

Fig. 5.12 Architecture of the prediction model of salinity in the estuary of Cananeia and Ilha Comprida

Table 5.1 Classifications used in the salinity model of the Ribeira River, according to the rule base of the Frame 5.9

Accumulated rain	Initial sal.	Flow	Final sal.
Low $= C_b$	Low $= SI_b$	Low $= V_b$	Very low $= SF_{ba}$
Average $= C_m$	Average low $= SI_{mb}$	Average $= V_m$	Low $= SF_b$
Average high $= C_{ma}$	Average $= SI_m$	Average high $= V_{ma}$	Average low $= SF_{mb}$
High $= C_a$	High $= SI_a$	High $= V_a$	Average $= SF_m$
Very high $= C_{at}$		Very high $= V_{at}$	

The variables are linguistic and each one of its values is a fuzzy number with triangular or trapezoidal membership functions (see Fig. 5.13a–c).

Analyzing the data set with the above mentioned variables, it is possible to establish a knowledge base with linguistic rules relating them, to estimate the value of the final salinity where this estimation is made by the defuzzification process using the center of gravity.

Rule Base

Each one of the rules (see Frame 5.9) has the following form:

R_4 - **If** *the accumulated precipitation of the region within a 1–3 day period is low* **and** *the flow of Ribeira river is high* **then** *the final salinity is low.*

R_{23} - **If** *the accumulated precipitation of the region within a 1–3 day period is average high* **and** *the initial salinity of the period is average low* **and** *the flow of Ribeira river is low* **then** *the final salinity is average low.*

Frame 5.9 outlines all the rules (rule base with three inputs and one output) and Table 5.1 shows the legend for the rule base.

As we did in Example 5.3, here we will illustrate, step by step, the Mamdani inference method for this application.

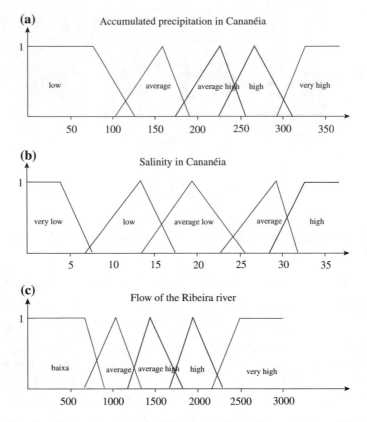

Fig. 5.13 Membership functions – **a** Rain; **b** Final and initial salinity and **c** Flow of the river

Inference

The inference process computes the output variable from the values of the input variables. The process uses the values of the membership degrees of the input variables to obtain the value of the membership degree of the output variable.

To illustrate Mamdani inference method for this problem, we will compute as follows:

- Consider the following input values: **rainfall** = 23 mm, **initial salinity** = 23 $^0/_{00}$[1] and **flow of the Ribeira river** = 1454 m^3/s, that is, the initial conditions are crisp;
- Each one of the initial values has a membership degree in relation to fuzzy subsets that define the three input variables. Thus, the rainfall value 23 mm belongs to the fuzzy subset "low" with membership degree $\varphi_{C_b}(23)$ according to the Fig. 5.13a, that is, $\varphi_{C_b}(23) = \varphi_{\text{low precipitation}}(23) = 1$.

---

[1] Symbol that means "for thousand".

	If accumulated rain **and**	Initial Sal **and**	Flow	**Then**	Final Sal
R_1	low	average low	average		average low
R_2	**low**	**average**	**average high**		**average low**
R_3	**low**	**average low**	**average high**		**low**
R_4	low	average low	high		low
R_5	low	low	high		average low
R_6	low	average	very high		low
R_7	low	average low	very high		average low
R_8	low	low	very high		average low
R_9	low	average	low		average
R_{10}	low	average	average		average low
R_{11}	low	low	low		low
R_{12}	average	average	low		average low
R_{13}	average	average low	low		average low
R_{14}	average	average	average		average low
R_{15}	average	average	average high		average low
R_{16}	average	average low	average		low
R_{17}	average	high	low		average
R_{18}	average	high	average		average low
R_{19}	average	high	average high		low
R_{20}	average	low	average		low
R_{21}	average	low	low		low
R_{22}	average high	average	low		average low
R_{23}	average high	average low	low		average low
R_{24}	high	average	low		average low
R_{25}	high	average low	low		low
R_{26}	very high	average	low		very low
R_{27}	very high	average low	low		very low
R_{28}	very high	low	low		very low

Frame 5.9: Rule base for forecasting the salinity in the estuary of Cananeia and Ilha Comprida

The initial salinity value, 23, belongs to the fuzzy subsets "average low" and "average" (Fig. 5.13b), with membership degree $\varphi_{SI_{mb}}(23) = 0.67$ and $\varphi_{SI_m}(23) = 0.25$, respectively. The flow value of the Ribeira river, $1454\,\mathrm{m^3/s}$ belongs to the fuzzy set "average high", with membership degree $\varphi_{V_{ma}}(1454) = 0.82$. Each combination of these sets driven by input values activates some rule of the knowledge base. In this case 2 rules were fired, namely, R_2 and R_3 of the rule base (Frame 5.9).

R_2 If the accumulated rainfall in the region within a 1–3 day period is *low* **and** the initial salinity of the period is *average* **and** the flow of the Ribeira river is *average high* **then** the final salinity will be *average low*.

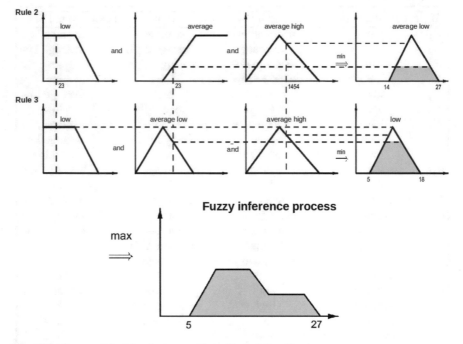

Fig. 5.14 Output of the Mamdani controller without defuzzification

R₃ **If** the accumulated rainfall in the region within a 1–3 day period is *low* **and** the initial salinity of the period is *average low* **and** the flow of the Ribeira river is *average high* **then** the final salinity will be *low*.

The Mamdani inference method aggregates the membership degrees related to each one of the input values using the **minimum** t-norm. Thus, for rules R_2 and R_3, we have, respectively

$$R_2 : \min \left\{ \varphi_{C_b}(23), \varphi_{SI_m}(23), \varphi_{V_{ma}}(1454) \right\} = \min[1; 0.25; 0.82] = 0.25.$$
$$R_3 : \min \left\{ \varphi_{C_b}(23), \varphi_{SI_{mb}}(23), \varphi_{V_{ma}}(1454) \right\} = \min[1; 0.67; 0.82] = 0.67.$$

The minimum aggregation operation is used for each one of the fired rules. The membership value obtained by each rule (0.25 for R_2 and 0.67 for R_3) will be projected onto the membership function of the output variable of the related rule in a way that only the values of the output membership that are less or equal to the output numbers, 0.25 for R_2 and 0.67 for R_3, are kept (see the dark regions in Fig. 5.14).

The outputs of each of the fired rules in turn are aggregated using the **maximum** t-conorm to obtain the general output of the Mamdani controller without defuzzification (Fig. 5.14). Finally, using the center of gravity method of defuzzification on the final fuzzy output, we obtain as crisp output the value 15.2 to represent the final salinity.

Table 5.2 Relations between the observed final salinity values and the estimated ones by the fuzzy model

Precipitation accumulated (mm)	Salinity initial $(^0/_{00})$	Flow river (m^3/s)	Salinity observed$(^0/_{00})$	Salinity modeled $(^0/_{00})$
13.6	14	2016	6	3.4
115	30	1163	18	17.7
148	24	763	18	17.6
31	18	1515	15	13.2
3	18	2273	8	7.6
320	26	687	5	3.4
110	20	938	13	14.4
180	18	800	16	15.8
102	25	584	25	23.5
123	30	469	26	24.2
23	23	1454	17	15.2

The Table 5.2 has all the values of the input variables, the values of the observed salinities and the values of the salinities obtained by the model. The results of the FRBS were very favorable, according to Sobrinho [13].

Summary and Final Comments

Because the ecosystem is very large, relating input variables with dynamic temporal patterns, statistical methods become difficult to adopt since the effort to obtain the data and construct statistical distributions is significant. In fuzzy modeling, with some data and expert knowledge, it is possible to construct a rule base that allows us to predict salinity. The rule base can be improved as new data are developed and/or obtained. The results in this example show the power of fuzzy system in the modeling ecological phenomena especially where the data and statistical demands are significant and/or difficult.

The next model uses the *Fuzzy Toolbox of Matlab 6.5*®, which has implemented the Mamdani method with defuzzification of the Center of Mass, as well as the TSK method.

5.6.2 Model 2 – Rate of Seropositive Transfer (HIV⁺)

Model 2 illustrates the use of fuzzy controllers in the **AIDS** epidemiological phenomena that is of concern of many public health units in many countries, including Brazil. The methodology that we present below was part of Jafelice's thesis [14, 15] and was developed with the goal to obtain the value of a parameter for a differential equation that models the time evolution of the number of symptomatic individuals in a seropositive population.

The number of researchers who study mathematical models of AIDS has substantially grown in the last years. The mathematical models to study the evolution of AIDS in a populations are, in general, given by a system of differential equations. In the simplest classical models the infected population is divided in asymptomatic and symptomatic individuals, whose conversion rate is given by a parameter λ, also known as the *incidence rate* [15].

The diagram below represents such a system with conversion rate λ.

$$\boxed{\text{Asymptomatic}} \overset{\lambda}{\Longrightarrow} \boxed{\text{Symptomatic}}$$

A statistical fit method given data is a traditional method by which the rate λ is computed. Our aim here is to present an alternative to this method using a fuzzy system which takes into account expert knowledge to estimate λ.

The study of AIDS by health experts takes into account two basic parameters: viral load (V) and the concentration of $CD4^+$ (the main lymphocyte attacked by the virus) of the seropositive individuals. These same experts also agree that the rate λ fundamentally depends on the viral load and on the level of $CD4^+$ of the seropositive population. However, to date, the establishment of such dependencies is very subjective. In this example we will suggest a way of establish this relation, considering the conversion rate λ depending on the viral load (v) and on the level (c) of $CD4^+$ of each individual of the seropositive population, that is, we show how to compute

$$\lambda = \lambda(v, c).$$

However, to begin, we are going to discuss a little how HIV in an individual works.

HIV mainly attacks the lymphocyte T of $CD4^+$ type in the bloodstream. The low concentration of the $CD4^+$ cells in the bloodstream has implications in the evolution of the HIV infection. When the virus comes into contact with the host's cell membrane, the RNA-viral is injected. In the cytoplasm the viral RNA serves as a model in the synthesis of a DNA chain that in turn serves as a model for an additional one, thus forming a DNA molecule with a double chain. This DNA with a double chain goes in the nucleus and incorporates its genetic information into the cell.

The strange DNA (pro-virus) may be indefinitely inactive and with the multiplication of the host cell, a copy of the altered DNA is taken to the replicated cells. For reasons not well understood, the pro-virus activates itself and starts the synthesis of new RNA molecules to form new viruses. This RNA, together with the viral proteases, guide both the synthesis of the capsule protein and the virus enzymes to create a new virus. Then, the host cell is destroyed.

The human defense system is formed by macrophages located at many places in the organism and is always looking for foreign a body. When they detect them, they send a first chemical alert sign that is recognized by lymphocytes T of $CD4^+$ type which in turn make them "be alert" and starts the activation of the immune system cells, namely, lymphocytes B. Those transform themselves into plasma cells to produce antibodies and the lymphocytes $CD8$ that recognize the infected cells and destroy them. Since the virus attacks the lymphocytes $CD4^+$, the general alarm is not given and so the immune activation is not started. The defense system is not notified and the immune system loses its effectiveness.

The $CD4^+$ cell counts in blood has implications for the evolution of the HIV infection because it is the marker of an immune deficiency and it is associated with certain clinical factors. The measure of cellular immunocompetence is the most useful factor to monitoring HIV infected patients and the most widely accepted one, although it is not the only one. Today, it is commonly believed that the amount of immunocompetence cells somehow regulates the proliferation of the virus and it is responsible for the retardation in the transfer of asymptomatic to symptomatic ones.

$CD4^+$ cell counts may be divided into four groups for the modeling, according to concentration per milliliter of blood draw from patient and the infection stages of HIV are classified according to these groups in the bloodstream[2] as follows:

(1) The stage of HIV characterized by **low risk** to develop AIDS, occurs when $CD4^+ > 0.5$ cell/ml;
(2) The stage of HIV characterized by appearance of signs of mild symptoms occurs when $0.2 < CD4^+ < 0.5$ cells/ml and this we classify as **moderate risk** to develop AIDS;
(3) An **moderately high risk** to develop AIDS occurs when $0.05 < CD4^+ < 0.2$ cells/ml;
(4) If $CD4^+ < 0.05$ cells/ml, we have a **high risk** to appear opportunistic diseases such as Kaposi sarcoma. If this the case, the possibility of survival is low.

There is a relation, on the other hand, between the HIV viral load and the possibility of developing AIDS. High viral loads greatly destroy $CD4^+$ lymphocytes and the immune system loses its defensive ability. A low viral load does not substantially affect the immune system. The following data are relevant for the construction of the model [14, 15]:

(a) There is a **low risk** of disease progression when there is a viral load under 10000 parts of RNA/ml, that is, $V < 10000$;
(b) If the viral load is between 10 thousand and 100 thousand parts of RNA/ml, that is, if $10000 < V < 100000$, there is a **moderate risk** of progression;
(c) If $V > 100000$, there is a **high risk** of progression.

Notice that in the parameters of interest – viral load (V) and level of $CD4^+$ – we do not have a single value that characterizes the group but a range of values. The boundaries of each of these classifications is not rigid and this is precisely how the experts in the field deal with HIV. For example, suppose there is one patient with $CD4^+ = 0.49$ cells/ml and there is another patient with $CD4^+ = 0.51$ cells/ml. One would be classifieds as having moderate risk for AIDS and the other low risk. However, it is not reasonable that individuals with $CD4^+$ equal to 0.49 cells/ml to be treated differently from the one with $CD4^+$ equal to 0.51 cells/ml. The uncertainties

---

[2]Source: Brazilian Health Ministery – http://www.aids.gov.br.

Inputs   *Outputs*

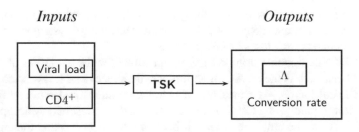

Fig. 5.15 Scheme of the TSK controller with 2 inputs and 1 output

of the viral load and the level of $CD4^+$ are not stochastic. They have their origin in a language that uses graduations to express expert knowledge.

The viral load V and the level of $CD4^+$ are typical cases of linguistic variables, since they are classified into groups with uncertain boundaries, that is, fuzzy boundaries. Thus, the assumed values of the viral load and the level of $CD4^+$ are fuzzy sets. As a consequence, the transfer rate will also be a linguistic variable Λ. The precise relationship $\lambda = \lambda(v, c)$ between the transfer rate Λ, the viral load V and the level of $CD4^+$ is not known since the relationship is understood and expressed linguistically. Fuzzy logic is an effective and natural way to evaluate this relationship. The scheme is depicted in Fig. 5.15.

Fuzzy Rule Base

The fuzzy rule base presented in Frame 5.10 was developed in collaboration with AIDS experts, researchers and physicians. A simple way to present a rule base is via table (Table 5.3). We can use either the Mamdani method or the TSK method to obtain $\lambda = \lambda(v, c)$. As an illustration, we compute λ using TSK method with constant consequent, that is, the values to which classification Λ belong are real numbers given by experts (as, for example, those given in Table 5.4).

R_1. If V is low (B) and $CD4^+$ is very low (MB) then Λ is strong (F);
R_2. If V is low (B) and $CD4^+$ is low (B) then Λ is average (M);
R_3. If V is low (B) and $CD4^+$ is average (M) then Λ is average (M);
R_4. If V is low (B) and $CD4^+$ is high average (MA) then Λ is average weak (Mf);
R_5. If V is low (B) and $CD4^+$ is high (A) then Λ is weak (f);
R_6. If V is average (M) and $CD4^+$ is very low (b) then Λ is strong (F);
R_7. If V is average (M) and $CD4^+$ is low (B) then Λ is strong (F);
R_8. If V is average (M) and $CD4^+$ is average (M) then Λ is average (M);
R_9. If V is average (M) and $CD4^+$ is average high (MA) then Λ is average weak (Mf);
R_{10} If V is average (M) e $CD4^+$ is high (A) then Λ is weak (f);
R_{11} If V is high (A) and $CD4^+$ is very low (MB) then Λ is forte (F);
R_{12} If V is high (A) and $CD4^+$ is low (B) then Λ is strong (F);
R_{13} If V is high (A) and $CD4^+$ is average (M) then Λ is average (M);
R_{14} If V is high (A) and $CD4^+$ is average high (MA) then Λ is average (M);
R_{15} If V is high (A) and $CD4^+$ is high (A) then Λ is average (M).

Frame 5.10: Rule base for the model of seropositive transfer rate

Table 5.3 Transfer rate Λ

		Level of $CD4^+$				
		MB	B	M	MA	A
Viral	B	F	M	M	Mf	f
Load	M	F	F	M	Mf	f
	A	F	F	M	M	M

Table 5.4 Classification of Λ

Level of Λ	Classification
$\Lambda = \lambda_1 = 0.00$	for f: Weak
$\Lambda = \lambda_2 = 0.15$	for Mf: Average weak
$\Lambda = \lambda_3 = 0.65$	for M: Average
$\Lambda = \lambda_4 = 1.00$	for F: Strong

Fig. 5.16 Viral load

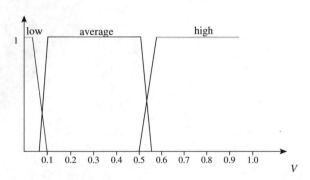

Fig. 5.17 Level of CD_4^+

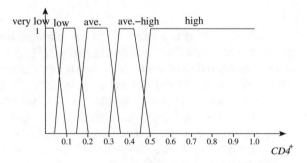

Membership Functions

The membership functions of the assumed fuzzy subsets by each one of the variables V, $CD4^+$ are modeled as trapezoidal. On the other hand, the values of conversion rates are singletons (See Figs. 5.16, 5.17 and 5.18).

Fig. 5.18 Crisp fuzzy subsets "conversion rate"

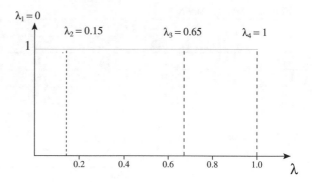

Fig. 5.19 Controller's output: surface of $\lambda(v, c)$

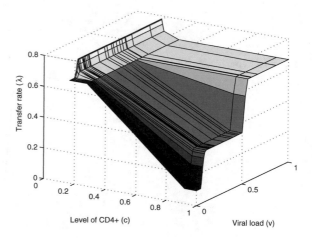

The TSK method to obtain λ from the rule base described previously and from the membership functions, generates a surface (Fig. 5.19). From this surface, we can suggest an analytic expression for $\lambda = \lambda(v, c)$. According to medical practice, the parameter most used to control and diagnose HIV^+ is the value of $CD4^+$. Thus, in a first approximation, we can simply use $\lambda = \lambda(c)$ as a transfer rate in the fuzzy model. According to the Fig. 5.19, for each viral load value $V = v$, we have $\lambda = \lambda(c)$, with configuration approximately piecewise linear as is shown in Fig. 5.20. The parameter c_{min} represents the minimum level of $CD4^+$ an individual becomes symptomatic and, c_M represents the level of $CD4^+$ from which the chances to becomes symptomatic is minimum.

We observe that if we were interested in studying the conversion rate as function of a viral load, $\lambda = \lambda(v)$, then it would be possible, especially in the particular case where there is no treatment. In this case, there is a discrete correlation between V and $CD4^+$. Moreover, as the viral load becomes large, the level of $CD4^+$ diminishes. Simple models of relations between viral load and $CD4^+$ level, $c = c(v)$, are suggested by analysis. One such relationship might be given by the equations:

Fig. 5.20 Conversion rate in function of $CD4^+$

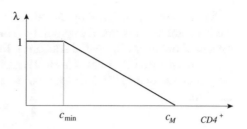

$$c(v) = \frac{r}{a + \beta v} \text{ or } c(v) = \lambda_0 + ae^{-\beta v},$$

so that, for this case, we have $\lambda = \lambda(v)$.

To conclude this example, we want to stress that the transfer rate obtained here from the information given by experts has strong biological meaning, since it depends on others parameters of the disease: viral load V and level of $CD4^+$. This is the difference from the classical case where this rate is generally given by a type of fit or simulations of the sample data.

5.6.3 Model 3 – Pharmacological Decay

Another application of fuzzy controllers in biomathematics is in pharmacokinetics. The first part uses a TSK model and the second part uses the Mamdani model. In the first part we model the dynamic of the state variable of interest, concentration versus time. In the second part we estimate the parameter of decay of the model equation using expert information.

A fundamental problem on pharmacology is to know how the concentration of a drug decays in the blood of a individual. The drug moves through the body by the bloodstream and it is known that different groups of tissue have more or less resistance to the circulation according to the amount of blood vessels. Tissues group rich in blood vessels are heart, lungs, liver, kidneys and brain. Groups of muscle tissues have an intermediate number of vessels. A small number of blood vessels occur in fat, skin and bones. These groups of tissues, together with physico-chemical properties of the drug, strongly influence the distribution, retention and disposal of the substance in the body [16]. The movement from one compartment group of tissue, for example, to another continuously modifies the concentration of drug in each compartment to achieve a dynamic equilibrium, when there is no more transfer of drug concentration between the compartments. In practice, the number of compartments corresponds to the number of compartments from which the data of drug concentration in the individual was collected and arranged in a logarithm scale. See, for example, Fig. 5.21b with two lines, one for each phase in the drug concentration collection process (distribution and elimination): $y_\alpha = b_1 - a_1 t$ and $y_\beta = b_2 - a_2 t$.

Most drugs are analyzed by bicompartimental or tricompartimentals models and the mathematical treatment to predict the blood concentration is usually given by a system of ordinary differential equations. In bicompartimental models we have two stages: the distribution phase (α - fast) and the elimination phase (β - slower) of the drug from the body [17]. The solution of this systems of differential equations has the form

$$C(t) = A_1 e^{-\alpha t} + A_2 e^{-\beta t}.$$

The example that we give was proposed by Menegotto and Barros [18] and is based on data extracted from [17] that plotted on a Cartesian plane of time t (in hours) *versus* the logarithm of concentration C. The data clearly indicates that it is a two-compartment pharmacokinetic model (see Fig. 5.21b). Thus, the traditional mathematical model is given by a system of two linear differential equations whose solution (which is the drug concentration in the individual at each time t) is

$$C(t) = 1.3e^{-0.173t} + 0.82e^{-0.0092t} \tag{5.11}$$

and the graphs of each phase for these data are

$$y_\alpha = 0.255 - 0.0278t \quad \text{and} \quad y_\beta = -0.086 - 0.004t.$$

Our aim now is to reproduce a fuzzy model of the bicompartimental system taking into account that the outputs are derived from these graphs. Since the outputs are linear functions, we adopted the TSK inference method where the antecedents are "low time" and "high time", using a triangular and trapezoidal fuzzy number, respectively.

There is a value t^* of great indecision in the phases (see Fig. 5.21a) which is

$$\varphi_{A_1}(t^*) = \varphi_{A_2}(t^*) = 0.5.$$

This time can be computed from the intersection of the lines y_α and y_β which in this case is $t^* \simeq 14.3$h. From this, we have the value $t = 28.6$ that appears in the formulas of φ_{A_1} and φ_{A_2}:

$$\varphi_{A_1}(t) = \begin{cases} 1 - \frac{t}{28.6} & \text{if } 0 \leq t \leq 28.6 \\ 0 & \text{if } t > 28.6 \end{cases}$$

and

$$\varphi_{A_2}(t) = \begin{cases} \frac{t}{28.6} & \text{if } 0 \leq t \leq 28.6 \\ 1 & \text{if } t > 28.6 \end{cases}.$$

The fuzzy rules are described below:

R_1 : If t is low(A_1), then $y_\alpha = \log C_\alpha = b_1 - a_1 t \Leftrightarrow C_\alpha = 10^{y_\alpha}$ (α-phase)

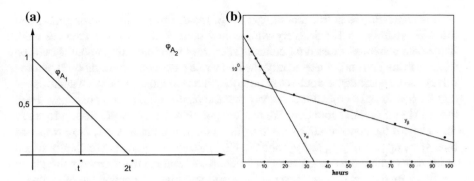

Fig. 5.21 **a** Antecedents. **b** Consequents y_α and y_β

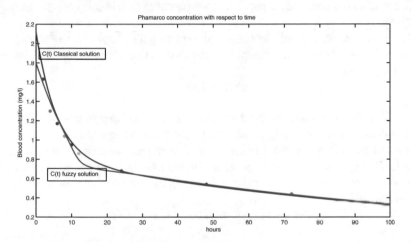

Fig. 5.22 Data, curves of the deterministic and fuzzy models

$$R_2 : \text{If } t \text{ is high } (A_2), \text{ then } y_\beta = \log C_\beta = b_2 - a_2 t \Leftrightarrow C_\beta = 10^{y_\beta} (\beta\text{-phase})$$

Thus, by the TSK inference method, formula (5.10), the drug concentration in the blood of the individual is given by

$$C(t) = \frac{\varphi_{A_1}(t)10^{y_\alpha} + \varphi_{A_2}(t)10^{y_\beta}}{\varphi_{A_1}(t) + \varphi_{A_2}(t)} \tag{5.12}$$

so that from the expressions of y_α, y_β, φ_{A_1} and φ_{A_2} we have

$$C(t) = \begin{cases} \left(1 - \frac{t}{28.6}\right) 10^{0.255 - 0.0278t} + \frac{t}{28.6} 10^{-0.086 - 0.004t} & \text{if } 0 \leq t \leq 28.6 \\ 10^{-0.086 - 0.004t} & \text{if } t > 28.6 \end{cases}, \tag{5.13}$$

whose graphical representation is found in Fig. 5.22.

It is interesting to notice that the graphs of the deterministic solution (5.11) and the TSK solution (5.12) are very similar and both of them fit the data set well. If the data generates three drug concentration response lines, the model should be tricompartimental and, consequently, the fuzzy rule base would be composed of three rules whose consequents would be given by each one of those lines. We want to stress that the idea is not to substitute the way that the pharmacological models have been treated via differential equation. We are just pointing out a new possibility to study the decay of the concentrations since from a practical point of view, drug response lines show up (namely, y_α and y_β) and the TSK inference method is excellently suited in the cases where the consequents are lines. An advantage that we can point out in the fuzzy method is that one does not demand any kind of knowledge of ordinary differential equations. The models that are based on fuzzy rules are very intuitive and TKS and Mamdani method, in particular, are part of available software (for example, Matlab).

Now suppose we are only interested in modeling the elimination of the drug. In this case, we are choosing just one phase. The elimination phase whose mathematical model is given by

$$C(t) = C_0 e^{-\lambda t},$$

where C_0 is the initial dose of the drug and λ is the decay rate in the organism.

The decay rate λ, generally is obtained by the fitting of data. The dose of the drug concentration is from the elimination rate and from particularities of the medicated individual. Suppose we have only renal elimination. The biological characteristic that influences the rate λ are: *urinary volume (v)*, *clearance of creatinine (c)* and *Ph serum (p)*, that is,

$$\lambda = \lambda(v, c, p) \Rightarrow C(t) = C_0 e^{-\lambda(v,c,p)t}.$$

The function λ, dependent on these three variable, which are the ones with medical interest since they can be measured in laboratory, was obtained by Lopes and Jafelice [19], together with an expert, a fuzzy rule base was developed. The input variables were *urinary volume*, *Clearance of creatinine* and *Ph serum* and the output was the *elimination rate* λ. Each input variable was assigned linguistic terms which in turn was translated into fuzzy sets according to the expert. Then, using the Mamdani inference method, it was possible to compute the decay rate.

The great advantage of this approach is that there is no need, in principle, for a data set to estimate λ. Besides, individuals with some problem, like renal incontinence, the concentration of the drug remains in the blood for a longer time compared with a normal individual. In this case, it is still possible to calibrate the right dose, since what is expected is that the drug remains in the body for a certain period of time until the administration of a new dose. Thus, it is possible to program the dosage taking into account the deficiencies of each patient.

References

1. G. Klir, B. Yuan, *Fuzzy Sets and Fuzzy Logic Theory and Applications* (Prentice-Hall, Upper Saddle River, 1995)
2. H.T. Nguyen, M. Sugeno, R. Tang, R. Yager (eds.), *Theoretical Aspects of Fuzzy Control*, in *IEEE International Conference on Fuzzy Systems 1993* (Wiley, New York, 1995)
3. H.T. Nguyen, E.A. Walker, *A First Course of Fuzzy Logic* (CRC Press, Boca Raton, 1997)
4. I.S. Shaw, M.G. Simões, *Controle e modelagem fuzzy* Editora Edgar Blucher Ltda, São Paulo (2001)
5. W. Pedrycz, F. Gomide, *An Introduction to Fuzzy Sets: Analysis and Design* (The MIT Press, Massachusets, 1998)
6. E.H. Mamdani, S. Assilian, An experiment in linguistic synthesis with a fuzzy logic controller. Int. J. Man-Mach. Stud. **7**, 1–13 (1975)
7. T. Takagi, M. Sugeno, Fuzzy identification of systems and its applications to modeling and control. IEEE Trans. Syst. Man Cybern. **15**, 116–132 (1985)
8. H.O. Aguiar Jr., *Lógica difusa: Aspectos práticos e aplicações* Editora Interciência Ltda (1999)
9. L. Weber, P.A.T. Klein, *Aplicação da lógica fuzzy em software e hardware* Ulbra, Canoas-RS (2003)
10. M. Missio, *Modelos de edp intregrados a lógica fuzzy e métodos probabilísticos no tratamento de incertezas: uma aplicação em febre aftosa em bovinos* Tese de Doutorado, IMECC-UNICAMP, Campinas (2008)
11. M.J.P. Castanho, *Construção e avaliação de um modelo matemático para predizer câncer de próstata e descrever seu crescimento utilizando a teoria dos conjuntos fuzzy* Tese de Doutorado, FEEC-UNICAMP, Campinas (2005)
12. G.P. Silveira, L.L. Vendite, L.C. Barros, Software desenvolvido a partir de um modelo matemático fuzzy para predizer o estágio patológico do câncer de próstata. Biomatemática **18**, 27–36 (2008)
13. R.P. Sobrinho, *Desenvolvimento de um sistema especialista fuzzy aplicado à previsão de variação da salinidade superficial no estuário lagunar de Cananeia Iguape e Ilha Comprida*, Relatório técnico, Prefeitura Municipal de Ilha Comprida (2001)
14. R.M. Jafelice, *Um estudo da dinâmica de transferência de soropositivos para aidéticos via modelagem fuzzy* Tese de Doutorado, FEEC-UNICAMP, Campinas (2003)
15. R.M. Jafelice, L.C. Barros, R.C. Bassanezi, F. Gomide, Fuzzy modeling in symptomatic HIV virus infected population. Bull. Math. Biol. **66**, 1597–1620 (2004)
16. A.C. Zanini, S. Oga, *Introdução à farmacologia* Editora Atheneu, São Paulo (1989)
17. F. Jamili, *Clinical Pharmacokinetics of Selected Classes of Drugs: Pharmacokinetic Compartments*, Available at http://www.pharmacy.ualberta.ca/pharm415/pharmaco.htm, Accessed on 15 June 2010
18. J. Menegotto, L.C. Barros, *Aplicação da teoria dos conjuntos fuzzy em modelos farmacocinéticos multicompartimentais* Technical report, IMECC - UNICAMP, Sorocaba, Brazil (2010)
19. W.A. Lopes, R.M. Jafelice, Fuzzy Modeling in the Elimination of Drugs, in *Proceedings of International Symposium on Mathematical and Computational Biology* (2005), pp. 339–355

Chapter 6
Fuzzy Relational Equations and Universal Approximation

All Knowledge should be useful and be involve the pratical.
(Sophists – 5th Century BCE)

Abstract This chapter presents the concepts of fuzzy relationships and fuzzy relational equations. These are applied to medical diagnosis and Bayesian inference. The notion of universal approximator with applications to dynamical systems, complete the chapter.

This chapter presents two topics that are theoretically distinct: *fuzzy relational equations* and *universal approximation*. The first topic extends the application of *generalized modus ponens* that was discussed in Chap. 4. The second topic deals with theoretical issues associated with the use of fuzzy sets to approximate functions. In particular, it allows us to connect fuzzy rule-based systems, that represent useful practical tools, with possible theoretical models of a certain phenomenon described as mathematical functions.

Although the main concepts and results concerning the relational equations that we present in this chapter may be regarded in other contexts such as image processing by means of fuzzy mathematical morphology and pattern recognition via fuzzy associative memories [1–4], they were specifically chosen in order to study *medical diagnoses*. In contrast, the ones concerning the universal approximation are geared to approximate any theoretical functional using fuzzy controllers. Such a fact has important consequences for ordinary differential equations where the direction fields (also called slope fields) are neither explicitly given nor totally known.

For didactical reasons, we opted to present these two subjects in the same chapter since that are based in Chaps. 4 and 5, respectively. The interested reader can find more information and details in the cited references of this chapter.

The *max–min* composition between binary fuzzy relations discussed in Chap. 3 play an important role in the first part of this chapter. However, other types of compositions between fuzzy relations are also used here. Next, we listed some of them based on t-norms, t-conorms, negations, and fuzzy implication.

© Springer-Verlag Berlin Heidelberg 2017
L.C. de Barros et al., *A First Course in Fuzzy Logic, Fuzzy Dynamical Systems, and Biomathematics*, Studies in Fuzziness and Soft Computing 347, DOI 10.1007/978-3-662-53324-6_6

6.1   Generalized Compositions of Fuzzy Relations

In the following definitions, $\mathcal{R}$ and $\mathcal{S}$ stand for binary fuzzy relations defined on $U \times V$ and $V \times W$, respectively; $\triangle$ stands for a t-norm; $\triangledown$ stands for a t-conorm; and $\Longrightarrow$ stands for a fuzzy implication.

Definition 6.1 The sup–t composition defines a fuzzy relation $\mathcal{R} \otimes^t \mathcal{S}$ on $U \times W$ whose membership function is given by

$$\varphi_{\mathcal{R} \otimes^t \mathcal{S}}(x, z) = \sup_{y \in V} \left[\varphi_{\mathcal{R}}(x, y) \triangle \varphi_{\mathcal{S}}(y, z) \right].$$

Example 6.1 If $\triangle = \min$ and $\sup = \max$, then we have the max–min composition:

$$\varphi_{\mathcal{R} \otimes^t \mathcal{S}}(x, z) = \varphi_{\mathcal{R} \circ \mathcal{S}}(x, z) = \max_{y \in V} \left[\varphi_{\mathcal{R}}(x, y) \wedge \varphi_{\mathcal{S}}(y, z) \right].$$

Definition 6.2 The inf–c composition yields a fuzzy relation $\mathcal{R} \otimes_c \mathcal{S}$ on $U \times W$ whose membership function is given by

$$\varphi_{\mathcal{R} \otimes_c \mathcal{S}}(x, z) = \inf_{y \in V} \left[\varphi_{\mathcal{R}}(x, y) \triangledown \varphi_{\mathcal{S}}(y, z) \right].$$

Example 6.2 If $\triangledown$ denotes the maximum t-conorm, then we have the $[\inf - \max]$ composition:

$$\varphi_{\mathcal{R} \otimes_c \mathcal{S}}(x, z) = \inf_{y \in V} \left[\varphi_{\mathcal{R}}(x, y) \vee \varphi_{\mathcal{S}}(y, z) \right].$$

Definition 6.3 The inf–implication defines a fuzzy relation $\mathcal{R} \otimes_{\Longrightarrow} \mathcal{S}$ on $U \times W$ whose membership function is given by

$$\varphi_{\mathcal{R} \otimes_{\Longrightarrow} \mathcal{S}}(x, z) = \inf_{y \in V} \left[\varphi_{\mathcal{R}}(x, y) \Longrightarrow \varphi_{\mathcal{S}}(y, z) \right].$$

We now (and for the remainder of the chapter) focus only in inf–implications based on R-implications (see Definition 4.4 of Chap. 4):

$$(x \Longrightarrow y) = \sup\{z \in [0, 1] : x \triangle z \leq y\}.$$

Example 6.3 A well-known example of R-implications is the Gödel's implication:

$$(x \Longrightarrow y) = g(x, y) = \sup\{w \in [0, 1] : x \wedge w \leq y\} = \begin{cases} 1 & \text{if } x \leq y \\ y & \text{if } x > y \end{cases}.$$

Since

$$(\varphi_{\mathcal{R}}(x, y) \Longrightarrow \varphi_{\mathcal{S}}(y, z)) = \begin{cases} 1 & \text{if } \varphi_{\mathcal{R}}(x, y) \leq \varphi_{\mathcal{S}}(y, z) \\ \varphi_{\mathcal{S}}(y, z) & \text{if } \varphi_{\mathcal{R}}(x, y) > \varphi_{\mathcal{S}}(y, z) \end{cases},$$

we have that $\varphi_{\mathcal{R} \otimes_{\Longrightarrow} \mathcal{S}}(x, z) \in \{1, \inf_{y \in V} [\varphi_{\mathcal{S}}(y, z)]\}$.

Similar to the previous comments concerning max–min composition in Chap. 3, it is worth to note that for finite universes the above compositions are obtained as products of matrices by replacing the sum and product operators by the maximum (minimum) and a t-norm (t-conorm or fuzzy implication), respectively.

Exercise 6.1 Let us consider the following binary fuzzy relations given by the matrices

$$\mathcal{R} = [\, 0.6 \; 0.6 \; 0.5 \,] \text{ and } \mathcal{S} = \begin{bmatrix} 0.9 & 0.6 & 1.0 \\ 0.8 & 0.8 & 0.5 \\ 0.6 & 0.4 & 0.6 \end{bmatrix}.$$

Determine the matrix form of the fuzzy relation $\mathcal{R} \otimes^t \mathcal{S}$ for each t-norm $\triangle$:

(a) $\triangle(x, y) = x \wedge y$;

(b) $\triangle(x, y) = xy$;

(c) $\triangle(x, y) = \max(0, x + y - 1)$;

(d) $\triangle(x, y) = \dfrac{xy}{x + y - xy}$;

(e) $\triangle(x, y) = \dfrac{xy}{2 - (x + y - xy)}$;

(f) $\triangle(x, y) = \begin{cases} x \wedge y & \text{if } \max(x, y) = 1 \\ 0 & \text{otherwise} \end{cases}$.

Exercise 6.2 For the fuzzy relations of Exercise 6.1, determine the matrix form of $\mathcal{R} \otimes_{\Longrightarrow} \mathcal{S}$ for the each one of the following implications:

(a) Gödel: $(x \Longrightarrow y) = g(x, y) = \begin{cases} 1 & \text{if } x \leq y \\ y & \text{if } x > y \end{cases}$;

(b) Goguen: $(x \Longrightarrow y) = g_n(x, y) = \begin{cases} 1 & \text{if } x \leq y \\ \frac{y}{x} & \text{if } x > y \end{cases}$.

Recall that the above implications represent R-implications

$$(x \Longrightarrow y) = \sup\{w \in [0, 1] : x \triangle w \leq y\}.$$

In particular, for $\triangle = \min$ we obtain the case (a) and for $\triangle = \text{product}$ we obtain the case (b).

Exercise 6.3 Verify that for any t-norm and for any fuzzy relations $\mathcal{R}$ and $\mathcal{S}$ the following equality holds

$$(\mathcal{R} \otimes^t \mathcal{S})^{-1} = \mathcal{S}^{-1} \otimes^t \mathcal{R}^{-1}$$

We next focus on the study of fuzzy relational equations. Firstly, we will present some methods for solving particular cases of relational equations. Secondly, we will investigate necessary conditions for existence of solution to such equations. For compositions in what follows have finite universes. Thus, the relations can be represented in matrix form.

6.2   Fuzzy Relational Equations

Let us consider the finite universes

$$U = \{u_1, u_2, \ldots, u_m\}, \ V = \{v_1, v_2, \ldots, v_n\} \text{ and } W = \{w_1, w_2, \ldots, w_p\}.$$

Relational equations deal with the problem of finding a matrix form of a binary fuzzy relation based on two other known ones. Here, we deal with *fuzzy relational equations* of the form

$$\mathcal{R} * \mathcal{X} = \mathcal{T} \text{ or } \mathcal{X} * \mathcal{R} = \mathcal{T},$$

where $\mathcal{R}$ and $\mathcal{T}$ denote the matrix form of two given binary fuzzy relations, "$*$" stands for any fuzzy relational composition, and $\mathcal{X}$ denotes the matrix form of the unknown fuzzy relation. For instance, solving equation

$$\mathcal{R} * \mathcal{X} = \mathcal{T}$$

means to find the matrix form of a binary fuzzy relation $\mathcal{X}$ in $V \times W$ assuming that the matrix forms $\mathcal{R}$ in $U \times V$ and $\mathcal{T}$ in $U \times W$ are known.

6.2.1   *Fuzzy Relational Equations with the* max–min *Composition*

Initially, let us investigate the case where the operation "$*$" is the max–min composition and the equation is given by

$$\mathcal{R} \circ \mathcal{X} = \mathcal{T}. \tag{6.1}$$

Assuming that the associated universes are finite, the fuzzy relations have matrix representations

$$\mathcal{R} = [r_{ij}], \ \mathcal{X} = [x_{jk}] \text{ and } \mathcal{T} = [t_{ik}]$$

where $r_{ij} = \varphi_{\mathcal{R}}(u_i, v_j), x_{jk} = \varphi_{\mathcal{X}}(v_j, w_k)$ and $t_{ik} = \varphi_{\mathcal{T}}(u_i, w_k)$. Since we are dealing with the max–min composition, solving (6.1) means to find $x_{jk} \in [0, 1]$ such that

$$\max_{1 \leq j \leq n} [\min(r_{ij}, x_{jk})] = t_{ik}, \tag{6.2}$$

for each $1 \leq i \leq m$ and $1 \leq k \leq p$.

Therefore, in order to investigate the solution of (6.1), the first thing to be done by us is to verify if such an equation system has solution. From (6.2) we have

$$\max_{1\le j\le n} [\min(r_{ij}, x_{jk})] = t_{ik} \implies \max_{1\le j\le n} r_{ij} \ge t_{ik}$$

for every i and k. Thus, follows immediately that if there exists a row i satisfying

$$\max_{1\le j\le n} r_{ij} < \max_{1\le k\le p} t_{ik}, \tag{6.3}$$

then there is no $\mathcal{X}$ that solves the equation. The last statement leads us to the following result:

Proposition 6.1 *If the above inequality (6.3) holds true, then the fuzzy relational equation (6.1) has no solution.*

Example 6.4 Consider the following relational equation

$$\mathcal{R} \circ \mathcal{X} = \mathcal{T} \iff \begin{bmatrix} 0.7 & 0.6 \\ 0.2 & 0.3 \end{bmatrix} \circ \begin{bmatrix} x_{11} & x_{12} \\ x_{21} & x_{22} \end{bmatrix} = \begin{bmatrix} 0.4 & 0.8 \\ 0.3 & 0.2 \end{bmatrix}.$$

In order to determine $\mathcal{X}$ we must solve the system of four equations

$$\begin{cases} \max[\min(0.7; x_{11}), \min(0.6; x_{21})] = 0.4 \\ \max[\min(0.2; x_{11}), \min(0.3; x_{21})] = 0.3 \\ \max[\min(0.7; x_{12}), \min(0.6; x_{22})] = 0.8 \\ \max[\min(0.2; x_{12}), \min(0.3; x_{22})] = 0.2 \end{cases} \tag{6.4}$$

Applying Proposition 6.1, we can easily verify that the system (6.4) has no solution because

$$\max[\min(0.7; x_{12}), \min(0.6; x_{22})] \le \max[0.7; 0.6] = 0.7 < 0.8 = \max t_{ik}.$$

Note that, whereas the two first equations of system (6.4) only have the variables x_{11} and x_{21}, the two last ones only have the variables x_{12} and x_{22}. This allows us to conclude that the relational equation

$$\begin{bmatrix} 0.7 & 0.6 \\ 0.2 & 0.3 \end{bmatrix} \circ \begin{bmatrix} x_{11} \\ x_{21} \end{bmatrix} = \begin{bmatrix} 0.4 \\ 0.3 \end{bmatrix}$$

has a solution, for instance

$$\mathcal{X}_1 = \begin{bmatrix} 0.4 \\ 0.3 \end{bmatrix}.$$

Besides $\mathcal{X}_1$, the reader can also observe that $\mathcal{X}_1$,

$$\mathcal{X}_2 = \begin{bmatrix} 0.1 \\ 0.4 \end{bmatrix} \text{ and } \mathcal{X}_3 = \begin{bmatrix} 0.4 \\ 0.4 \end{bmatrix}$$

are also solutions of the same relational equation. In this way, a relational equation may have many possible solutions. Furthermore, in this example, $\mathcal{X}_3$ is the maximal of them, that is, its components are greater or equal to the corresponding components of any other solution of the given equation.

Solutions such as $\mathcal{X}_3$, that is, with x_{ij} as great as possible, are said to be *maximal*. Thus, a maximal solution is the fuzzy relation that solves the given equation where each element has the greatest degree of membership.

Exercise 6.4 Solve the following relational equation

$$
\begin{bmatrix} 0.2\ 0.9\ 0.1 \\ 0.1\ 0.2\ 0.8 \\ 0.9\ 0.1\ 0.2 \end{bmatrix} \circ \begin{bmatrix} x_1 \\ x_2 \\ x_3 \end{bmatrix} = \begin{bmatrix} 0.8 \\ 0.2 \\ 0.3 \end{bmatrix}.
$$

Verify if this equation has more than one solution. In this case, determine the maximal solution.

Let us complete this section by observing that there is a method for solving (6.1) that also can be used to solve relational equations with the variables on the left side of $\mathcal{R}$:

$$
\mathcal{Y} \circ \mathcal{R} = \mathcal{T}.
$$

From Exercise 6.3, we have that $(\mathcal{Y} \circ \mathcal{R})^{-1} = \mathcal{T}^{-1} \Longleftrightarrow \mathcal{R}^{-1} \circ \mathcal{Y}^{-1} = \mathcal{T}^{-1}$. Thus, the solution of equation $\mathcal{Y} \circ \mathcal{R} = \mathcal{T}$ is the inverse (the transpose of the matrix) of the solution of $\mathcal{R}^{-1} \circ \mathcal{X} = \mathcal{T}^{-1}$, where $\mathcal{X} = \mathcal{Y}^{-1}$, which is the typical case (6.1).

Exercise 6.5 Solve the equation

$$
[\,x_1\ x_2\,] \circ \begin{bmatrix} 0.7\ 0.6 \\ 0.2\ 0.3 \end{bmatrix} = [\,0.5\ 0.5\,].
$$

6.2.2 Fuzzy Relational Equations with the sup–t Composition

This subsection generalizes (6.1) by using other compositions besides max–min. Moreover, we will enunciate the main result concerning these relational equations.

We now consider any of the compositions presented in Sect. 6.1. Hence, the equation of interest is

$$
\mathcal{R} \otimes^t \mathcal{X} = \mathcal{T}. \tag{6.5}
$$

Similar to the max–min case, the set of equations

$$
\mathcal{X} \otimes^t \mathcal{R} = \mathcal{T}
$$

can be solved using a method that solves (6.5) since we have

$$(\mathcal{R} \otimes^t \mathcal{X})^{-1} = \mathcal{X}^{-1} \otimes^t \mathcal{R}^{-1}.$$

Therefore, let us focus only on equations of the form (6.5), where $\mathcal{R}$ is in $U \times V$ and $\mathcal{T}$ is in $U \times W$ are two known relations and $\mathcal{X}$ is the binary relation in $V \times W$ to be determined such that Eq. (6.6) below holds true,

$$\mathcal{R} \otimes^t \mathcal{X} = \mathcal{T}. \tag{6.6}$$

In contrast with the max–min case, here, we will not investigate necessary conditions for existence of solutions of (6.5). This study is analogous to that done in Sect. 6.2.1. However, we will prove a result that indicates how to obtain a solution of equation (6.5), if it exists.

Theorem 6.2 *Given a t-norm $\triangle$ and fuzzy relations $\mathcal{R}$ and $\mathcal{T}$ defined in $U \times V$ and $U \times W$, respectively, if the equation $\mathcal{R} \otimes^t \mathcal{X} = \mathcal{T}$ has a solution, then its maximal solution is $\mathcal{D} = \mathcal{R}^{-1} \otimes_{\Longrightarrow} \mathcal{T}$, where the implication is given by*

$$(x \Longrightarrow y) = \sup\{z \in [0, 1] : x \triangle z \le y\}.$$

Proof The reader can find the proof of this theorem in [5]. ∎

The next corollaries follow from the above theorem.

Corollary 6.3 *If $\mathcal{D} = \mathcal{R}^{-1} \otimes_{\Longrightarrow} \mathcal{T}$ is not a solution of equation $\mathcal{R} \otimes^t \mathcal{X} = \mathcal{T}$, then it has no solution.*

Corollary 6.4 *If there exists a solution of (6.5) for $\triangle = \wedge$, that is, if there exists a solution of the equation $\mathcal{R} \circ \mathcal{X} = \mathcal{T}$ with the minimum t-norm, then $\mathcal{D} = \mathcal{R}^{-1} \otimes_g \mathcal{T}$ is its maximal solution, where g is the Gödel's implication.*

Corollary 6.5 *If there exist a solution of (6.5) for $\triangle = $ product, that is, if there exist a solution of the equation $\mathcal{R} \otimes^t \mathcal{X} = \mathcal{T}$ with the product t-norm, then $\mathcal{D} = \mathcal{R}^{-1} \otimes_{g_n} \mathcal{T}$ is its maximal solution, where g_n denotes the Goguen's implication.*

Exercise 6.6 Use the above corollaries to verify if the following relational equation

$$\begin{bmatrix} 0.9 & 0.3 & 1.0 \\ 0.8 & 0.8 & 0.5 \\ 0.6 & 0.4 & 0.7 \end{bmatrix} \otimes^t \begin{bmatrix} x_1 \\ x_2 \\ x_3 \end{bmatrix} = \begin{bmatrix} 0.6 \\ 0.4 \\ 0.5 \end{bmatrix}$$

has solution. If it exists, exhibit one of them for each of the following t-norm: $\triangle$:

(a) $\triangle = \min$
(b) $\triangle = $ product.

The next subsection proposes a diagnostic model that indicates the potential of relational equations in application. Specifically, we will make use of Corollary 6.4 to illustrate such potential.

6.2.3 *Mathematical Modelling: Medical Diagnosis*

The following experiment [6] was performed to see if a fuzzy model is useful to obtain diagnostics of diseases. The basic idea for a medical diagnosis is to relate symptoms or patients' signs with possible diseases according to an expert's medical knowledge. This application can be summarized in an input-output system:

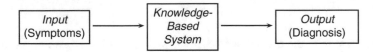

Let us consider the following universal sets:

$U =$ set of patients;
$V =$ set of symptoms;
$W =$ set of diseases.

Specifically, we deal with childhood illnesses where we have knowledge of four patients P_1, P_2, P_3, and P_4, with symptoms $s_1, s_2, s_3, s_4, s_5, s_6, s_7, s_8, s_9, s_{10}$, and s_{11}, that were diagnosed with d_1, d_2, d_3, and d_4, where:

$s_1 =$ fever;	$s_5 =$ ganglion;	$s_9 =$ photophobia;
$s_2 =$ headache;	$s_6 =$ coryza;	$s_{10} =$ dry cough;
$s_3 =$ sore throat;	$s_7 =$ conjunctivitis;	$s_{11} =$ vomit
$s_4 =$ exanthema;	$s_8 =$ strawberry tongue;	

and

$d_1 =$ scarlet fever; $d_2 =$ rubella; $d_3 =$ measles; $d_4 =$ flu.

These data will draw upon the knowledge base which will be described in terms of fuzzy relations.

We want to obtain a fuzzy relation $\mathcal{D}$ such that $\mathcal{S} \circ \mathcal{D} = \mathcal{T}$, where $\mathcal{S}$ and $\mathcal{T}$ are respectively the matricial forms of the fuzzy relations of symptoms and patients defined in $U \times V$ and $U \times W$.

Knowledge Base – Building of Fuzzy System

The knowledge base is composed of the fuzzy relations $\mathcal{S}$ and $\mathcal{T}$ whose matrices are given below in a tabular form:

In this example, the data in each one of the above tables were obtained from the literature (such a fact allows us to use data corresponding to diseases that may not be diagnosed any more). However, expert's data can be used in the model.

Table 6.1 Matrix of the relation S: patients and their symptoms

$P\backslash s$	s_1	s_2	s_3	s_4	s_5	s_6	s_7	s_8	s_9	s_{10}	s_{11}
P_1	0.8	0.4	0.5	0.8	0.2	0.1	0.1	0.9	0.1	0.1	0.4
P_2	0.3	0.1	0.4	0.8	0.9	0.2	0.1	0.1	0.1	0.1	0.3
P_3	0.8	0.3	0.5	0.8	0.1	0.2	0.9	0.1	0.6	0.3	0.6
P_4	0.8	0.7	0.7	0.2	0.1	0.9	0.1	0.1	0.1	0.9	0.4

Table 6.2 Matrix of the relation T: diagnostic pattern

$P\backslash d$	d_1	d_2	d_3	d_4
P_1	0.9	0.3	0.4	0.2
P_2	0.3	0.9	0.1	0.1
P_3	0.4	0.1	0.9	0.3
P_4	0.2	0.1	0.3	0.9

Table 6.3 Matrix of the Relation $\mathcal{D} = \mathcal{S}^{-1} \otimes_g \mathcal{T}$: symptoms and diagnoses

$s\backslash d$	d_1	d_2	d_3	d_4
s_1	0.2	0.1	0.1	0.1
s_2	0.2	0.1	0.3	0.2
s_3	0.2	0.1	0.1	0.1
s_4	0.3	0.1	0.1	0.1
s_5	0.3	1.0	0.1	0.1
s_6	0.2	0.1	0.1	0.1
s_7	0.4	0.1	1.0	0.3
s_8	1.0	0.3	0.4	0.2
s_9	0.4	0.1	1.0	0.3
s_{10}	0.2	0.1	0.3	1.0
s_{11}	0.2	0.1	0.1	0.1

We have that $\mathcal{D} = \mathcal{S}^{-1} \otimes_g \mathcal{T}$ using Corollary 6.4 and the matrices of Tables 6.1 and 6.2, where the matrix $\mathcal{D}$ is given in Table 6.3. Thus, each element of the relation $\mathcal{D}$ indicates the degree of connection of each symptom with the diseases under consideration. For instance, the value $d_{23} = 0.3$ indicates that, on a range from **zero** to **one**, the symptom s_2 (headache) is related to the disease d_3 (measles) with degree 0.3. It is important to note that the *matrix of diagnoses* $\mathcal{D} = \mathcal{S}^{-1} \otimes_g \mathcal{T}$ was obtained applying Corollary 6.4 that solves the relational equation $\mathcal{S} \circ \mathcal{X} = \mathcal{T}$. In other words, the diagnosis of each patient P_i in the knowledge base, that were mathematically translated by the matrices $\mathcal{S}$ and $\mathcal{T}$, can be retrieved by means of relation $\mathcal{D}$. For example, let us use the matrix $\mathcal{D}$ to obtain the diagnosis of patient P_1 from the associated symptoms.

The mathematical model to obtain a diagnosis is $\mathcal{S} \circ \mathcal{D}$, according to formula (3.3), so that we can obtain the first patient's diagnosis by calculating $\mathcal{P}_1 \circ \mathcal{D}$ where $\mathcal{P}_1$ denotes the matrix of symptoms:

$$
\mathcal{P}_1 \circ \mathcal{D} =
\begin{bmatrix}
0.8 \\
0.4 \\
0.5 \\
0.8 \\
0.2 \\
0.1 \\
0.1 \\
0.9 \\
0.1 \\
0.1 \\
0.4
\end{bmatrix}^{\top}
\circ
\begin{bmatrix}
0.2 & 0.1 & 0.1 & 0.1 \\
0.2 & 0.1 & 0.3 & 0.2 \\
0.2 & 0.1 & 0.1 & 0.1 \\
0.3 & 0.1 & 0.1 & 0.1 \\
0.3 & 1.0 & 0.1 & 0.1 \\
0.2 & 0.1 & 0.1 & 0.1 \\
0.4 & 0.1 & 1.0 & 0.3 \\
1.0 & 0.3 & 0.4 & 0.2 \\
0.4 & 0.1 & 1.0 & 0.3 \\
0.2 & 0.1 & 0.3 & 1.0 \\
0.2 & 0.1 & 0.1 & 0.1
\end{bmatrix}
= \begin{bmatrix} 0.9 & 0.3 & 0.4 & 0.2 \end{bmatrix}.
$$

and $v^{\top}$ stands for the transpose of the vector v.

The resulting matrix is composed of membership degrees for each of the diseases with respect to first patient. Indeed, since the matrix $\mathcal{P}_1$ is a relation in $U \times V$ (patients $\times$ symptoms) and $\mathcal{D}$ is a relation in $V \times W$ (symptoms $\times$ diseases), the composition of $\mathcal{P}_1$ with $\mathcal{D}$ yields a relation in $U \times W$ (patients $\times$ diseases). Similarly, we can obtain diagnoses for other patients

Exercise 6.7 Solve the items below.

(a) Show that if a mathematical model for diagnosis is given by equation $\mathcal{S} \otimes^t \mathcal{X} = \mathcal{T}$ with the product t-norm, then the diagnostic matrix is given by $\mathcal{D} = \mathcal{S}^{-1} \otimes_{g_n} \mathcal{T}$, where g_n denotes the Goguen's implication (hint: use Corollary 6.5)
(b) For (a), repeat the above replacing the minimum t-norm by product t-norm.
(c) Compare the result obtained in (b) with the ones in the above application using the *max-min* operation.

The interested reader can find more applications in [7, 8].

Two important properties of the fuzzy relation $\mathcal{D}$ are discussed below. Let $\mathcal{D} = \mathcal{S}^{-1} \circ \mathcal{T}$. The following properties hold true:

(p_1) $\mathcal{D}$ "retrieves" the diagnoses of the patients in the knowledge base.
(p_2) Diagnoses of new patients can be incorporated in the knowledge base and thus increasing the capacity of obtaining more diagnoses by means of the fuzzy relation $\mathcal{D}$, as happens with an experienced doctor.

These two properties of the fuzzy relation $\mathcal{D}$ validate its use in diagnostic formulation.

Property (p_1) is the main characteristic of so called *Expert Systems*. Expert systems are those that **mimic** human experts. Property (p_2), that permits update the knowledge base, is the one that characterizes *Neural Networks*. Neural networks are systems that **learn** in the sense of incorporating new situations in its knowledge base and thus are analogous to the human systems (see [9, 10]).

Let us conclude this section by recalling that several relational equations have no solution, mainly because they do not satisfy the necessary conditions given by inequality (6.3). In this case, we use the notion of approximate solution for the given equation (see [5, 11]).

Fundamentally, an approximate solution of equation (6.1) is a solution of another fuzzy relational equation in which the relation $\mathcal{R}$ is slightly expanded whereas $\mathcal{T}$ is slightly reduced in order to satisfy the inequality (6.3). For this case with respect to medical diagnostics, we can postulate (even though intuitively) that the relational equation would satisfy inequality (6.3) whenever the matrix $\mathcal{T}$ (dataset) is composed of at least an instance of each disease. In other words, whenever there exists at least one element in each column of $\mathcal{T}$ close to 1. In our case, patients P_1, P_2, P_3, and P_4 had scarlet fever, rubella, measles, and flu, respectively.

The diagnostic matrix $\mathcal{D}$ is given in terms of a fuzzy implication in which $\mathcal{T}$ is implicated — $\mathcal{D} = \mathcal{S}^{-1} \otimes_{\Longrightarrow} \mathcal{T}$ $(\mathcal{D} = \mathcal{S}^{-1} \Longrightarrow \mathcal{T})$. Thus, intuitively the condition (6.3) is automatically satisfied. In other words, the largest values of $\mathcal{D}$ are greater or equal to the largest values of $\mathcal{T}$ so that the values of an implication are at least equal to the implicated values.

Finally, the choice of the relational equation $\mathcal{S} \otimes^t \mathcal{X} = \mathcal{T}$ as a medical diagnostic model was made by means of logical coherence: symptoms imply treatment $((\mathcal{S}^{-1} \Longrightarrow \mathcal{T}))$. Hence, we chose the equation whose solution is $\mathcal{D} = \mathcal{S}^{-1} \otimes_{\Longrightarrow} \mathcal{T}$.

More detailed studies concerning this subject can be found in [5, 11–14].

6.3 Fuzzy Relational Equation and Bayesian Inference

The purpose of this section is to interpret the solution of (6.5) from the Bayesian viewpoint by considering membership functions as possibility distributions of variables (see Chap. 7). In the classical stochastic case, Bayes's rule is useful to revise a distribution $g(x)$ (called priori) in light of new information concerning the variable of interest X. Such information is derived from a variable Y that is related to X. Thus, they are incorporated into Bayes's model by means of a probability density represented by $f(y \mid x)$. It is worth noting that, on the one hand, $f(y \mid x)$ represents a likelihood function of X for a fixed y. On the other hand, $f(y \mid x)$ is the conditional probability of Y given $X = x$.

After correcting $g(x)$, we obtain a "new" distribution $\eta(x \mid y)$ called the posteriori probability distribution of X. Here, the main issue is to obtain $\eta(x \mid y)$ given the priori distribution $g(x)$ and likelihood $f(y \mid x)$. The classical proposal due to Bayes [15, 16] is

$$\eta(x \mid y) = \frac{f(y \mid x)g(x)}{\int_X f(y \mid x)g(x)}. \tag{6.7}$$

The possibilistic rule of Bayes "emerges" as a solution to the fuzzy relational equation of the form (6.5) where the variable is the posteriori distribution. Note that this approach is quite different from the stochastic approach where the formula

(6.7) is "postulated" as the way to correct the priori distribution $g(x)$. In order to address our issue of interest, we will suppose that the relational equations always have solutions.

Although we are dealing of possibility distributions and not of membership functions of fuzzy sets, there is a close relation between these functions (see Sect. 7.1.3 of Chap. 7) that allows us to use some results from fuzzy set theory in possibility theory such as relational equations.

According to Equation (6.6), given fuzzy relations A and B respectively in the universal sets $U \times V$ and $U \times W$, when it exists, it is known [5, 12] that the maximal (or less specific) solution of

$$A \otimes^t Z = B \tag{6.8}$$

is the fuzzy relation R in $V \times W$ whose membership function is

$$\begin{aligned}
\varphi_R(v, w) &= \inf_{u \in U} (\varphi_{A^{-1}}(v, u) \Longrightarrow \varphi_B(u, w)) \\
&= \inf_{u \in U} (\varphi_A(u, v) \Longrightarrow \varphi_B(u, w))
\end{aligned} \tag{6.9}$$

where A^{-1} denotes the inverse of A (i.e. $\varphi_{A^{-1}}(v, u) = \varphi_A(u, v)$) and "$\Longrightarrow$" denotes the residual fuzzy implication, that is,

$$(a \Longrightarrow b) = \sup\{z \in [0, 1] : a \triangle z \leq b\}. \tag{6.10}$$

Let us consider the particular case where A and B are fuzzy sets (or unary relations) in U and V, respectively. In this case, the membership function of the solution R of (6.8) (when it exists) is given by

$$\begin{aligned}
\varphi_R(u, v) &= (\varphi_A(u) \Longrightarrow \varphi_B(v)) \\
&= \sup\{z \in [0, 1] : \varphi_A(u) \triangle z \leq \varphi_B(v)\}
\end{aligned} \tag{6.11}$$

where $\triangle$ stands for a $t - norm$.

On the one hand, once that R is given by an implication, we can apply the typical interpretation of a conditional $\varphi_R(u, v)$ which corresponds to the result of the implication pair

$$(\varphi_A(u), \varphi_B(v))$$

where $\varphi_B(v)$ denotes the membership degree of v in B given u in A where the membership degree of A is $\varphi_A(u)$. We use the notation $\varphi_R(u, v) = \varphi_{B|A}(v \mid u)$ if R stands for the solution in (6.11). On the other hand, $\varphi_R(u, \cdot)$ is a function with respect to variable v for a given u in A with membership degree of $\varphi_A(u)$. Thus, let us denote $\varphi_R(u, \cdot)$ using the symbol $\varphi_{B|A}(\cdot \mid u)$ where $\varphi_{B|A}(v \mid u)$ indicates the membership degree of v in B given u in A with membership degree of $\varphi_A(u)$.

Using the above comments, the compositional rule of inference (3.2) can be rewritten as

$$\varphi_{B^*}(v) = \sup_{u \in U} \left(\varphi_A(u) \, \triangle \, \varphi_{B|A}(u \mid v) \right). \tag{6.12}$$

As we discussed in Chap. 3, B^* does not necessarily equals B since Eq. (6.12) may not have a solution [12]. For each $v \in V$, the following functional equation

$$\varphi_{B^*}(v) \, \triangle_1 \, \varphi_S(v, u) = \varphi_A(u) \, \triangle_2 \, \varphi_R(u, v), \quad \forall u \in U, \tag{6.13}$$

is equivalent to the relational equation with the arguments given explicitly

$$\varphi_{B^*}(v) \, \otimes^t \, \varphi_S(v, u) = \varphi_A(u) \, \triangle_2 \, \varphi_R(u, v) \, \forall u \in U \tag{6.14}$$

where S denotes an unknown fuzzy relation. If a solution of (6.14) exists, then the membership function of S according to (6.11) is given by

$$\varphi_S(v, u) = (\varphi_{B^*}(v) \implies (\varphi_A(u) \, \triangle_2 \, \varphi_R(u, v))). \tag{6.15}$$

Remarks

1. The t-norms $\triangle_1$ and $\triangle_2$ in (6.11) may be different;
2. Given the above interpretation of (6.11), the membership function $\varphi_S(v, u)$ in (6.15) represents a typical conditional membership $\varphi_S(u \mid v)$;
3. Recall that $\varphi_R(u, v) = \varphi_{B|A}(v \mid u)$ in (6.15) for a given fixed v represents the "correction" of a priori $\varphi_A(u)$ according to the Bayesian approach;
4. Similar to remark 3, $\varphi_{B|A}(v \mid u)$ can be interpreted as a "likelihood" and not as a "conditional of v given u" since u is the variable;
5. The option to adopt an operation of type $\otimes^t$ ($= sup - t$) in the left-side of (6.14) is due to the max-min theories which deal with "central measures" such as the mathematical expectation.

6.3.1 Possibility Distribution and Bayesian Inference

We will make use of all previous notation and results concerning fuzzy relational equations by replacing membership functions by possibility distributions. In this context, (6.8) has the form

$$X \otimes^t Z = Y \tag{6.16}$$

and Eq. (6.15), according to *Remark 3*, has the form

$$\pi_\triangle(x \mid y) = \left(\pi_Y^*(y) \implies \left(\pi_X(x) \, \triangle \, \pi_{Y|X}(y \mid x) \right) \right) \tag{6.17}$$

where $(a \implies b)$ denotes a residual implication as in (6.10) and

$$\pi_Y^*(y) = \sup_{x \in X} \pi_X(x) \, \triangle \, \pi_{Y|X}(y \mid x). \tag{6.18}$$

Based on Remarks 2–4, we can interpret the term $\pi_X(x) \bigtriangleup \pi_{Y|X}(y \mid x)$ as an update of $\pi_X(x)$ from the likelihood function $\pi_{Y|X}(y \mid x)$ that was adjusted according to some historical record such as datasets, expert's knowledge, *etc.*. The term $\pi_{Y^*}(y) = \sup_x \pi_X(x) \bigtriangleup \pi_{Y|X}(y \mid x)$ operates as a normalization constant. Finally, given X and Y, if (6.16) has solution, then $\pi_\triangle(x \mid y)$ and $\pi_{(Y|X)}(y \mid x)$ must have their arguments interchanged such as in formula (6.17). Such a fact directly arises from fuzzy relational equations theory and perfectly matches Bayesian methodology. Based on these observations, we will consider (6.17) as a possibilistic general formula of Bayes for an arbitrary t-norm $\bigtriangleup$.

Let us leave as an exercise for the reader the task of verifying that for the minimum t-norm ($\bigtriangleup = \wedge = \min$) we have

$$\pi_\wedge(x \mid y) = \begin{cases} 1 & \text{if } \pi_Y^*(y) = \pi_X(x) \wedge \pi_{Y|X}(y \mid x) \\ \pi_X(x) \wedge \pi_{Y|X}(y \mid x) & \text{if } \pi_Y^*(y) > \pi_X(x) \wedge \pi_{Y|X}(y \mid x) \end{cases}.$$

For product t-norm ($\bigtriangleup = ``\cdot"$), Eq. (6.17) is given by (6.21) which is discussed below. In this case, the above interpretation of (6.17) is more apparent if compared to the classical equation of Bayes (see Eq. (6.7)).

Remark For the product t-norm, we will use the notation $\pi(x \mid y)$ instead of $\pi_{(\cdot)}(x \mid y)$.

6.3.2 Possibilistic Rule of Bayes

Let us focus only on solutions for (6.17) given by residual implications. These solutions, when they exist, are less specific than any other solution, that is, they are maximal solutions. In particular, let us study maximal solutions of equation (6.17) for several t-norms.

- In the case where $\bigtriangleup = \cdot$, i.e., the product t-norm, (6.10) has the form

$$(a \Longrightarrow b) = \begin{cases} 1 & \text{if } a \leq b \\ \frac{b}{a} & \text{if } a > b \end{cases}. \tag{6.19}$$

Therefore, since

$$\pi_Y^*(y) = \sup_{x \in X} \pi_X(x) \bigtriangleup \pi_{Y|X}(y \mid x) \geq \pi_X(x) \bigtriangleup \pi_{Y|X}(y \mid x), \tag{6.20}$$

we have that (6.17) can be rewritten as follows

$$\pi(x \mid y) = \frac{\pi_X(x)\pi_{Y|X}(y \mid x)}{\sup_{x \in X} \pi_X(x)\pi_{Y|X}(y \mid x)}. \tag{6.21}$$

The analogy between the formula (6.21) and the Bayes's rule (6.7) is evident and suggest naming (6.21) the possibilistic rule of Bayes. For the product t-norm, Eqs. (6.17) and (6.21) are equivalent which implies that we can use one or the other to obtain the posteriori distribution $\pi(x \mid y)$.

It is worth noting that if Y is less specific than X, that is, $\pi_Y \geq \pi_X$, then the likelihood given by means of residual implication satisfies $\pi_{Y|X} \equiv 1$. Consequently, the posteriori distribution $\pi_\triangle(x \mid y)$ coincides with the a priori $\pi_X(x)$. Such a fact also occurs in the stochastic case and means that the variable Y is not able to improve the information contained in X. For a deeper study of this subject and its applications we recommend the interested reader to consult [17–19].

The next section deals with another sense of approximation which is different from the above one discussed for relational equations.

6.4 Universal Approximation

Mathematical methods, in general, that yield conclusions (*outputs: y*) from a given information (*inputs: x*), are given by functions: $y = f(x)$. Usually, these methods require mathematically "precise" data and functions. However, the use of fuzzy sets with fuzzy logic allows us to extend these input-ouput systems. Fuzzy controllers arise as a typical example in this context. The usual mathematical modeling of a input-output system is one where the inputs and outputs are real numbers and the knowledge base is given by means of a function.

Example 6.5 The function that relates the side l of a square with its perimeter p is given by $p = 4l$. In this case, we have the following input-output pairs (in meters):

Input (l)	Output (p)
1	4
2	8
3	12

This example deals with a ideal situation where the procedure, which associates each input to an output, is given by a mathematical function. In this case, the knowledge base is summarized by the function $p(l) = 4l$. However, even for this simple case, outputs are only produced from precise inputs (real numbers). For instance, what is the perimeter of a square whose length "*around 3 m*"? The impossibility of producing a suitable output for such a question by a crisp model is due to classical mathematical model's inability to deal with imprecise or ambiguous information as input. In general, we have two options to deal with this kind of situation. The first option consists of electing a real number as input, eliminating the uncertainty of the input. In our context, this approach consists of applying a defuzzification technique on the input in order to obtain a real number thus allowing the use of classical mathematics. The second option consists of increasing the knowledge base in order to include such a input. For example, for the above input, an expert could provide a linguist output such as "*around 12 m*".

The imprecisions, such as those above, are present only in the inputs and outputs, but not in the knowledge base which must be designed and adjusted in order to understand each uncertain input. However, there are situations in which the knowledge base contains several imprecisions due to the possibility of dealing with partial information or misinformation, mainly when they are provided by experts. This is the case when the system is produced by means of linguistic terms. When the imprecisions are mathematically modeled using fuzzy tools such as fuzzy sets and fuzzy logic, then the resulting input-output system is said to be a **Fuzzy System**.

The inputs in Example 6.5 have the form "*around*" so that we could model them as triangular fuzzy numbers (as in Chap. 2). Suppose that the knowledge base is given as before, that is, given by the function $\widehat{p} = 4\widehat{l}$, where $\widehat{l}$ stands for the fuzzy number "*around l*", we can use the extension principle of Zadeh as well as the multiplication of a real number by a fuzzy number to obtain a fuzzy number as the output having the form "*around*"

Fuzzy logic demonstrates its usefulness and indeed its contribution to situations where the knowledge base is composed of a collection of rules of the form *if ... then* .... Obviously, connectives, implications and fuzzy relations play a fundamental role in this context.

6.4.1 Approximating Capability

Let us consider a fuzzy system that associates each input $x \in X$ with an unique output $y \in Y$. In Chap. 5, we presented several examples of fuzzy systems most notably fuzzy controllers. Example 5.3 corresponds to a fuzzy system with two inputs and one output: each pair of real numbers (x, y) is associated with a real number u. Thus, the corresponding fuzzy system defines a function $f^* : \mathfrak{D} \subset \mathbb{R}^2 \longrightarrow \mathbb{R}$. Such a property can also be found in Model 5.6.2 (HIV). In contrast, the controller of Model 5.6.1 (Salinity) yields a function $g^* : \mathfrak{D} \subset \mathbb{R}^3 \longrightarrow \mathbb{R}$.

Note that each one of these examples produces a mapping from an input domain X to an output range Y. This is a typical characteristic of rule-based fuzzy systems and is essential for the following discussion concerning the approximation of a (theoretical) function which describes a certain phenomenon.

The great utility of fuzzy systems (fuzzy controllers) in the study of approximation is the fact that we can replace the corresponding (theoretical) function, that may be hard to deal with due to some difficulties such as only having partial knowledge of it, by a fuzzy system with a certain degree of reliability. For instance, what could we propose as a (theoretical) function for the problem of forecasting of surface salinity presented in Model 5.6.1?

The above examples used either the Mamdani inference method or the TSK inference method. Therefore, we chose the minimum t-norm and maximum t-conorm in these cases. However, in these examples, we can also employ other types of controllers as well as other t-norms and t-conorms. Generally, each function f^* given by a fuzzy system depends on:

(a) the membership functions of the fuzzy sets of the rule base;
(b) the t-norm and t-conorm used;
(c) the method of defuzzification adopted.

The next observation is geared to help the reader, mainly those with a certain experience in numerical simulation, to understand mathematically the role played by fuzzy systems (especially by fuzzy controllers).

For each set of data pairs (x_i, y_i), $1 \leq i \leq r$, with $x_i \in X$ and $y_i \in Y$, the application of the ordinary least square method yields a function $f_r^* : X \longrightarrow Y$. Let f be an unknown (theoretical) function that satisfies $y_i = f(x_i)$ for $i = 1, \ldots, r$. Thus, it seems reasonable to assume that the adjusted function f_r^* approximates f when the number of data r increases. In other words, the more the information of f the better its approximation f_r^* will be.

Analogously, fuzzy systems are given by data pairs (A_i, B_i) of the form "if x is A_i then y is B_i", where A_i and B_i are fuzzy sets of X and Y, respectively. Based on the above properties (a), (b), and (c), a fuzzy system yields a function f_r^* where r denotes the number of rules in the rule base. To present the main result of this section, which establishes the approximation of a theoretical function (f) by a sequence of fuzzy systems, let us require that the rule base must contain the graph of the function f. Now suppose that the rule base is given as in Frame 6.1.

$$\boxed{\begin{array}{l} R_1\text{: "If } x \text{ is } A_1 \text{ then } y \text{ is } B_1\text{"} \\ \text{or} \\ \qquad R_2\text{: "If } x \text{ is } A_2 \text{ then } y \text{ is } B_2\text{"} \\ \text{or} \\ \qquad \vdots \qquad\qquad \vdots \\ \text{or} \\ \qquad R_r\text{: "If } x \text{ is } A_r \text{ then } y \text{ is } B_r\text{"} \end{array}}$$

Frame 6.1: Rule Base for approximating the theoretical function f

The graphical representation of each one of the rules is called a *granule*. Figure 6.1 graphically depicts the granules corresponding to the above rules.

The graph of Fig. 6.1 illustrates how a fuzzy system can approximate a function. As mentioned above, it is necessary that the granules of a rule base contain the graph of the theoretical function to be approximated.

Generally, a class of objects **B** approximates a class **A** if for each element of **A** there exists an element in **B** such that they are close enough. In this case, mathematically speaking, **B** is said to be dense in **A**. For example, the set of rational numbers $\mathbb{Q}$ is dense in the set of real numbers $\mathbb{R}$, which means that any real number can be approximated by a rational number. Another example is the set of polynomials that is

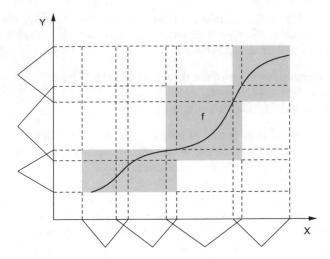

Fig. 6.1 Granules and theoretical function f

dense in the set of continuous functions as established in Weierstrass's well-known theorem. In addition, a neural network can approximate any continuous function defined in a compact universe [9].

Next, let us present two important results from a theoretical point of view concerning the study of approximation of continuous functions by means of a fuzzy systems or, more specifically, fuzzy controllers. Before this, some notation is introduced which will help in the understanding of the results we present. Let $\mathcal{F}$ be the class of the functions $f_r^* : \mathbb{R}^n \longrightarrow \mathbb{R}$ obtained from a fuzzy system:

$$
f_r^*(x_1, x_2, \ldots, x_n) = \frac{\displaystyle\sum_{j=1}^{r} y_j \, \triangle \, (\varphi_{A_{1j}}(x_1) \, \triangle \, \cdots \, \triangle \, \varphi_{A_{nj}}(x_n))}{\displaystyle\sum_{j=1}^{r} \varphi_{A_{1j}}(x_1) \, \triangle \, \cdots \, \triangle \, \varphi_{A_{nj}}(x_n)},
\tag{6.22}
$$

where r is the number of rules and $\varphi_{A_{1j}}, \ldots, \varphi_{A_{nj}}$ are the corresponding membership functions of the fuzzy sets A_{ij}, $1 \leq i \leq n$ and $1 \leq j \leq r$, and $\triangle$ is a t-norm.

Theorem 6.6 (Nguyen and Walker) *If membership functions are given by Gaussians, and if $\triangle$ is the minimum t-norm or the product t-norm, then the class $\mathcal{F}$ (obtained from fuzzy systems) is dense in the set of the continuous functions defined in a compact set (such as a closed real interval).*

Proof The proof of this theorem can be found in [20].   ■

The above theorem can be interpreted as follows. For each continuous function f (in our context, a "theoretical" function f) there exists a sequence of functions f_r^*, obtained by fuzzy systems, that are sufficiently close of f. Furthermore, Theorem 6.6 has a special importance for fuzzy controllers of type TSK where the outputs are not defuzzified and the functions f_r^* have the form of Eq. (6.22).

Theorem 6.7 (Nguyen and Walker) *Suppose that the membership functions, which compose the rule base, are continuous with bounded support (such as triangular and trapezoidal fuzzy sets). If both t-norm and t-conorm are continuous and a defuzzification method such as center of gravity or mean of maximum is adopted, then the class $\mathcal{F}$ of the functions f_r^* is dense in the class of the continuous functions defined in compact sets.*

Proof The proof of this theorem can be found in [20]. ∎

The central idea in these theorems is that the greater the number of rules r, the closer the output of the controller and the expected theoretical function value are. The more rules, the narrower the supports of the fuzzy sets in the rule base are and thus the smaller the granules which cover the graph of the theoretical function are (see Fig. 6.1).

Note that the above result is similar to the theorem of Weierstrass if we replace the degrees of the polynomial (n) by the number of rules (r). The approximating capability is fundamental in certain areas of mathematics such as **numerical analysis** and approximation theory, implying that the fuzzy controllers can play an important role in these areas.

Next, let us illustrate the potential of the approximating capability of the fuzzy controllers by means of certain evolutionary systems.

6.5 Applications of Fuzzy Controllers in Dynamic Systems

This section highlights the approximation property of fuzzy controllers for applications in dynamic systems. Furthermore, we propose a method to solve classical dynamic systems by means of fuzzy controllers.

A classical dynamic system has the form

$$x_{t+1} = F(x_t) \iff x_{t+1} - x_t = f(x_t) \tag{6.23}$$

for the discrete case and

$$\frac{dx}{dt} = f(x) \tag{6.24}$$

for the continuous case.

The field f, in both cases, represents **rates of change** or **variation** and is central in the study of these systems. However, if f is not explicitly given or, worse, if f is partially known based only on certain characteristics of a given phenomenon, then, how can we study the evolution of the system? The usual approach consists in assuming that f is a given mathematical expression that satisfies certain properties.

We propose a rule-based fuzzy linguistic model derived from certain characteristics of the phenomenon. The inputs are the **state variables** whereas the outputs are the **state variations**. This is a necessity in applying fuzzy controllers to dynamic systems. From the modeling point of view, such a procedure is reasonable when the available information is incomplete and the phenomenon is partially understood. Since the formulation of the rules is based on the knowledge about the phenomenon, we expect that the resulting function f_r of the controller (Sect. 6.3.1) to be able to capture such a knowledge.

We can study the solution of the differential equation by replacing the theoretical field f by f_r

$$x_{t+1} - x_t = f_r(x_t) \tag{6.25}$$

for the discrete case and the differential equation

$$\frac{dx}{dt} = f_r(x) \tag{6.26}$$

for the continuous case. Depending on the mathematical properties of f (for example, continuity) and the chosen methodology, we expect that the solutions of (6.25) and (6.26) respectively to converge to the solutions of (6.23) and (6.24) since f_r converges to f when the number of rules (r) increases. In some cases the function f_r is explicitly given (see Theorem 6.6, [21, 22], and the references therein). For instance, f_r can be given by a rational form – quotient of polynomials (see [23]). In this cases, (6.25) and/or (6.26) may have analytical solutions.

Next, we will provide some details concerning the method we employ here. However, in Chap. 9 we will present a more detailed development of the application of fuzzy controllers to dynamic systems.

Suppose that a certain phenomenon can be modeled by the following initial value problem (IVP)

$$\begin{cases} \frac{dx}{dt} = f(t, x) \\ x(t_0) = x_0 \end{cases} \tag{6.27}$$

where the solution is

$$x(t) = x_0 + \int_{t_0}^{t} f(s, x(s))ds. \tag{6.28}$$

Let us consider a fuzzy controller with r rules that describe the characteristics of the field f, that is, our rules produce a function f_r. Now, suppose that $f_r \xrightarrow[r \to \infty]{} f$, as discussed in Sect. 6.3.1. Further, suppose that the function f_r satisfies the necessary conditions such that the IVP

$$\begin{cases} \frac{dx}{dt} = f_r(t, x) \\ x(t_0) = x_0 \end{cases} \tag{6.29}$$

has the solution

$$x_r(t) = x_0 + \int_{t_0}^{t} f_r(s, x(s)) \mathrm{d}s. \tag{6.30}$$

An interesting question that arises in this context is, under what conditions do you have

$$x_r \xrightarrow[r \to \infty]{} x \text{ if } f_r \xrightarrow[r \to \infty]{} f ?$$

That is, under what conditions does the convergence of the functions f_r to f imply that their integrals converge to the integral of f?

The answers to these kinds of questions are typically found in area of mathematical analysis, for instance, in theorems of monotonic convergence as well as Lebesgue's dominated convergence theorem. An answer to the above question concerning the compact sets a the real line can be found in [21].

In order to study the presented method, besides supposing that $x_r \xrightarrow[r \to \infty]{} x$, let us assume that each function f_r has sufficient properties to ensure that the problem (6.29) is well-defined and has a solution given by (6.30). Finally, since the function f_r of a fuzzy controller is usually given in a tabular form, let us use classical numerical methods to obtain numerical solutions of (6.29), that is, the method will provide a sequence $\{x_r\}_n$ that approximates x_r. Because $x_r \xrightarrow[r \to \infty]{} x$, and $\{x_r\}_n \xrightarrow[n \to +\infty]{} x_r$, we expect that $\{x_r\}_n \xrightarrow[r \to \infty]{n \to \infty} x$. Basically, this is the method that we employ to estimate solutions of ordinary differential equations using fuzzy controllers when we are dealing with partial information of the direction field (see the first example of Sect. 8.1.5 in Chap. 8). In addition to this method for continuous models, we will study an analogous methodology for the discrete system in Chap. 9.

References

1. E. Esmi, P. Sussner, S. Sandri, Tunable equivalence fuzzy associative memories. Fuzzy Sets Syst. **292**, 242–260 (2015)
2. P. Sussner, M.E. Valle, Implicative fuzzy associative memories. IEEE Trans. Fuzzy Syst. **14**(6), 793–807 (2006)
3. M.E. Valle, P. Sussner, A general framework for fuzzy morphological associative memories. Fuzzy Sets Syst. **159**(7), 747–768 (2008)
4. M.E. Valle, P. Sussner, Storage and recall capabilities of fuzzy morphological associative memories with adjunction-based learning. Neural Netw. **24**(1), 75–90 (2011)
5. G. Klir, B. Yuan, *Fuzzy Sets and Fuzzy Logic Theory and Applications* (Prentice-Hall, Englewood Cliffs, 1995)
6. R.C. Bassanezi, H.E. Roman, *Relaciones Fuzzy: Optimizacion de Diagnostico Medico*. Anais do Encontro Nacional de Ecologia (Rio de Janeiro), LNCC. (1989), pp. 115–124
7. J.C.R. Pereira, P.A. Tonelli, L.C. Barros, N.R.S. Ortega, Defuzzification in medical diagnosis. Adv. Log. Artif. Intell. Robot. **85**, 202–207 (2002)

8. J.C.R. Pereira, P.A. Tonelli, L.C. Barros, N.R.S. Ortega, Clinical sings of pneumonia in children: association with and prediction od diagnosis by fuzzy sets theory. Braz. J. Med. Biol. Res. **37**, 1–9 (2004)
9. C.M. Bishop, *Neural Networks for Pattern Recognition* (Oxford University Press, Oxford, 1995)
10. P. Sussner, E. Esmi, *Constructive Morphological Neural Networks: Some Theoretical Aspects and Experimental Results in Classification.* Constructive Neural Networks (Springer, Berlin, 2009), pp. 123–144
11. W. Wangning, Fuzzy reasoning and fuzzy relational equations. Fuzzy Sets Syst. **20**, 67–78 (1986)
12. W. Pedrycz, F. Gomide, *An Introduction to Fuzzy Sets: Analysis and Design* (The MIT Press, Cambridge, 1998)
13. E. Sanchez, Resolution of composite fuzzy relation equations. Inf. Control **30**, 35–47 (1976)
14. M. Wergenknecht, K. Hartmann, On the construction of fuzzy eigen soluyions in given regions. Fuzzy Sets Syst. **20**, 55–65 (1996)
15. D.C. Montgomery, *Forecasting and Time Series Analysis* (St. Louis: McGraw-Hill, New York, 1976)
16. A. Min, C. Czado, Bayesian model selection for D-vine pair-copula constructions. Can. J. Stat. **39**(2), 239–258 (2011)
17. F. Bacani, *Modelos de predição utilizando lógica fuzzy: uma abordagem inspirada na inferência bayesiana.* Dissertação de Mestrado, IMECC-UNICAMP, Campinas, 2012
18. F. Bacani, L.C. Barros, *Application of Prediction Models Using Fuzzy Sets: A Bayesian Inspired Approach* (2016) (submitted for publication)
19. L.C. Barros, F. Bacani, E.E. Laureano, Equação relacional fuzzy e inferência bayesiana, in *Proceedings of Second Brazilian Conference on Fuzzy Systems* (Brazil, 2012)
20. H.T. Nguyen, E.A. Walker, *A First Course of Fuzzy Logic* (CRC Press, Boca Raton, 1997)
21. M.R.B. Dias, L.C. Barros, Differential equations based on fuzzy rules, in *IFSA/EUSFLAT Conference* (2009), pp. 240–246
22. J.D.M. Silva, *Análise de estabilidade de sistemas dinâmicos p-fuzzy com aplicações em bio-matemática.* Tese de Doutorado, IMECC-UNICAMP, Campinas (2005)
23. H.T. Nguyen, M. Sugeno, R. Tang, R. Yager (eds.), Theoretical aspects of fuzzy control, in *IEEE International Conference on Fuzzy Systems 1993* (Wiley, New York, 1995)

Chapter 7
Measure, Integrals and Fuzzy Events

In every field of knowledge, there is a tendency for the quantitative, for the measure. So, it can be stated that the scientific study of each branch of knowledge begins when a measure is introduced and the study of quantitative variation is the evolution of the qualitative.

(B. J. Caraça)

Abstract This chapter reviews classical measure theory including probability and Lebesgue measures. This discussion is followed by fuzzy measures, Sugeno measures, and possibilistic measures in order to understand the integration of Lebesgue, Choquet and Sugeno. These concepts are used in the development of fuzzy expected value. Lastly, the chapter closes with a discussion of the concepts of fuzzy event, the probability of a fuzzy event, dependence of fuzzy events, independence of fuzzy events, together with the concepts of random linguistic variables and random fuzzy variables.

The main objective in this chapter is to discuss questions related to the mathematical formulations of certain types of qualitative subjectivities and their measurements. We seek to discuss and clarify some differences and similarities between probability theory and possibility theory. Intuitively, the probability of an event is related to its occurrence. A possibility distribution function is related to the identification of the event itself. In a random experiment, the uncertainty ends at the time the event occurs. In the possibilistic case, the question remains. The event is not totally clear; it has uncertain boundaries. For example, in the probabilistic case, after tossing a coin, we have no doubts about the outcome: heads or tails. In the possibilistic case, doubt occurs even after the coin is tossed if one cannot clearly see the coin.

The axiomatic foundation of possibility theory lies in fuzzy measure. Moreover, we will use fuzzy measures as the basis for fuzzy integration and fuzzy expectation. We use these in various application found subsequently. Consequently we begin this chapter with fuzzy measure.

© Springer-Verlag Berlin Heidelberg 2017
L.C. de Barros et al., *A First Course in Fuzzy Logic, Fuzzy Dynamical Systems, and Biomathematics*, Studies in Fuzziness and Soft Computing 347, DOI 10.1007/978-3-662-53324-6_7

7.1 Classic Measure and Fuzzy Measure

Measure theory is a major area of mathematical analysis. The notion of measure generalizes the usual concepts of length, area, volume, etc. A probability measure is a typical case of a measure, where range is restricted to the interval [0, 1]. As we shall see, fuzzy measures also have the same range. The classical measure of interest in this chapter is the probability measure. The reader interested in general measure theory can see, for example, [1] or [2] among others.

7.1.1 Probability Measure

Probability measures have been frequently been used to make predictions. Many experiments analyze random events. In this case, the stochastic approach associates each random experiment to a sample space. For each sample space the occurrence of event is studied.

The measure of the chance of occurrence of an event is its probability which is represented by a real number in the interval [0, 1]. For experiments with a finite number of outcomes, the probability of an event is defined as the ratio between the number of favorable cases divided by the number of a possible cases in the sample space. An axiomatic definition of probability was developed by Kolmogorov [3].

As already mentioned, the central idea in the definition of probability is to associate each event of a sample space a number in the interval [0, 1] which indicates its likelihood of occurrence. Thus, the probability is simply a real function of sets, a set-value function. Formally, a function of sets is a probability measure if it satisfies some properties, specific to measures and its domain is called σ-algebra.

Definition 7.1 Let Ω be a sample spaces. A family $\mathcal{A}$ of subsets of Ω is called σ-algebra if it satisfies the following axioms:

(σ_1) The empty set $\emptyset$ is in $\mathcal{A}$;
(σ_2) If a event A belongs to $\mathcal{A}$, then its complement $A' = \Omega - A$ also belongs to $\mathcal{A}$;
(σ_3) If the event $A_1, A_2, \ldots$ belong to $\mathcal{A}$, then their union also belongs to $\mathcal{A}$.

As consequence of the axioms of a σ-algebra $\mathcal{A}$ it follow that:

(σ_4) The sample space Ω belongs to $\mathcal{A}$;
(σ_5) If the events $A_1, A_2, \ldots$ belong to $\mathcal{A}$, then the intersection of events must belong to $\mathcal{A}$.

Thus, we have

$$
\begin{cases}
(\sigma_1) & \emptyset \in \mathcal{A} \\
(\sigma_2) & A \in \mathcal{A} \Longrightarrow A' \in \mathcal{A} \\
(\sigma_3) & A_1, A_2, \ldots, A_i, \ldots \in \mathcal{A} \Longrightarrow \bigcup_{i \in \mathbb{N}} A_i \in \mathcal{A} \\
(\sigma_4) & \Omega \in \mathcal{A} \\
(\sigma_5) & A_1, A_2, \ldots, A_i, \ldots \in \mathcal{A} \Longrightarrow \bigcap_{i \in \mathbb{N}} A_i \in \mathcal{A}.
\end{cases}
\tag{7.1}
$$

An example of a σ-algebra is the set of all subsets of Ω called the power set of omega $\Omega : \mathcal{P}(\Omega) = \{A : A \subset \Omega\}$.

Definition 7.2 Given the domain $\mathcal{A}$, a probability measure P must satisfy the following axioms:

(P_1) For every event A of $\mathcal{A}$, the probability measure $P(A)$ is a real number between 0 and 1;

(P_2) The probability measure of the sample space Ω is 1;

(P_3) The probability of the union of events that are pairwise disjoint is the sum of each probability

This is formally written as:

$$
\begin{cases}
(P_1) & \forall A \in \mathcal{A} \Longrightarrow 0 \le P(A) \le 1; \\
(P_2) & P(\Omega) = 1; \\
(P_3) & \text{If } A_1, A_2, \ldots, A_i, \ldots \in \mathcal{A} \text{ and } A_i \cap A_j = \emptyset, i \ne j, \\
& \quad \text{then } P\left(\bigcup_{i \in N} A_i\right) = \sum_{i \in \mathbb{N}} P(A_i)
\end{cases}
\tag{7.2}
$$

Property P_3 is called sigma-additivity. As consequence of the axions of probability measure we have:

(P_4) $P(\emptyset) = 0$; because $\Omega = \Omega \cup \emptyset \cup \emptyset \cup \ldots$. Then, it follows that $P(\Omega) = P(\Omega) + \Sigma P(\emptyset)$. Therefore, $P(\emptyset) = 0$.

(P_5) If $A \subseteq B$ then $P(A) \le P(B)$ (*monotonicity*);

(P_6) $\forall A \in \mathcal{A}, P(A') = 1 - P(A)$ (*complement*), where A' is the complement of A;

(P_7) $\forall A, B \in \mathcal{A}, P(A \cup B) = P(A) + P(B) - P(A \cap B)$ (*additivity*);

(P_8) If $A_1 \subseteq A_2 \subseteq \ldots \subseteq A_i \subseteq \ldots$ then $P\left(\bigcup_{i \in N} A_i\right) = \lim_{i \to \infty} P(A_i)$ (*continuity*);

(P_9) If $A_1 \supseteq A_2 \supseteq \ldots \supseteq A_i \supseteq \ldots$ then $P\left(\bigcap_{i \in N} A_i\right) = \lim_{i \to \infty} P(A_i)$ (*continuity*).

Probability measures are σ-additive. However, sigma-additivity of probability measures excludes many intuitive ways that measures operate. The next example illustrate how strong the requirement of sigma-additivity is.

Example 7.1 Suppose that we want to measure the productivity of a group of workers in an industry. Let $\mu(A)$ represent the productivity of the subgroup A of workers. In this case, it is unreasonable to require that $\mu(A)$ is necessarily additive, that is, $\mu(A \cup B) = \mu(A) + \mu(B)$, for $A \cap B = \emptyset$. It may occur that $\mu(A \cup B) < \mu(A) + \mu(B)$ if there is an incompatibility between the operation of subgroup A and subgroup B. Or it may occur that $\mu(A \cup B) > \mu(A) + \mu(B)$ if there is synergy between the subgroups A and B.[1]

Many areas where phenomena must be "measured " are not sigma-additive as illustrated by the example. So it is unreasonable to always expect additivity. In the 1950s, Choquet [5] used the concept of *capacity measure* in problems of mechanics. Such measures do not require σ-additivity in the definition of a classic measure.

In summary, measures of uncertainty need to also have a place for non-additive functions. The question is what types of uncertainties are needed in a mathematical model? While this question is difficult to answer, what is clear, is that non-additive measures are needed in many models of uncertainty.

7.2   Fuzzy Measure

Sugeno in 1974 [6] proposed the concept of fuzzy measure by replacing axiom P_3 of the definition of probability measure by the continuity property P_7. This text calls the measure with this change the *Sugeno measure*.

Definition 7.3 (*Sugeno Measure*) Let $\mathcal{A}$ be a σ-algebra on $\Omega \neq \emptyset$. A set-valued function $\mu_S : \mathcal{A} \rightarrow [0, 1]$ is called a *Sugeno Measure* if

 (i) $\mu_S(\emptyset) = 0$ and $\mu_S(\Omega) = 1$;
 (ii) $\forall A, B \in \mathcal{A}$, if $A \subseteq B$, then $\mu_S(A) \leq \mu_S(B)$;
 (iii)   If $A_1 \subseteq A_2 \subseteq \ldots \subseteq A_i \subseteq \ldots$ then $\mu_S \left(\bigcup_{i \in \mathbb{N}} A_i \right) = \lim_{i \to \infty} \mu_S(A_i)$;
 (iv)   If $A_1 \supseteq A_2 \supseteq \ldots \supseteq A_i \supseteq \ldots$ then $\mu_S \left(\bigcap_{i \in \mathbb{N}} A_i \right) = \lim_{i \to \infty} \mu_S(A_i)$.

The Sugeno measure is also called in many texts (see Klir/Yuan pp. xxx) a *fuzzy measure*. The basic propriety that any measure must have for a theory of integration is monotonicity. With a Sugeno Measure, it is possible to extend the scope of mathematical modeling to encompass non-additive uncertainties.

The definition of fuzzy measure is not always the same in the literature. For example it is very common to demand measures to be monotonic and positive. However, among the several various definitions, what is common is the requirement of monotonicity and that a measure of empty set is null. The capacity measure of Choquet (see [5]) is such an example. This text will adopts the following definition of fuzzy measure.

---

[1] Adapted from Murofushi [4].

Definition 7.4 Let $\mathcal{A}$ be a $\sigma-$algebra on $\Omega \neq \emptyset$. A set-valued function $\mu : \mathcal{A} \longrightarrow$ [0, 1] is called a *fuzzy measure* if

(i) $\mu(\emptyset) = 0$ and $\mu(\Omega) = 1$;
(ii) $\mu(A) \leq \mu(B)$ whenever $A \subseteq B$.

The Sugeno measure is a particular fuzzy measure.

Example 7.2 Let $\mathcal{A}$ be a σ-algebra and the function $g_\lambda : \mathcal{A} \longrightarrow$ [0, 1] satisfying:

(1) $g_\lambda(\Omega) = 1$;
(2) $g_\lambda(A \cup B) = g_\lambda(A) + g_\lambda(B) + \lambda g_\lambda(A) g_\lambda(B)$, for some $\lambda > -1$, if $A \cap B = \emptyset$.

We show that g_λ is a fuzzy measure. Indeed it is enough to check that $g_\lambda(\emptyset) = 0$ and $g_\lambda(A) \leq g_\lambda(B)$ if $A \subseteq B$.

- $1 = g_\lambda(\Omega) = g_\lambda(\Omega \cup \emptyset) = g_\lambda(\Omega) + g_\lambda(\emptyset) + \lambda g_\lambda(\Omega) g_\lambda(\emptyset) =$
  $= 1 + g_\lambda(\emptyset) + \lambda g_\lambda(\emptyset)$,
  This means that,

$$1 = 1 + g_\lambda(\emptyset) + \lambda g_\lambda(\emptyset) \iff (1 + \lambda)g_\lambda(\emptyset) = 0.$$

Then, from (2), follows that $g_\lambda(\emptyset) = 0$ because $\lambda > -1$.
- If $A \subseteq B$ then $B = A \cup (B - A)$ and $A \cap (B - A) = \emptyset$

$$\begin{aligned} g_\lambda(B) &= g_\lambda(A \cup (B - A)) \\ &= g_\lambda(A) + g_\lambda(B - A) + \lambda g_\lambda(A) g_\lambda(B - A) \\ &= g_\lambda(A) + [1 + \lambda g_\lambda(A)] g_\lambda(B - A). \end{aligned}$$

However, $[1 + \lambda g_\lambda(A)]g_\lambda(B - A) \geq 0$. Thus, $g_\lambda(B) \geq g_\lambda(A)$.

Exercise 7.1. Show that for $\lambda = 0$, g_λ is a Sugeno measure if, and only if, g_λ is a probability measure (Suggestion: see Proposition 1.4 in [7, 8]).

Example 7.3 Consider a pack of n wolves, i.e., the set $\Omega = \{x_1, x_2, \ldots, x_n\}$. For each element of Ω we attribute a number $p_i \in [0, 1]$ for degree of predation. Predation p_i will be dependent on age (puppy, young, adult, old). Let's define a function g in the set $\mathscr{P}(\Omega)$, the power set of Ω, to be the "potentiality of predation in a hunt".

The potential predation for the whole pack is maximum, that is,

$$g(\Omega) = g(\{x_1, x_2, \ldots, x_n\}) = 1.$$

For each one of the subgroups A and B, with $A \cap B = \emptyset$, it is possible that

$$g(A \cup B) = g(A) + g(B) + \lambda g(A)g(B) \text{ for any } \lambda > -1.$$

According to Example 7.2, the potential of predation, given by g, is a fuzzy measure.

Let us further explore Example 7.3 by investigating the power of fuzzy measures to model the phenomenon "predation", evaluating the performance of the participation of younger wolves in a hunt:

- if they do not contribute very much (sometimes capture the prey but sometimes scare away the prey), then we choose λ in the interval $(-1, 0)$;
- if they moderately contribute to the hunt (do not startle the prey) we have $\lambda = 0$;
- if they strongly contribute to the hunt (capture and run the prey towards stronger wolves), then we consider $\lambda > 0$.

Another concept that is typically studied in the context of fuzzy set theory is *possibility*. This subject was introduced by Zadeh and has grown both in its theory and in its applicability.

Possibility measures are special measure within evidence theory (see Klir and Yuan [9]) and so are associated with probability theory.

7.3   Possibility Measure

In 1978 Zadeh published the first article on possibility measure [10]. This article brings to the fore an important discussions dealing with the theoretical, semantic, and practical distinctions between possibility and probability. One of these distinction is with respect to an affirmation, seemingly naive, but quite common in day-to-day usage, "a fact is possible but unlikely". This suggests that, whatever concept we use for possibility (a measure that we denote by Π), we need have $\Pi(A) \geq P(A)$. Currently, this inequality has been much debated and is often called the *Principle of Consistency* (see Klir and Yuan [9]).To introduce the concept of a possibility measure, it is interesting to bring up a few preliminary reflections.

Suppose that for a given problem we wish to get the value of a parameter ω_0. However, the only information available is that the value belongs to certain space Ω. This partial knowledge about ω_0 indicates that some model of uncertainty should be used to estimate ω_0. If for some reason it is known that all elements of Ω are equally possible, then it is possible to assume a uniform distribution in Ω to estimate ω_0. However, from the point of view of possibility theory all elements of Ω have the same degree of possibility.

Now, if there is gradation associated with the information (given by a specialist, for example), that is, there are elements more plausible than others in Ω, how does one treat such information? Again, the stochastic treatment suggests the adoption of a probability distribution and use it in order to obtain ω_0. From a fuzzy set theory point of view, the information of a specialist in fuzzy sets theory, is treated by mean membership functions where the expert indicates which of the elements of Ω must be given more or less "weight" according to their knowledge. The adoption of a mathematical model designed a priori or constructed together with a expert is a key difference between probability theory and possibility in the mathematical treatment of uncertainties.

In summary, for stochastic theory, the available information is treated by probability density functions. In possibility theory it is via a possibility measure. The possibility function will be function viewed as a *distribution of possibilities* on Ω. Note that, formally, φ is a typical derived from a membership function of a fuzzy subset of Ω.

The following example illustrates a typical way information is treated by expert which can be modeled by a possibility distribution.

Example 7.4 In the proposition "*X is a small number*", consider that *small number* is given by a fuzzy subset of non-negative integer numbers. In this case, we have a possibility distribution (not formally defined yet) instead of a probability distribution for X because in the absence of a survey on what a "small number "is among a population, this concept in not probabilistic. That is, it is still possible to say to what degree an integer n conforms to the subjective notion of *small numbers* without a survey. This degree can be given by a number, $\varphi_X(n)$ which indicates a "tendency " of n to be small and $\varphi_X : N \to [0, 1]$ is interpreted as a possibility distribution of X on the set of natural numbers. On the other hand, how does one obtain $P(n)$ for the probability of n?

We present a short summary of the theory of possibilities.

Definition 7.5 A *possibility distribution* on the set $\Omega \neq \emptyset$ is a function $\varphi : \Omega \to$ $[0, 1]$ satisfying $\sup_{\omega \in \Omega} \varphi(\omega) = 1$.

We note that any normal fuzzy subset of Ω can be used to define a possibility distribution on Ω. However, as Zadeh [11] points out, the semantics of the entity being modeled is associated with information deficiency or lack of information, or incomplete information.

Definition 7.6 Let $\mathcal{A}$ be a σ−algebra on $\Omega \neq \emptyset$. A set-valued function $\Pi : \mathcal{A} \to$ $[0, 1]$ is called a *possibility measure* if it satisfies:

(a) $\Pi(\emptyset) = 0$ and $\Pi(\Omega) = 1$;
(b) For any family $\{A_{i \in \mathbb{J}}\}$ of subsets on Ω follows

$$\Pi \left(\bigcup_{i \in \mathbb{J}} A_i \right) = \sup\{\Pi(A_i) : i \in \mathbb{J}\},$$

where $\mathbb{J}$ is an index set.

Note that, given the possibility measure Π, this induces a possibility distribution function, φ_Π on Ω through its restriction on the elements of Ω, in other words, $\varphi_\Pi(\omega) = \Pi(\{\omega\})$. On the other hand, given a possibility distribution function, this measure induces a possibility over Ω given by

$$\Pi(A) = \begin{cases} \sup_{\omega \in A} \varphi(\omega) & \text{if } A \neq \emptyset \\ 0 & \text{if } A = \emptyset \end{cases},$$

for all $A \in \mathcal{A}$.

It follows from the definition of possibility measure that, for any subsets A, B $\in \mathcal{A}$,

$$\Pi(A \cup B) = \max \{\Pi(A), \Pi(B)\}.$$

Moreover, $\Pi(A) \leq \Pi(B)$ whenever $A \subseteq B$. Thus, any possibility measure is a fuzzy measure.

We next look at the differences between the probability and possibility distribution by considering the following example.

Example 7.5 [2]After a few days lost in the desert a man finds an oasis with two water sources. The first source has a sign written: "the probability of the water being contaminated is 0.02 ". That is, $p(A) = 0.02$. At the second source the inscription on the sign reads: "the degree of possible contamination of this source is 0.02 ", i.e., $\Pi(A) = 0.02$. The question to be answered is which source should the individual choose.

We observed that the question in this case is not just a semantic matter but of health because if the individual drinks water from the first source, there is great chance that she or he will drink clean water, but there is a 2 % risk of being poisoned. If the person chooses the second source, she or he is not completely sure of drinking potable water and her or his only risk is something like diarrhea or headache.

Note that only posteriori analysis is it possible be sure of the content of each source. The process of inference is a rational effort to predict the unknown. What should be debated is what kind of knowledge best instructs decision making. It may be noted by this example has the two logical structures resulting in two distinct processes of knowledge acquisition, two epistemological alternatives. What is the better informed approach to knowledge, chance or trend? Chance/probability affirms that the water is or is not contaminated indicating whether or not the water is drinkable. The second source indicates the degree of contamination which is the level of contamination.

Probability and degrees of possibility have distinct natures in their interpretations. Although both are expressed by values between **zero** and **one** and both indicate uncertainty, probability assesses and describes the **chance** of a particular event to occur, whereas possibility measures the **tendency of an event** (to occur).

The following example continues our discussion of the difference the between probability and possibility, though stressing that not all fuzzy membership functions can be interpreted as a possibility distribution.

Example 7.6 (*Epidemiology*) In epidemic studies it is a very common concern to know how strong the infectiousness of a disease is, that is, how many people are infected by an infectious element. This is closely related to the parameter, $\beta \in [0, 1]$ which indicates the rate at which susceptible individuals become infected. Biologically, the parameter β, called the *transmission coefficient rate*, is directly linked to the chance of disease transmission to occur when there is contact between a susceptible and an infected individual.

---

[2]Adapted from Bezdek [12].

This parameter is evaluated in classical models (deterministic) by a kind of average obtained from the population and, thereby, all infecting individuals have the same "power" to infect susceptible individuals. It is as if we were to assume homogeneity in the class of those infected. However, this assumption is a very naive one since it is quite reasonable to expect the opposite, that is, there exist individuals with greater power to transmit the disease than others. The reasons for this are quite different (see Sadegh-Zadeh [13]). One of those, which will be the only one considered here, is the viral load that can be modeled by $\beta = \beta(v)$ where v represents the the viral load which the infectious individual possesses. Given the considerations made so far, the parameter β can be seen as a membership function of some fuzzy subset over a universe in which the viral load assumes its values. Since v can be translated into a number, its domain is the set of nonnegative real numbers. Thus,

$$\beta : \mathbb{R}^+ \to [0, 1].$$

The number $\beta(v)$ just reflects the degree to which that β is related to v, that is, the effect of v on the parameter β. Knowing the value v_0 of the viral load we have an effect on the value of β.

So far we have not considered any kind of uncertainty. No information about the viral load was given in obtaining v_0 and thus we have no indication that the function β corresponds to a possibility distribution. However, from an expert of the disease in question, we may obtain information such as v_0 belongs to the interval $[v_{\min}, v_{\max}]$. In this case, we can think of a mathematical model in an attempt to evaluate v_0, in a selected space for the parameter in question. In addition to which the space the parameter belongs, we know that there are values of $v \in [v_{\min}, v_{\max}]$ that are more plausible than others, given by "weights" $\rho(v) \in [0, 1]$. With this, it possible to establish a *possibility distribution*

$$\rho : [v_{\min}, v_{\max}] \to [0, 1]$$

for v in an attempt to evaluate v_0.

This function ρ can be directly "built" by the specialist according to their empirical knowledge or from data. Such a function need not be a probability density distribution known a priori. Further, ρ is not necessarily a probability density distribution - its integral can be different than 1. This discussion points out differences between possibilistic and stochastic methods in obtaining an estimation of the parameter v_0.

We can say that the probability density distribution is to the probability measure what the possibility distribution is to the possibility measure. For example, consider $A \subset \Omega = \mathbb{R}$. If for any $v \in [v_{\min}, v_{\max}]$ we have $\rho(v) = 1$, then the possibility distribution ρ induces a possibility measure Ω given by

$$\Pi(A) = \begin{cases} \sup_{v \in A} \rho(v) & \text{if } A \neq \emptyset \\ 0 & \text{If } A = \emptyset \end{cases}.$$

Fig. 7.1 Relationships of
fuzzy measures

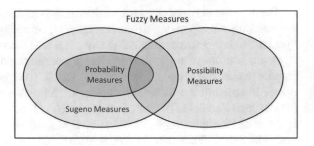

It is not difficult to see that, in this case, Π is also a possibility measurement.

If $\int_{\Omega} \rho(v)dv = 1$, then ρ is a probability density distribution that induces a probability measure on Ω, given by

$$P(A) = \int_A \rho(v)dv.$$

It is not difficult to see that P is also a Sugeno measure. However Π is not a Sugeno measure [14]. On the other hand, in any finite space the concepts of possibility measure and Sugeno measure are equivalent (see [14, 15]).

Figure 7.1 summarizes the relationships among the measures we discussed above. The following subsection concludes our discussion about measures.

7.4 Probability/Possibility Transformations

It is essential find a way to transform possibility to probability vice versa in many practical problems. For example, we may wish to construct a possibility function from a set of statistical data or the reverse, that is, to construct a probability density function from a possibility distribution. Also, in many cases, it may be interesting to compare the information obtained from the two methods applied to the same phenomenon.

All the methods in the literature used to transform probability into possibility, or vice versa, have something in common, they all obey the *Principle of Consistency*, commented at the beginning of Sect. 7.1.3, that is

$$P(A) \leq \Pi(A) \text{ for all } A \subseteq \Omega.$$

Here we focus only on the method of transformation between probability and possibility in the case in which Ω is a finite space. Thus, we suppose that $\Omega = \{\omega_1, \omega_2, \ldots, \omega_n\}$, and that

$$\Pi(\omega_1) \geq \Pi(\omega_2) \geq \ldots \geq \Pi(\omega_n) \text{ and } P(\omega_1) \geq P(\omega_2) \geq \ldots \geq P(\omega_n).$$

The simplest transformation, and the only one discussed here, is:

$$\text{(a)} \quad \Pi(\omega_i) = \frac{P(\omega_i)}{P(\omega_1)} \quad \text{and} \quad \text{(b)} \quad P(\omega_i) = \frac{\Pi(\omega_i)}{\sum\limits_{i=1}^{n} \Pi(\omega_i)}.$$

The example below is a summary of a study made by Castanho [16] in her doctoral thesis.

Example 7.7 (*Diagnosis of Prostate Cancer*) The physician, in the process of diagnosing, evaluates the stage of prostate cancer to indicate a proper treatment. It is known that treatments, such as surgery or radiotherapy, have a high chance of cure if the cancer is confined to the organ. To evaluate the stage of the prostate cancer the physician has reviewed information provided by clinical examinations (rectal examination and/or imaging, blood test that measures the level of prostate specific antigen (PSA) which is a substance that increases with the increase of the tumor, and biopsy). A biopsy of the tumor is classified by the Gleason Score according to the degree of differentiation of cells (tumor aggressiveness).

Combining these three variables (rectal exam, PSA, biopsy) and using data in the urological literature, there are several tables that indicate the likelihood of the patient being at a particular developmental stage of the disease (incursions into the prostatic capsule, vesicles seminal, and pelvic lymph nodes). These ratings are clearly subjective. The boundaries between each of these stages are fuzzy, which suggests treating them as linguistic variables as we saw in Chap. 4.

Castanho [16] developed a system based on fuzzy rules to obtain the stage of the disease using the linguistic variables associated with the type of the incursions. In this system the output variable (disease stage) is modeled by means of fuzzy sets. For every real value that represents the system output there is a corresponding degree of membership of the fuzzy set that describes a stage of the disease. The proposition "stage of the disease is confined ", for example, allows one to see this level as a possibility of the disease to be confined to the prostate. Accordingly, this proposition defines a possibility distribution in the set of individuals.

The same phenomenon with information given in probabilistic terms (probability tables) can be transformed into a possibilistic distribution using the method initially proposed by [16, 17]. Consistency needs to be checked. For example, suppose a patient has the following pre-surgical data: clinical state classified as *palpable*; limited to *less than half of one lobe* (a *lobe* is each of the two parts in which a prostate is anatomically subdivided); PSA level equal to 5.3 ng/ml (ng means nanogram) and Gleason biopsy degree of 7.0. According to the rule-based system, the possibility of this patient having cancer confined to the prostate is 0.60; that he has capsular involvement is 0.93 and incursion into the vesicle and/or lymph nodes is 0.11. Using the transformation

$$P(\omega_i) = \frac{\Pi(\omega_i)}{\displaystyle\sum_{i=1}^{n} \Pi(\omega_i)},$$

we obtain the following probabilities: 0.36; 0.57 and 0.07, respectively. In the probability tables of Partin (see [16]) we found 0.33; 0.52 and 0.14 respectively. At least for this case, we can say that the results given in terms of probability indicating the likelihood results is about the same as that obtained from a possibilistic approach.

Castanho et al. [16, 18] developed a method she called the ROC-Fuzzy which is an adaptation of the classic Roc Curve (*Receiver Operating Characteristic*), used in signal systems and also in medicine to assess the power of a test. More recently, Silveira [19] redid the study of Castanho to compare the fuzzy method with nomograms of Katan [20] and developed a software system to help the urologist in similar ways as those of traditional nomograms.

The reader can find other possibility to probability transformations in various texts of fuzzy logic [9, 16, 21–24]. Let us close this section by commenting that, in an effort to obtain an expected value that estimates a certain parameter, as discussed in Example 7.6, beyond the concept of measure, we need the notion of integral, similar to what is done in the classical case.

Briefly, we can draw a parallel among the methodologies of fuzzy and stochastic in order to obtain values that estimate parameters for example. In the stochastic case, from a randomized experiment, we have a density distribution function that in turn induces a probability measure. From this measure we can construct integrals and then in the possibilistic case, which can be constructed from expert knowledge or constructed from a set of statistical data, we have a possibility distribution function which induces a possibility measure.

The idea is to construct a fuzzy integral from the fuzzy measure and finally obtain an expected value. Thus, in the following section we will focus our study on several kinds of integrals.

7.5   Fuzzy Integrals

The above presented a short justification of the need to study the concept of integral, although both in mathematics or most commonly in the exact sciences, such a concept does not need any motivation. Its importance in the theoretical disciplines of mathematical analysis is no less than that in applied mathematical analysis where the integral is used in various types of problems such as the calculation of volumes, areas, energy, work to mention a few uses. This section presents some concepts and properties of integrals with respect to both classical and fuzzy measures.

7.5.1 Lebesgue Integral

We will next show the basic idea of how to construction of the Lebesgue integral with respect to an abstract measure, without being concerned with more theoretical issues such as the existence of the integral. This will serve as a model for integration from fuzzy measure which is the main concern of this section. The basic idea is the following: given the fact that *all positive functions f are limits of a sequence of simple functions*, we initially define the Lebesgue integral for simple functions. Therefore, the integral of an arbitrary positive function f is defined as the limit of integrals of these simple functions that converge to f.

Suppose that $g : \Omega \to [0, \infty)$ is a simple function,

$$g(\omega) = \sum_{i=1}^{k} \alpha_i \chi_{A_i}(\omega),$$

with A_i, $1 \le i \le k$, a countable partition of Ω and χ_{A_i} the characteristic function of A_i.

Definition 7.7 Let μ be a (σ-additive) measure in Ω. The *Lebesgue Integral* of the simple function g over Ω, with respect to the (classic) measure μ, is given by

$$\int_{\Omega} g \, d\mu = \sum_{i=1}^{k} \alpha_i \mu(A_i). \tag{7.3}$$

Example 7.8 Consider that g is given by only three distinct (positive) values: α_1, α_2, and α_3. Then,

$$g(\omega) = \alpha_1 \chi_{A_1}(\omega) + \alpha_2 \chi_{A_2}(\omega) + \alpha_3 \chi_{A_3}(\omega), \quad \forall \omega \in \Omega.$$

Therefore

$$\int_{\Omega} g \, d\mu = \alpha_1 \mu(A_1) + \alpha_2 \mu(A_2) + \alpha_3 \mu(A_3).$$

Note that each parcel $\alpha_i \mu(A_i)$ can be seen as a "area" and the integral of g is the total area defined by its graph. Figure 7.2 illustrates the Lebesgue integral of g.

On the other hand, the area mentioned above, which gives the Lebesgue integral of g, can be obtained by partitioning on the vertical axis α. From this point of view, this area is given by

$$\mu\{\omega \in \Omega : g(\omega) > 0\}(\alpha_1 - 0) + \mu\{\omega \in \Omega : g(\omega) > \alpha_1\}(\alpha_2 - \alpha_1)$$
$$+ \mu\{\omega \in \Omega : g(\omega) > \alpha_2\}(\alpha_3 - \alpha_2) =$$
$$= \int_{0}^{\alpha_3} \mu\{\omega \in \Omega : g(\omega) > \alpha\} \, d\alpha$$

where the latter corresponds to the Riemann integral of the function $h(\alpha) = \mu\{\omega \in \Omega : g(\omega) > \alpha\}$ with respect to α. Thus, we obtain

$$\int_{\Omega} g \, \mathrm{d}\mu = \int_{0}^{\alpha_3} \mu\{\omega \in \Omega : g(\omega) > \alpha\} \, \mathrm{d}\alpha.$$

This example can be generalized to any simple function, that is,

$$\int_{\Omega} g \, \mathrm{d}\mu = \sum_{i=0}^{\infty} \mu\{\omega \in \Omega : g(\omega) > \alpha_i\}(\alpha_{(i+1)} - \alpha_i)$$

$$= \int_{0}^{\infty} \mu\{\omega \in \Omega : g(\omega) > \alpha\} \, \mathrm{d}\alpha. \qquad (7.4)$$

According to we have said above, a positive function $f : \Omega \to [0, \infty)$ is the limit of a sequence of simple functions. The Lebesgue integral with respect to (classical) measure μ is the limits of the integrals of these simple functions. Hence, and from (7.4) we have

$$\int_{\Omega} f \, \mathrm{d}\mu = (\text{"area" defined by the graph of } f \text{ over } \Omega)$$

$$= \int_{0}^{\infty} h(\alpha) \, \mathrm{d}\alpha \qquad (7.5)$$

with $h(\alpha) = \mu\{\omega \in \Omega : f(\omega) > \alpha\}$. Formula (7.5) indicates that the abstract Lebesgue integral of f can be obtained from the Riemann integral of the function that provides a measure of the "levels" of f (see Fig. 7.3).

An immediate consequence of Formula (7.5) is that if $X : \Omega \to [0, \infty)$ is a random variable in Ω with probability measure P, then

$$E(X) = \int_{\Omega} X \, \mathrm{d}P = \int_{0}^{\infty} P[X > x] \, \mathrm{d}x,$$

where $E(X)$ is the expected value of X and

Fig. 7.2 Lebesgue integral
of a simple function

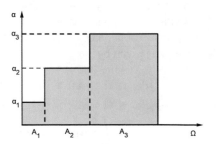

$$[X > x] = \{\omega \in \Omega : X(\omega) > x\}.$$

This is a widely used result in the calculation of expected value of random variables and it serves as a motivation for the Choquet Integral, which has also been used in the theory of fuzzy integrals since the Choquet integral, requires no additivity in the measure. Note that if X is a random variable with $X(\omega) \geq 0$, $\forall \omega \in \Omega$, it follows that $E(X) = \int_0^\infty (1 - F(x))\, dx$ where $F(x) = P(X \leq x)$ is cumulative distribution function of X. For discrete case, we have

$$E(X) = \sum_{n=0}^\infty P(X > n) = \sum_{n=1}^\infty P(x \geq n).$$

7.5.2 Choquet Integral

The Choquet Integral, being one that does not require an additive measure, brings us closer to our construction of integrals with fuzzy measure. Thus, it is presented next.

Definition 7.8 The *Choquet Integral* of the $f : \Omega \to [0, \infty)$ with the respect to a measure, not necessarily additive, μ, is given by:

$$(C) \int_\Omega f\, d\mu = \int_0^\infty \mu\{\omega \in \Omega : f(\omega) > \alpha\}\, d\alpha.$$

Note that if μ is not additive, some properties of the Lebesgue integral no longer apply. The main property is that of linearity, which means, if μ is not additive then it may happen that

$$(C) \int_\Omega (af + g)\, d\mu \neq a \left[(C) \int_\Omega f\, d\mu \right] + (C) \int_\Omega g\, d\mu.$$

Fig. 7.3 Riemann Integral of the function $h = \mu\{\omega \in \Omega : f(\omega) > \alpha\}$ and Lebesgue Integral of the function f

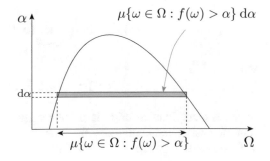

Intuitively, to obtain the Choquet Integral of a function

$$f : \Omega \to [0, \infty),$$

one only uses the concept of Riemann integral on the levels of f which are defined in the range of that function, the real numbers. Choquet has used this concept of integral with respect to the capacity measure (which is not additive) in studies of mechanics [5]. Recently, Sugeno has been proposed calculus theory based on Choquet Integral [25, 26].

7.5.3   Sugeno Integral

The Sugeno integral was introduced in the early 70 s and was called fuzzy integral [6]. The fuzzy integral was created to defuzzify fuzzy numbers using a measure that was not necessarily σ-additive.

The definition given here is for functions whose range is the interval [0, 1] so that it is applicable to fuzzy membership functions. However, this concept can be used for more general functions where the range is the set of positive real numbers. Thus, the requirement that the range of the function be [0, 1] could be set aside [27].

Definition 7.9 Let $f : \Omega \to [0, 1]$ be a function and μ a fuzzy measure on Ω. The *Sugeno Integral* of f on Ω with respect to μ is the number

$$
\begin{aligned}
(S) \int_\Omega f \, d\mu &= \sup_{0 \leq \alpha \leq 1} [\alpha \wedge \mu\{\omega \in \Omega : f(\omega) \geq \alpha\}] \\
&= \sup_{0 \leq \alpha \leq 1} [\alpha \wedge \mu\{\omega \in \Omega : f(\omega) > \alpha\}].
\end{aligned}
\tag{7.6}
$$

A first observation to be made is that the Sugeno integral can be formally obtained by replacing the sum by **supremum** (sup) and the product by **minimum** ($\wedge$) in the Lebesgue integral (or the Choquet integral) with respect to the measure. If A is a classic subset of Ω, then

$$(S) \int_A f \, d\mu = \sup_{0 \leq \alpha \leq 1} [\alpha \wedge \mu(A \cap H(\alpha)],$$

where

$$H(\alpha) = \mu\{\omega \in \Omega : f(\omega) \geq \alpha\}$$

is called *level function of f*. It is interesting to note that $H : [0, 1] \longrightarrow [0, 1]$ is a non-increasing and continuous function almost everywhere [15]. This observation will be useful in understanding the following results.

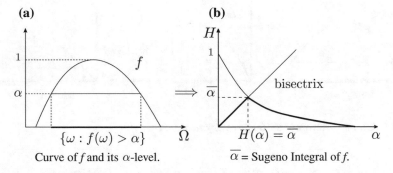

(a)

1

α

$\{\omega : f(\omega) > \alpha\}$ Ω

Curve of f and its α-level.

(b)

H

1

$\overline{\alpha}$ bisectrix

$H(\alpha) = \overline{\alpha}$ α

$\overline{\alpha}$ = Sugeno Integral of f.

Fig. 7.4 Illustration of Theorem 7.1

Theorem 7.1 *Let $f : \Omega \longrightarrow [0, 1]$ be a function (typically a membership function) and μ a fuzzy measure on Ω. If the function $H(\alpha) = \mu\{\omega \in \Omega : f(\omega) \geq \alpha\}$ has a fixed point $\overline{\alpha}$, then*

$$(S) \int_\Omega f \, d\mu = \overline{\alpha} = H(\overline{\alpha}). \tag{7.7}$$

In other words, the Sugeno Integral of f coincides with the fixed point of H, if it exists.

Proof The proof of this theorem can be found in [6]. ∎

The Fig. 7.4 is an illustration of this theorem.

The part of the curve in Fig. 7.4b indicates the value of $[\alpha \wedge H(\alpha)]$, for $\alpha \in [0, 1]$, and has as the supremum the value $\overline{\alpha}$, which is the intersection of the 45° line, $y = x$, with the graph of $H(\alpha)$ and therefore, $\overline{\alpha}$ is the fixed point of $H(\alpha)$.

Example 7.9 Let F be a fuzzy subset of $\mathbb{R}$ whose membership function $f : \mathbb{R} \to [0, 1]$ is given by $f(x) = -4x^2 + 4x$. Then,

$$[F]^\alpha = \left\{x \in \mathbb{R} : -4x^2 + 4x \geq \alpha\right\} = \left[\frac{1 - \sqrt{1 - \alpha}}{2}, \frac{1 + \sqrt{1 - \alpha}}{2}\right].$$

If we consider the usual Lebesgue measure m of the line which is, obviously, also a fuzzy measure, then

$$m([F]^\alpha) = \frac{1 + \sqrt{1 - \alpha}}{2} - \frac{1 - \sqrt{1 - \alpha}}{2} = \sqrt{1 - \alpha} = H(\alpha).$$

Therefore,

$$(S) \int_\mathbb{R} f \, dm = \sup_{0 \leq \alpha \leq 1} \left[\alpha \wedge \sqrt{1 - \alpha}\right].$$

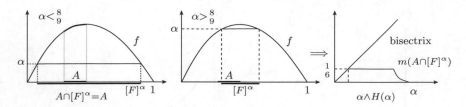

Fig. 7.5 Geometric layout of the Sugeno integral of f on A

The function $H(\alpha) = m([F]^{\alpha}) = \sqrt{1-\alpha}$, which associates to each α-level its measure, is monotone and decreasing and, in this case, it is continuous. By the Theorem 7.1, we have (Fig. 7.5)

$$(S) \int_{\mathbb{R}} f \, dm = H(\overline{\alpha}) = \overline{\alpha} = \frac{-1 + \sqrt{5}}{2}$$

because

$$H(\overline{\alpha}) = \overline{\alpha} \iff \sqrt{1-\overline{\alpha}} = \overline{\alpha} \implies \overline{\alpha} = \frac{-1 + \sqrt{5}}{2}.$$

Now, consider $A = \left[\frac{1}{3}, \frac{1}{2}\right]$. Then

$$m(A \cap [F]^{\alpha}) = \begin{cases} \dfrac{1}{6} & \text{if } \alpha \leq \dfrac{8}{9} \\ \dfrac{\sqrt{1-\alpha}}{2} & \text{if } \dfrac{8}{9} \leq \alpha \leq 1 \end{cases} \implies$$

$$[\alpha \wedge m(A \cap [F]^{\alpha})] = \begin{cases} \alpha & \text{if } \alpha \leq \dfrac{1}{6} \\ \dfrac{1}{6} & \text{if } \dfrac{1}{6} < \alpha \leq \dfrac{8}{9} \\ \dfrac{\sqrt{1-\alpha}}{2} & \text{if } \dfrac{8}{9} < \alpha \leq 1 \end{cases} \implies \int_{\left[\frac{1}{3}, \frac{1}{2}\right]} f \, dm = \frac{1}{6}.$$

We leave to the reader the task of obtaining

$$(C) \int f \, d\mu; \text{ and } \left| (C) \int f \, d\mu - (S) \int f \, d\mu \right|$$

for f from Example 7.9.

Theorem 7.2 *Let $f : \Omega \to [0, 1]$ be a function (typically a membership function) and μ a (classic) measure on Ω. Then,*

$$\left| (S) \int_{\Omega} f \, d\mu - \int_0^1 H(\alpha) \, d\alpha \right| \le \frac{1}{4}. \tag{7.8}$$

Note that $\int_0^1 H(\alpha) \, d\alpha = \int_0^1 \mu\{\omega \in \Omega : f(\omega) \ge \alpha\} \, d\alpha$ is the Choquet integral of the function f.

Proof We will only sketch the proof. The complete proof may be found in [6]. Let $\overline{\alpha} = H(\overline{\alpha})$ be the fixed point of $H(\alpha)$. Then,

$$\left| (S) \int_{\Omega} f \, d\mu - \int_0^1 H(\alpha) \, d\alpha \right| = \left| \overline{\alpha} - \int_0^1 H(\alpha) \, d\alpha \right| =$$

$$\left| \int_0^{\overline{\alpha}} 1 \, d\alpha - \left[\int_0^{\overline{\alpha}} H(\alpha) \, d\alpha + \int_{\overline{\alpha}}^1 H(\alpha) \, d\alpha \right] \right|.$$

It follows that

$$\left| \int_0^{\overline{\alpha}} (1 - H(\alpha)) \, d\alpha - \int_{\overline{\alpha}}^1 H(\alpha) \, d\alpha \right| \le \int_0^{\overline{\alpha}} (1 - H(\alpha)) \, d\alpha \le$$

$$\int_0^{\overline{\alpha}} (1 - H(\overline{\alpha})) \, d\alpha = \int_0^{\overline{\alpha}} (1 - \overline{\alpha}) \, d\alpha = (1 - \overline{\alpha})\overline{\alpha} \le \frac{1}{4},$$

since that $\overline{\alpha} \in [0, 1]$. ∎

Remark The penultimate inequality above is valid because H is a decreasing function. Importantly, it is not possible to reduce the maximum difference of $\frac{1}{4}$ appearing in the above theorem. This means that there are functions f for which this difference is reached [28].

Properties of the Sugeno Integral

The Sugeno integral is not linear, similar to the Choquet integral. Moreover, both are monotone, that is,

$$(S) \int_{\Omega} f \, d\mu \le (S) \int_{\Omega} g \, d\mu \text{ if } f \le g.$$

Below are several properties of the Sugeno integral whose proofs can be found in [6].

Let $f : \Omega \longrightarrow [0, 1]$ and $g : \Omega \longrightarrow [0, 1]$ be functions, μ a fuzzy measure on Ω, and A and B subsets of Ω. Then the following properties hold:

(i) If $f(x) = k$, then $(S) \int_A f \, d\mu = k \wedge \mu(A)$;

(ii) If $f \le g$, then $(S) \int_A f \, d\mu \le (S) \int_A g \, d\mu$;

(iii) $(S)\displaystyle\int_A (f \vee g)\, \mathrm{d}\mu \geq (S)\displaystyle\int_A f\, \mathrm{d}\mu \vee (S)\displaystyle\int_A g\, \mathrm{d}\mu;$

(iv) $(S)\displaystyle\int_A (f \wedge g)\, \mathrm{d}\mu \leq (S)\displaystyle\int_A f\, \mathrm{d}\mu \wedge (S)\displaystyle\int_A g\, \mathrm{d}\mu;$

(v) If $A \subset B$, then $(S)\displaystyle\int_A f\, \mathrm{d}\mu \leq (S)\displaystyle\int_B f\, \mathrm{d}\mu;$

(vi) $(S)\displaystyle\int_{A \cup B} f\, \mathrm{d}\mu \geq (S)\displaystyle\int_A f\, \mathrm{d}\mu \vee (S)\displaystyle\int_B f\, \mathrm{d}\mu;$

(vii) $(S)\displaystyle\int_{A \cap B} f\, \mathrm{d}\mu \leq (S)\displaystyle\int_A f\, \mathrm{d}\mu \wedge (S)\displaystyle\int_B f\, \mathrm{d}\mu;$

where $f \vee g$ and $f \wedge g$ are, respectively, the maximum and minimum of the functions f and g.

The Lebesgue integral was used to obtain the expected value of a random variable with respect to a probability measure. In the same manner, we will use the Sugeno integral to obtain the fuzzy expected value *FEV* of an uncertainty variable with respect to a fuzzy measure.

Definition 7.10 Let $X : \Omega \to [0, 1]$ be an uncertainty variable (typically given by a membership function) and μ a fuzzy measure on Ω. The *fuzzy expected value* of X is the real number

$$FEV(X) = (S)\int_\Omega X\, \mathrm{d}\mu = \sup_{0 \leq \alpha \leq 1} [\alpha \wedge \mu\{\omega \in \Omega : X(\omega) \geq \alpha\}]. \qquad (7.9)$$

The following result was stated by Sugeno [6] and it is a consequence of Theorem 7.2.

Corollary 7.3 *Let $X : \Omega \to [0, 1]$ be a normalized random variable (which is typically given by a membership function) and P a probability measure on Ω. Then,*

(a) (Sugeno)

$$| FEV(X) - E(X) | \leq \frac{1}{4}.$$

(b)

$$FEV(X) \leq \sqrt{E(X)}.$$

Proof (a) Recall that, given the fuzzy measure

$$FEV(X) = (S)\int_\Omega X\, \mathrm{d}P$$

and

$$E(X) = \int_\Omega X\, \mathrm{d}P = \int_0^1 P\{\omega \in \Omega : X(\omega) \geq \alpha\}\, \mathrm{d}\alpha = \int_0^1 H(\alpha)\, \mathrm{d}\alpha.$$

The result follow from Theorem 7.2.

(b) Note that $0 \leq E(X) \leq 1$. From the Chebyshev inequality [7, 8]

$$H(\alpha) = P\{\omega : X(\omega) \geq \alpha\} \leq \frac{1}{\alpha}E(X),$$

which implies that

$$FEV(X) = \sup_{0 \leq \alpha \leq 1} [\alpha \wedge H(\alpha)] \leq \sup_{0 \leq \alpha \leq 1} \left[\alpha \wedge \frac{1}{\alpha}E(X)\right] = \bar{\alpha},$$

where $\bar{\alpha}$ is the solution $\alpha = \frac{1}{\alpha}E(X)$.

Therefore, $\bar{\alpha} = \sqrt{E(X)}$, hence the result follows. ∎

This corollary legitimizes the use of fuzzy expected value instead of the classical expected value when the uncertainty of the studied phenomenon is not coming solely from randomness, but of different possibilities for the variable of interest.

Because $FEV(X)$ is a fixed point of the function $H : [0, 1] \rightarrow [0, 1]$, fixed point theorems such as Banach's contraction mapping theorem or Brouwer's fixed point theorem [29] can help one to estimate $FEV(X)$.

The following are some examples of random variables with density function distribution f for which the difference between $FEV(X)$ and $E(X)$ is smaller than $\frac{1}{4}$. First, it is worth remembering the following identities [7, 8].

(a) $H(\alpha) = P\{\omega \in \Omega : X(\omega) \geq \alpha\} = \int_{\alpha}^{1} f(x)\,dx;$

(b) $E(X) = \int_{\Omega} X\,dP = \int_{R} xf(x)\,dx.$

(c) If $g : \mathbb{R} \rightarrow \mathbb{R}$, then, for the random variable $g(X)$, we have that

$$E(g(X)) = \int_{\Omega} g(X)dP = \int_{\mathbb{R}} g(x)f(x)dx, \tag{7.10}$$

where X a is continuous random variable with density f. In particular,

$$E(X) = \int_{\Omega} X dP = \int_{\mathbb{R}} xf(x)dx.$$

In the case that X is discrete, we have that

$$E(g(X)) = \sum_{i} g(x_i)P[X = x_i], \tag{7.11}$$

with $P[X = x_i] = P\{\omega \in \Omega : X = x_i\}$. In particular,

$$E(X) = \sum_{i} x_i P[X = x_i].$$

(d) In the case that X is continuous

$$P\{\omega \in \Omega : X(\omega) \geq t\} = \int_t^\infty f(x)dx. \qquad (7.12)$$

In particular, if $\alpha \in [0, 1]$,

$$H(\alpha) = P\{\omega \in \Omega : X(\omega) \geq \alpha\} = \int_\alpha^1 f(x)dx.$$

Example 7.10 (*Uniform Distribution*) Suppose that the random variable $X : \Omega \to$ [0, 1] has a uniform distribution, that is, its probability density function is given by

$$f(x) = \begin{cases} 1 \text{ if } 0 \leq x \leq 1 \\ 0 \text{ otherwise} \end{cases}.$$

It is easy to see that $E(X) = \int_0^1 xf(x)\, dx = \dfrac{1}{2}$. On the other hand,

$$H(\alpha) = P\{\omega \in \Omega : X(\omega) \geq \alpha\} = \int_\alpha^1 f(x)\, dx = 1 - \alpha.$$

Now, since $FEV(X)$ is the solution of $H(\alpha) = \alpha$ or $1 - \alpha = \alpha$, this means $\overline{\alpha} = \frac{1}{2}$. In this example it follows that $FEV(X) = E(X) = \frac{1}{2}$. Therefore, $|FEV(X) - E(X)| = 0$.

Example 7.11 (*β Distribution*) Let the random variable $X : \Omega \to [0, 1]$ have a β distribution where its density function probability is given by

$$f(x) = \frac{1}{\beta(a, b)}x^{a-1}(1 - x)^{b-1}, \quad x \in [0, 1].$$

It is known that [7, 8] the stochastic expected value of X is given by

$$E(X) = \frac{a}{a + b}.$$

By means of numerical methods we have obtained the fuzzy expected values $FEV(X)$ for some parameters a and b of the β distribution, which are shown in Table 7.1.

Note that for any value of the parameters a and b, the difference between $FEV(X)$ and $E(X)$ is less than or equal to 0.25 which is according to Sugeno's Theorem and $FEV(X) \leq \sqrt{E(X)}$. Furthermore, if $a = b$ in the β distribution, then the stochastic and fuzzy expected value coincide. Actually, this result was proved for a more general case [30].

Table 7.1 A few values of E(X) and FEV(X) for beta distribution (β)

a	b	|a−b|	E(X)	FEV(X)	|E(X)-FEV(X)|
1	1	0	0.5000	0.5000	0.0000
1	2	1	0.3333	0.3820	0.0486
1	3	2	0.2500	0.3177	0.0677
1	4	3	0.2000	0.2755	0.0755
2	1	1	0.6667	0.6180	0.0486
2	2	0	0.5000	0.5000	0.0000
2	3	1	0.4000	0.4278	0.0278
2	4	2	0.3333	0.3773	0.0440
3	1	2	0.7500	0.6823	0.0677
3	2	1	0.6000	0.5722	0.0278
3	3	0	0.5000	0.5000	0.0000
3	4	1	0.4286	0.4472	0.0186
4	1	3	0.8000	0.7245	0.0755
4	2	2	0.6667	0.6227	0.0440
4	3	1	0.5714	0.5528	0.0186
4	4	0	0.5000	0.5000	0.0000

Theorem 7.4 *Let $X : \Omega \to [0, 1]$ be a random variable with density function $f :$ $[0, 1] \to [0, 1]$ that is symmetrical in relation to $x = \frac{1}{2}$, that is, $f(x) = f(1 - x)$ for all $x \in [0, 1]$. Then, $FEV(X) = E(X)$.*

Proof From $f(x) = f(1 - x)$ we have

$$\int_0^{\frac{1}{2}} f(x)\, dx = \int_0^{\frac{1}{2}} f(1 - x)\, dx = \int_1^{\frac{1}{2}} -f(x)\, dx = \int_{\frac{1}{2}}^1 f(x)\, dx.$$

On the other hand,

$$\int_0^1 f(x)\, dx = 1 = \int_0^{\frac{1}{2}} f(x)\, dx + \int_{\frac{1}{2}}^1 f(x)\, dx \Longrightarrow$$

$$\int_0^{\frac{1}{2}} f(x)\, dx = \int_{\frac{1}{2}}^1 f(x)\, dx = \frac{1}{2}$$

and $H(\alpha) = P\{\omega \in \Omega : X(\omega) \geq \alpha\} = \int_\alpha^1 f(x)\, dx.$

Therefore,

$$H(\frac{1}{2}) = \int_{\frac{1}{2}}^1 f(x)\, dx = \frac{1}{2}$$

and, consequently, $FEV(X) = \frac{1}{2}$. Now, it is known that the stochastic expected value in this case is $\frac{1}{2}$ for any symmetric random variable which coincides with the median. Thus, the theorem is proved.   ∎

This section ends with a method to obtain $FEV(X)$ in the case where X is an uncertain variable that assumes only a finite number of values.

Theorem 7.5 *Suppose that the variable $X : \Omega \to [0, 1]$ assumes only $n + 1$ values $\{x_i\}_{1 \leq i \leq n+1}$ and*

$$\mu_i = \mu\{\omega \in \Omega : X(\omega) \geq x_i\}, i = 1, \ldots, n,$$

(excluding $\mu = 1$ and $\mu = 0$).
   Then,

$$FEV(X) = \int_{\Omega} X \, d\mu = \text{median of } A,$$

where $A = \{x_1, x_2, \ldots, x_{n+1}, \mu_1, \ldots, \mu_n\}$ sorted in ascending order.

Proof See [31, Theorem 4.2.3].   ∎

Remember that the median of a ordered sequence $\{a_n\}_{n \in N}$ is defined by

$$\text{med}(\{a_n\}) = \begin{cases} a_{(n+1)/2} & \text{if } n \text{ is odd} \\ \dfrac{[a_{n/2} + a_{(n/2)+1}]}{2} & \text{if } n \text{ is even} \end{cases} .$$

Example 7.12 Suppose the fuzzy set of people with an *"excellent income"* in a certain enterprise, is given by:

- 1 person earns per hour U\$ 23.00 $\longrightarrow \alpha_5 = 0.40$
- 2 people earn per hour U\$ 24.00 $\longrightarrow \alpha_4 = 0.50$
- 4 people earn per hour U\$ 24.20 $\longrightarrow \alpha_3 = 0.55$
- 2 people make per hour U\$ 24.50 $\longrightarrow \alpha_2 = 0.60$
- 3 people make per hour U\$ 30.00 $\longrightarrow \alpha_1 = 1.00$

where α_i indicates the degree to which each person has an "excellent income".
   Suppose that $\mu(S) = \frac{\#S}{\#\Omega} = \frac{\#S}{12}$, where $\#S$ is the number of elements of S.

$$\mu\{\omega \in \Omega : X \geq \alpha\} = \begin{cases} 1 = \mu_0 \ \text{if } 0 \leq \alpha \leq \alpha_5 \\[2mm] \dfrac{11}{12} = \mu_1 \ \text{if } \alpha_5 < \alpha \leq \alpha_4 \\[2mm] \dfrac{9}{12} = \mu_2 \ \text{if } \alpha_4 < \alpha \leq \alpha_3 \\[2mm] \dfrac{5}{12} = \mu_3 \ \text{if } \alpha_3 < \alpha \leq \alpha_2 \\[2mm] \dfrac{3}{12} = \mu_4 \ \text{if } \alpha_2 < \alpha \leq \alpha_1 \\[2mm] 0 = \mu_5 \ \text{if } \alpha_1 < \alpha \leq 1 \end{cases}.$$

Therefore,

$$FEV(X) = \int_\Omega X \, d\mu$$
$$= \text{med}\left\{ \frac{3}{12} \, ; 0.40 \, ; \frac{5}{12} ; \, 0.50 \, ; \, 0.55 \, ; \, 0.60 \, ; \, \frac{9}{12} \, ; \frac{11}{12}, 1 \right\}$$
$$= 0.55,$$

where "med" is the median. Also note that the arithmetic mean in this case is 0.65.

The Sugeno integral, in Example 7.12, gives a good indication of the data, since the extreme value of $U\$30,00$ does not affect the result. On the other hand, the classical arithmetic mean is significantly affected by the extreme values.

7.6 Fuzzy Events

Historically, some researchers argue that the theories of probability and fuzzy are somehow 'competitors'. The notion of fuzzy events, introduced by Zadeh [11], indicates precisely the opposite. This concept illustrates the potential of the combination of the two theories: fuzzy, treating the identification of the event; and probabilistic, dealing with the occurrence of the same. Since then, several authors have devoted themselves to the study of this subject both from a theoretical standpoint as well as applications. Massad et al. [32] applied the concept of fuzzy event to assess the risk of being infected HIV for very sexually active, sexually active, and less sexually active individuals. Unlike Zadeh, Buckley [33] considers the probability $P(A)$ of an event A as a fuzzy number, that is, $P(A) \in \mathcal{F}(\mathbb{R})$. However, this text, with the except in Subsection 7.3.3 which deals with fuzzy random variables, follows the approach of Zadeh where A is fuzzy and $P(A)$ is a real number. Let $(\Omega, P, \mathcal{A})$ be a probability space, that is, Ω is a non-empty set, $\mathcal{A}$ is a σ-algebra and P is a probability measure.

Definition 7.11 A *fuzzy event* in Ω is simply a fuzzy subset of Ω whose α-levels are in the σ-algebra $\mathcal{A}$.

A classic event A satisfies the above definition and, therefore, can be regarded as a fuzzy event. In this case, the characteristic function of A is a discrete random variable $\chi_A : \Omega \to \{0, 1\}$. On the other hand, if A is a fuzzy set, its membership function $\varphi_A : \Omega \to [0, 1]$ is a random variable which is not discrete. The question that arises is how to calculate the probability of A?

7.6.1 Probability of Fuzzy Events

The point we made above is that fuzzy looks at the identification of an event since fuzzy is about the gradualness of a set whereas probability looks at the level of occurrence of an event.

Let's start with the classic case where the sample space is finite with equiprobable elementary events. Suppose $\Omega = \{\omega_1, \omega_2, \ldots, \omega_n\}$, so that each element has equal probability of $\frac{1}{n}$. It is known that A is an event with m elements, then

$$P(A) = \frac{m}{n} \tag{7.13}$$

defines a probability Ω.

Given the event A, its characteristic function $\chi_A : \Omega \to \{0, 1\}$ yields the number of positive cases as

$$m = \sum_i \chi_A(\omega_i).$$

Therefore

$$P(A) = \frac{\sum_i \chi_A(\omega_i)}{n}.$$

By extension, if A is fuzzy, and knowing the membership function $\varphi_A : \Omega \to [0, 1]$, the "number of favorable cases" is

$$m = \sum_i \varphi_A(\omega_i),$$

so that

$$P(A) = \frac{\sum_i \varphi_A(\omega_i)}{n}. \tag{7.14}$$

Of course, in this case, m is no longer necessarily an integer.

Example 7.13 Consider $\Omega = \{1, 2, 3, 4, 5, 6, 7, 8, 9, 10\}$ to be the sample space and the finite fuzzy event (see notation in Chap. 1)

$$A = \frac{0.1}{1} + \frac{0.25}{2} + \frac{0.25}{3} + \frac{0.0}{4} + \frac{0.8}{5} + \frac{0.0}{6} + \frac{0.0}{7} + \frac{0.8}{8} + \frac{0.0}{9} + \frac{1.0}{10}.$$

Calculating $P(A)$ and $P(A')$ from (7.14) we have,

$$P(A) = \frac{\displaystyle\sum_i \varphi_A(\omega_i)}{10} = \frac{0.1 + 0.25 + 0.25 + 0.8 + 0.8 + 1.0}{10} = 0.32,$$

and, remembering that $\varphi_{A'}(\omega_i) = 1 - \varphi_A(\omega_i)$ it follows that

$$A' = \frac{0.9}{1} + \frac{0.75}{2} + \frac{0.75}{3} + \frac{1.0}{4} + \frac{0.2}{5} + \frac{1.0}{6} + \frac{1.0}{7} + \frac{0.2}{8} + \frac{1.0}{9} + \frac{0.0}{10}$$

so that

$$P(A') = \frac{\displaystyle\sum_i \varphi_{A'}(\omega_i)}{10}$$

$$= \frac{0.9 + 0.75 + 0.75 + 1.0 + 0.2 + 1.0 + 1.0 + 0.2 + 1.0}{10}$$

$$= 0.68.$$

Note that this result was expected, since $P(A') = 1 - P(A) = 1 - 0.32 = 0.68$.

Now, any other event B, with the same number of positive cases m as A, is equally probable as A. This is because, according to formula (7.13), what matters is the ratio between m and the number of possible cases n, regardless which elements are part of A or B.

The number of positive cases m in the classic case can be obtained through counting methods of combinatorial analysis, permutation, arrangement and/or combination. As the reader may already know, clearly these principles do not take into account "qualities" of the elements forming part of the event. However, for the fuzzy case, if A is unknown, the number of favorable cases is not so easy to obtain as a gradual set.

Thinking about the adaptation of counting methods to the fuzzy case, one should take into consideration "the quality of each element" of the fuzzy event. For the number of favorable cases, what can be done is "relativize" the "contribution" of each element in order to determining the total number of positive cases m.

Let A be a fuzzy event with α being its α-*level*, where

$$\alpha_1 > \alpha_2 > \ldots > \alpha_k > \alpha_{k+1} = 0.$$

It follows that $[A]^{\alpha_1} \subset [A]^{\alpha_2} \subset \ldots \subset [A]^{\alpha_k} \subset [A]^0$. The number of favorable cases is

$$m = \alpha_1 m_1 + \alpha_2(m_2 - m_1) + \ldots + \alpha_k(m_k - m_{k-1})$$

or

$$m = (\alpha_1 - \alpha_2)m_1 + (\alpha_2 - \alpha_3)m_2 + \ldots + \alpha_k m_k,$$

where each m_i is the number of favorable cases associated with the classic set $[A]^{\alpha_i}$, which may be obtained by conventional counting methods since $[A]^{\alpha_i}$ is a classical set.

Thus, (7.13) becomes

$$P(A) = \frac{\displaystyle\sum_{i=1}^{k}(\alpha_i - \alpha_{i+1})m_i}{n}, \tag{7.15}$$

which gives us a formula for a probability associated with a fuzzy set. For example, the above fuzzy event A, has

$$m = (1.0 - 0.8)1 + (0.8 - 0.25)3 + (0.25 - 0.1)5 + (0.1 - 0.0)6 = 3.2$$

and

$$P(A) = \frac{3.2}{10} = 0.32.$$

Although our interest is the case where the event A is given so that its membership function φ_A is known, we will explore expression (7.15) a bit more.

Formula (7.15) can be rewritten as

$$P(A) = \sum_{i=1}^{k}(\alpha_i - \alpha_{i+1})\frac{m_i}{m} = \sum_{i=1}^{k}(\alpha_i - \alpha_{i+1})P([A]^{\alpha_i})$$

$$= \sum_{i=1}^{k}(\alpha_i - \alpha_{i+1})P[\varphi_A \geq \alpha_i] = \int_{\Omega} \varphi_A dP \tag{7.16}$$

Formulas (7.15) and (7.16) indicate that, for the finite case, $P(A)$ is exactly the expected value of the random variable φ_A. More generally, if A is any classic event (finite or not), its characteristic function is a discrete random variable since $\chi_A : \Omega \to \{0, 1\}$ and in this case

$$E(\chi_A) = 1 \cdot P(\chi_A = 1) + 0 \cdot P(\chi_A = 0) = P(A).$$

The above comments suggest the following definition.

Definition 7.12 Let $(\Omega, P, \mathcal{A})$ be a probability space and let A be a fuzzy event with membership function $\varphi_A : \Omega \to [0, 1]$. The probability of A is given by the expected value of φ_A, that is

$$P(A) = E(\varphi_A).$$

It is opportune to observe that the fuzzy expected value of φ_A, $E(\varphi_A)$, is also well-defined since $\varphi_A : \Omega \to [0, 1]$. Moreover, it's an exercise for the reader to prove that if A is a classical event then

$$E(\chi_A) = P(A).$$

To explore the concepts presented here, we will consider real-valued events, that is, those that are subsets (classical or fuzzy) of real line $\mathbb{R}$ equipped with some probability measure. Thus, to calculate $P(A)$, we will avail ourselves of the comments made just before Example 7.10. Specifically, formulas (7.10) and (7.11) suggest that $\mathbb{R}$ is a sample space whose measure P is induced by the probability distribution of a random variable X.

Suppose that X is a random variable and A is a fuzzy real-valued event with membership function $\varphi_A : \mathbb{R} \to [0, 1]$. Then, the probability of A is given by

$$P(A) = E(\varphi_A) = E(\varphi_A(X)) = \sum_i \varphi_A(x_i)P(X = x_i) \qquad (7.17)$$

if X is discrete, and if X is continuous

$$P(A) = E(\varphi_A) = E(\varphi_A(X)) = \int_{\mathbb{R}} \varphi_A(x)f(x)dx = \int_{suppA} \varphi_A(x)f(x)dx \qquad (7.18)$$

where f is the probability density function of X.

Figure 7.6 illustrates the probability $P(A)$, of the A event for the two cases: classic and fuzzy.

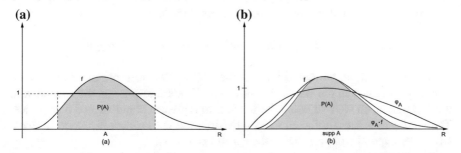

Fig. 7.6 **a** Exhibits a classical event, probability density function f, and $P(A) = $ *probability of A*. **b** Exhibits a fuzzy event, probability density function f, and $P(A) = $ *probability of A*

Firstly, in Fig. 7.6, $P(A)$ may be interpreted as the "area" bounded by the graph f and the support of A. In the fuzzy case, $P(A)$ is the "area" under the graph $\varphi_A \cdot f$ and the support of A. Both cases are depicted by the gray areas.

It is not difficult to see that $P(A)$, as defined in (7.18) above, satisfies the axioms of probability. For example,

$$P(\emptyset) = E(\varphi_\emptyset) = \int_\mathbb{R} 0 \cdot f(x)dx = 0$$

and

$$P(\Omega) = E(\varphi_\mathbb{R}) = \int_\mathbb{R} 1 \cdot f(x)dx = 1.$$

The other properties are left as an exercise for the reader. Remember that

$$\varphi_{A\cup B}(x) = \frac{\varphi_A(x) + \varphi_B(x) + |\varphi_A(x) - \varphi_B(x)|}{2}$$

and

$$\varphi_{A\cap B}(x) = \frac{\varphi_A(x) + \varphi_B(x) - |\varphi_A(x) - \varphi_B(x)|}{2}.$$

7.6.2 Independence Between Fuzzy Events

The concept of independence between fuzzy events necessarily involves the conditional probability. To extend the classical notion of conditional probability as it relates to the fuzzy case, we must rethink the mathematical modeling of simultaneous occurrence of two events A and B. For the classical case, the simultaneous occurrence is given by the intersection $A \cap B$. However, to extend this concept to the fuzzy case, the function must involve the characteristic function $\chi_{A\cap B}$. As we know, any *t-norm* can model the conjunction "and", in particular, we are thinking of the *t-norms* of *product* and *minimum*. For these cases we have

$$\chi_{A\cap B}(x) = \chi_A(x) \cdot \chi_B(x) \quad and \quad \chi_{A\cap B}(x) = \chi_A(x) \wedge \chi_B(x),$$

so that, in principle, we could adopt either "·" or "∧" to represent conjunction. The most common in the classical case is "·". We are interested in the extension to the fuzzy case, so we will adopt the *product* to represent simultaneous occurrence. The *minimum* is closely linked to membership and the *product* to the occurrence, which correspond with our choice for non-fuzzy events.

The classical case, where A and B are events of Ω with $P(B) > 0$, is

$$P(A|B) = \frac{P(AB)}{P(B)} = \frac{E(\chi_A \cdot \chi_B)}{E(\chi_B)}. \tag{7.19}$$

A is said to be independent of B if the occurrence of B does not interfere with the probability of A, that is, if $P(A|B) = P(A)$. The notation AB instead of $A \cap B$ is not by chance. It comes from the fact that we choose $\chi_A . \chi_B$ to represent $\chi_{A \cap B}$.

Therefore, A independent of B if, and only if,

$$\frac{E(\chi_A \cdot \chi_B)}{E(\chi_B)} = E(\chi_A) \Leftrightarrow E(\chi_A \cdot \chi_B) = E(\chi_A) \cdot E(\chi_B) \tag{7.20}$$

or

$$P(AB) = P(A)P(B).$$

Formula (7.20) above makes it possible to see that A is independent of B if, and only if, B is independent of A. Moreover, A and B are independent if, and only if, the random variables χ_A and χ_B are uncorrelated, that is, the correlation coefficient $\rho = 0$. As a matter of fact, χ_A and χ_B are independent random variables whereas A and B are independent events. This fact is a consequence of χ_A and χ_B being discrete and taking on just two values (see Exercise 7.8). In general, random variables that are not correlated are not necessarily independent (see Exercise 7.9).

Definition 7.13 Consider A and B, two fuzzy events of $\mathbb{R}$, with $P(B) > 0$ ($\Leftrightarrow$ $E(\varphi_B) > 0$). In view of (7.19), the conditional probability of A given B is defined by

$$P(A|B) = \frac{P(AB)}{P(B)} = \frac{E(\varphi_A . \varphi_B)}{E(\varphi_B)}. \tag{7.21}$$

As in the classical case, A is said to be independent of B if the occurrence of B does not interfere with probability of A, that is, if $P(A|B) = P(A)$. From (7.21), A independent of B if, and only if,

$$\frac{E(\varphi_A \cdot \varphi_B)}{E(\varphi_B)} = E(\varphi_A) \Leftrightarrow E(\varphi_A \cdot \varphi_B) = E(\varphi_A) \cdot E(\varphi_B). \tag{7.22}$$

Therefore, since the probabilities do not cancel, A and B are independent if, and only if, the random variables φ_A and φ_B are uncorrelated. Here unlike the classical case, the independence between A and B is not equivalent to independence between φ_A and φ_B. Of course, if φ_A and φ_B are independent, then A and B will be. But the reciprocal is not necessarily true (see Exercise 7.9).

According to Eq. (7.21), $P(B|B)$ may not equal 1 if B is not a crisp set. Such a fact is criticized by some authors [34] that prefer to adopt the minimum t-norm instead of the product t-norm in formula (7.21). However, the classical notion of independence can not be generalized to the fuzzy domain by means of formula (7.22) if we use the minimum t-norm. In addition, it is not obvious that we should have $P(B|B) = 1$ for a fuzzy event B since $P(A|B)$ represents chance of elements of A occurring in fuzzy set B but it is not clear which are the elements of B. Note that, from (7.21), $P(B|B) = 1$ holds if B is crisp.

The next subsection is a rapid look at a topic known in the literature as fuzzy random variable. From a random experiment, there are at least two ways to introduce the study of fuzzy random variables: the first is connected with the recognition of the uncertainty in the outcome of the experiment. The second, beyond the recognition of the uncertainty, deals with the mechanism of the experiment itself being uncertain; the way in which the events are drawn from the sample, for example. Although comments are made regarding the second theme, we will emphasize the first case. For this, unlike the latter, it follows that the probability of a fuzzy event is not necessarily a real number.

7.6.3   Random Linguistic Variable and Fuzzy Random Variable

The idea here is to explore the concept of linguistic variable assuming it is also random. Variables with these two characteristics will be called linguistic random variables or fuzzy random variables depending on the range of the variable in question. As we presented in the previous subsection, a random variable X induces a probability measure on $\mathbb{R}$. Hence, the question that arises [11] is how to calculate the probability

$$P(X \text{ is } A),$$

where A is a linguistic term, for example, *tall*, *low*, *very tall* ..., modeled as a real fuzzy event A.

This issue has already been addressed in previous subsections in an informal manner. From the point of view of classical theory, $P(X \text{ is } A) = P(X \in A)$, the above the question is translated into

$$P(X \in A) = \begin{cases} \sum_{x_i \in A} P[X = x_i] = \sum_i \chi_A(x_i)P[X = x_i] \\ \int_A f(x)dx = \int_{\mathbb{R}} \chi_A(x)f(x)dx \end{cases},$$

depending whether or not X is a discrete or continuous variable. Regardless, $P(X \in A) = E(\chi_A)$.

Thus, it is natural to define $P(X \text{ is } A)$ as

$$P(X \text{ is } A) = E(\varphi_A) = P(A),$$

where A is a real fuzzy set modeling the linguistic term of interest. This line of investigation leads us to the concept of linguistic random variable since we are translating $P(X \text{ is } A)$ into a real number.

Now, if we understand that $P(X \text{ is } A) = P(X = A)$, then we must give a meaning to the identity $X = A$, since originally X takes on real values (numbers) and A is a fuzzy event of the sample space $\mathbb{R}$. It is precisely here that the notion arises of a fuzzy random variable, as we will explained below.

Formally, a fuzzy random variable is simply a function

$$X : \Omega \to \mathcal{F}(\mathbb{R}).$$

Clearly we see that this concept extends the concept of random variable since $\mathbb{R} \subset \mathcal{F}(\mathbb{R})$.

Note that originally $X : \Omega \to \mathbb{R}$ so that to consider $X = A$, it must follow that $X : \Omega \to \mathcal{F}(\mathbb{R})$. Therefore, there is an abuse of notation since the range of the original variable has changed. Thus, we are dealing, in fact, with another variable $\hat{X} : \Omega \to \mathcal{F}(\mathbb{R})$ whose probability density is $F : \mathcal{F}(\mathbb{R}) \to \mathcal{F}(\mathbb{R})$, since by definition of density, this must be a subset of the range of the random variable. Thus, while the density function f of X induces a probability in $\mathbb{R}$, F induces a probability measure in $\mathcal{F}(\mathbb{R})$. In this approach, the probability of a fuzzy event happens to be a fuzzy number.

Without extending the theme of the fuzzy random variable, both $\hat{X}$ and F may be obtained by fuzzification of the functions X and f, via Zadeh extension principle, for example. To distinguish both cases, the first we call a random variable and the second a linguistic fuzzy random variable. For a study on the various approaches to fuzzy random variable the reader may consult [35].

Continuing with our study of the linguistic random variables, a case of interest is the calculation of $P(X$ is $A^*)$, in which A^* is an event obtained by some fuzzy modifier (Sect. 4.5) of the event A. Like in Chap. 4, here we will also only deal with powers of modifiers for the sole purpose of clarifying the main ideas of this theme and exploring their potential application in obtaining membership functions. Clearly, for a particular application, other modifiers should be taken into account.

Assuming that $A^* = A^s$, that is, $\varphi_{A^*} = (\varphi_A)^s$,

$$P(X \text{ is } A^*) = E(\varphi_{A^*}) = E(\varphi_A^s).$$

A case of particular interest is when $s = 2$:

$$P(A^2) = E(\varphi_A^2),$$

which is the second moment of φ_A, and

$$P(A^2) - [P(A)]^2 = E(\varphi_A^2) - [E(\varphi_A)]^2 = Var(\varphi_A),$$

where $Var(Y)$ is the variance of the random variable Y. By abuse of notation, we sometimes write $Var(A)$ instead of $Var(\varphi_A)$.

According to Jensen's inequality [7, 8], it follows that, for a restrictive modifier ($s > 1$, for example $s = 2$),

$$E(X^s) - [E(X)]^s \geq 0,$$

since in this case the modifier is given by the concave function $m(x) = x^s$.

A possible application of the above study is the "construction" of A and A^*, that is, in constructing of φ_A and φ_{A^*}. The problem becomes one of getting the parameters (s is one of the parameters) for the distributions of possibilities for A and A^*. For this case, from principles such as *maximum likelihood* (see [36]), we may think of the parameters as being based on one or two principles below:

(a) $P(A^*)$ is maximum (*maximum likelihood*);
(b) $Var(\varphi_{A^*})$ is minimal (*smaller variance*).

Of course, other methods, such as least squares, polynomial interpolation or even statistical inference methods can be used for the distribution of the possibility of A and A^*.

Another area of application is the estimation of parameters of a given density distribution, assuming that a fuzzy set A is given with membership function φ_A. Such a set may be provided by a specialist or by a dataset. The parameter in question can be estimated from classical statistical parametric techniques. Of course one can also use non-parametric techniques for estimating the density function. The interested reader can consult [37].

Before going to the exercises, we call the reader's attention to the difference between the concepts of independence for fuzzy sets seen here and in Section 4.6. In Chap. 4 independence is given by the possibility measure which is technically related to the conditional membership function of each of the membership functions of the fuzzy sets involved (see Sect. 4.6.2). Furthermore, independence between fuzzy events, seen in this section, is given by the probability measure and technically, involves the expected value of membership functions of the fuzzy sets in question as can be seen in the formula (7.22).

The following example illustrates the concepts presented in this section. Both in this example and in the exercises, the random variables that appear are linguistics and the probabilities of events are real numbers.

Example 7.14 A manufacturer produces parts, 5 % of which are faulty. For a sample of 10 parts, consider X to be the number of faulty parts. Calculate:

(a) $P(X \leq 1)$;
(b) $P(X$ is small), with "small" being the triangular fuzzy number $(0; 0; 2)$;
(c) $P(A \cap B)$, where A and B are the events of (a) and (b), respectively;
(d) $P(A \cup B)$;
(e) $P(B|A)$;
(f) Are A and B independent?

Solutions

X has binomial distribution with $n = 10$ and $p = 0.05$ (see [36]).

(a) It follows that
$$\varphi_A(x) = \begin{cases} 1 \text{ if } 0 \leq x \leq 1 \\ 0 \text{ otherwise} \end{cases}.$$

Then, by the formula (7.17),

$$P(A) = \sum_i \varphi_A(x_i)P(X = x_i) = \varphi_A(0)P(X = 0) + \varphi_A(1)P(X = 1)$$

$$= 1 \cdot P(X = 0) + 1 \cdot P(X = 1) = \binom{10}{0} 0.95^{10} + \binom{10}{1} 0.95^9 \cdot 0.05^1$$

$$= 0.91.$$

(b)

$$\varphi_B(x) = \begin{cases} 1 - \frac{x}{2} & \text{if } 0 \le x \le 2 \\ 0 & \text{otherwise} \end{cases}.$$

Therefore,

$$P(B) = \sum_i \varphi_B(x_i)P(X = x_i) = \varphi_B(0)P(X = 0) + \varphi_B(1)P(X = 1)$$

$$+ \varphi_B(2)P(X = 2) = 1 \cdot P(X = 0) + \frac{1}{2}P(X = 1) + 0 \cdot P(X = 2)$$

$$= \binom{10}{0} 0.95^{10} + \frac{1}{2} \binom{10}{1} 0.95^9 \cdot 0.05^1 = 0.7563.$$

(c) $\varphi_{A \cap B}(x) = \min[\varphi_A(x), \varphi_B(x)]$. Therefore,

$$P(A \cap B) = \sum_i \varphi_{A \cap B}(x_i)P(X = x_i) = \varphi_{A \cap B}(0)P(X = 0)$$

$$+ \varphi_{A \cap B}(1)P(X = 1) + \varphi_{A \cap B}(2)P(X = 2)$$

$$= 1 \cdot P(X = 0) + \frac{1}{2} \cdot P(X = 1) + 0 \cdot P(X = 2) = 0.7563.$$

(d) $P(A \cup B) = P(A) + P(B) - P(A \cap B) = 0.7563 + 0.91 - 0.7563$

$$= 0.91.$$

(e) $P(B|A) = \dfrac{P(AB)}{P(A)} = \dfrac{E(\varphi_A \varphi_B)}{E(\varphi_A)} =$

$$\frac{\varphi_A(0)\varphi_B(0)P(X = 0) + \varphi_A(1)\varphi_B(1)P(X = 1) + \varphi_A(2)\varphi_B(2)P(X = 2)}{0.91}$$

$$= \frac{1 \cdot P(X = 0) + 0.5 \cdot P(X = 1)}{0.91} = \frac{0.7563}{0.91} \ne 0.7563 = P(B).$$

(f) According to (e), A and B are not independent events.

Exercise 7.1 Repeat the previous example assuming X has binomial distribution with $n = 8$ and $p = 0.02$.

Exercise 7.2 Calculate the probability of the fuzzy event in Example 7.12.

Exercise 7.3 In a telephone call center, N calls arrive according to a Poisson distribution, with average $\lambda = 8$ calls per minute. Knowing the probability law of a Poisson distribution is given by

$$P(N = k) = \frac{e^{-\lambda}\lambda^k}{k!},$$

determine what is the probability that in a minute we have:

(a) Ten or more calls;
(b) Less than nine call;
(c) A *small* number of calls, where *small* is the fuzzy set given by the triangular fuzzy number $(0; 0; 9)$;
(d) A *low average* number of calls, where *low average* is the fuzzy event given by trapezoidal fuzzy number $(0; 1; 4; 9)$;
(e) $P(C|B)$ and $P(D|B)$, with A, B, C and D being the events respectively from the a), b), c), and d) above.

Exercise 7.4 Suppose that the time T of the duration of some disease is an exponential random variable $(T \sim exp(\lambda))$ with the parameter $\lambda = \frac{1}{5}$, that is, its density is given by

$$f(t) = \begin{cases} \frac{1}{5}e^{-\frac{t}{5}} & \text{if } t \geq 0 \\ 0 & \text{if } t < 0 \end{cases}.$$

Calculate:

(a) The expected value of T;
(b) $P(M)$ where M is the event "average" given by the triangular fuzzy set $(0; 5; 8)$;
(c) $P(M/B)$ where B is the event "low" given by the triangular fuzzy set $(0; 0; 8)$;
(d) Are M and B independent?

Exercise 7.5 Suppose that $X \sim exp(1)$, that is, X is a random variable with exponential distribution with the parameter $\lambda = 1$.

(a) Calculate $P(A)$, where A is the triangular fuzzy number $(0; 1; 1)$.
(b) Calculate $P(C)$ with

$$\varphi_C(x) = \begin{cases} x - x^2 & \text{if } 0 \leq x \leq 1 \\ 0 & \text{otherwise} \end{cases}.$$

(c) Repeat the (a) assuming $X \sim N(0, 1)$.

Exercise 7.6 Suppose that X has a uniform distribution between $[0, 1]$, A is the fuzzy event with membership function

$$\varphi_A(x) = a \in [0, 1],$$

and B is a triangular fuzzy number $(0; 0; 1)$. Calculate:

(a) $P(A)$ and $P(B)$;
(b) $P(A \cap B)$ and $P(AB)$;
(c) Are A and B independent?
(d) Let C be the event of Exercise 7.6 (b), check if A and C are independent. What about B and C?

Exercise 7.7 Show that if X and Y take on only the values 0 or 1, then X and Y are not correlated if, and only if, they are independent.

Exercise 7.8 Suppose that both X and Y assume the values -1, 0 and 1, with joint distribution

$$P_{XY}(-1, -1) = P_{XY}(-1, 1) = P_{XY}(1, -1) = P_{XY}(1, 1) = P_{XY}(0, 0) = \frac{1}{5}.$$

Show that X and Y are not correlated ($\rho = 0$), nor are they independent.

Exercise 7.9 Show that if X and Y are normal distributions, then X and Y are not correlated if, and only if, they are independent.

Exercise 7.10 Prove that:

(a) $P(A \cap B) \geq P(AB)$;
(b) $P(A|B) = 0$, if A and B are mutually empty, that is, $A \cap B = \emptyset$.

Exercise 7.11 Consider $X \sim U[0, 2]$ and the triangular fuzzy number $(0; 0; \delta)$, with $0 < \delta \leq 2$. Calculate:

(a) δ so that $P(A)$ is maximum;
(b) $s > 0$ so that $P(A^*)$ is maximum with $A^* = A^s$ and A is the fuzzy set given in a);
(c) $Var(\varphi_A)$ and $Var(\varphi_{A^*})$.

Exercise 7.12 Consider the triangular fuzzy number $A = (0; 0; 2)$ and X a triangular random variable whose density is given by

$$f(x; \theta) = \begin{cases} \frac{1}{\theta^2}(\theta - |x - 1|) & \text{if } x \in [1 - \theta, 1 + \theta] \\ 0 & \text{if } x \notin [1 - \theta, 1 + \theta] \end{cases}.$$

Calculate:

(a) $\theta > 0$ so that $P(A)$ is maximum;
(b) Plot the graph of the density found in the previous item.

We end this section by commenting that we have been dealing with phenomena that exhibit both types of uncertainties discussed herein. Generally, we are interested in the dynamics of these phenomena. The methodology we have used involves coupling methods of statistical simulation and fuzzy controllers, specifically of the Mamdani type. The fuzzy sets that form the rule base are used to simulate the dynamics of interest. However, the entries to these systems are extracted using a method of statistical simulation (Monte Carlo, for example), taking into account a priori distribution. Thus, we can look to the antecedent of fuzzy sets as fuzzy events. Missio [38] used this methodology to study the evolution of hoof-and-mouth disease in Mato Grosso do Sul. Gomes [39] used the same methodology to study the evolution Dengue in the city of Campinas, São Paulo, Brazil.

References

1. R.G. Bartle, *The Elements of Real Analysis* (Wiley, New York, 1964)
2. C.S. Honig, *A integral de Lebesgue e suas aplicações*. 11º Colóquio Brasileiro de Matemática (Poços de Caldas), IMPA – Instituto de Matemática Pura e Aplicada (1977)
3. A.N. Kolmogorov, S.V. Fomin, *Introductory Real Analysis* (Prentice-Hall, Englewood Cliffs, 1970)
4. T. Murofushi, M. Sugeno, An interpretation of fuzzy measures and choquet's integral as an integral with respect to a fuzzy measure. Fuzzy Sets Syst. **29**, 201–227 (1989)
5. G. Choquet, Theory of capacities. Ann. Inst. Fourier **5**, 131–295 (1955)
6. M. Sugeno, *Theory of fuzzy Integrals and Applications*. Ph.D. thesis, Tokyo Institute of Technology, Tokyo (1974)
7. B. James, *Probabilidade: um curso de nível intermediário*. Instituto de Matemática Pura e Aplicada, Rio de Janeiro (1981)
8. S.M. Ross, *A First Course in Probability* (Pearson Prentice Hall, Englewood Cliffs, 2010)
9. G. Klir, B. Yuan, *Fuzzy Sets and Fuzzy Logic Theory and Applications* (Prentice-Hall, Englewood Cliffs, 1995)
10. G. Klir, B. Yuan, Fuzzy sets as a basis for a theory of possibility. Fuzzy Sets Syst. **1**, 3–28 (1978)
11. G. Klir, B. Yuan, Probability measures of fuzzy events. J. Math. Anal. Appl. **23**, 421–427 (1968)
12. J. C. Bezdek, Fuzzy models – what are they, and why? Trans. Fuzzy Syst. **1**(1), 1–6 (1993) (Editorial)
13. K. Sadegh-Zadeh, Fundamentals of clinical methodology: 3. nosology. Artif. Intell. Med. **17**, 87–108 (1999)
14. M.L. Puri, D.A. Ralescu, A possibility measure is not a fuzzy measure. Fuzzy Sets Syst. **7**(3), 311–313 (1982)
15. R.C. Bassanezi, L.C. Barros, A simple model of life expectancy with subjective parameters. Kybernets **7**, 91–98 (1995)
16. M.J.P. Castanho, *Construção e avaliação de um modelo matemático para predizer câncer de próstata e descrever seu crescimento utilizando a teoria dos conjuntos fuzzy*. Tese de Doutorado, FEEC-UNICAMP, Campinas (2005)
17. M.J.P. Castanho, F. Hernandes, A.M. De Ré, S. Rautenberg, A. Billis, Fuzzy expert system for predicting pathological stage of prostate cancer. Expert Syst. Appl. **40**(2), 466–470 (2013)
18. M.J.P. Castanho, L.C. Barros, A. Yamakami, L.L. Vendite, Fuzzy receiver operating characteristic curve: an option to evaluate diagnostic tests. IEEE Trans. Inf. Technol. Biomed. **11**(3), 244–250 (2007)

19. G.P. Silveira, *Aplicação da Teoria de Conjuntos Fuzzy na predição do estadiamento patológico do Câncer de Próstata*. Dissertação de Mestrado, IMECC-UNICAMP, Campinas (2007)
20. A.J. Stephenson, M.W. Kattan, Nomograms for prostate cancer. J. Urological Oncol. **98**, 39–46 (2006)
21. M.R. Civanlar, H.J. Trussel, Constructing membership functions using statistical data. Fuzzy Sets Syst. **18**, 1–13 (1986)
22. D. Dubois, H. Prade, *Fuzzy Sets and Systems – Theory and Applications* (Academic Press, Inc., New York, 1980)
23. D. Dubois, H. Prade, Properties of measures of information in evidence and possibility theories. Fuzzy Sets Syst. **24**(2), 161–182 (1987)
24. T. Sudkamp, On probability-possibility transformations. Fuzzy Sets Syst. **51**, 73–81 (1992)
25. T. Sudkamp, A note on derivatives of functions with respect to fuzzy measures. Fuzzy Sets Syst. **222**, 1–17 (2013)
26. T. Sudkamp, A way to choquet calculus. IEEE Trans. Fuzzy Syst. **23**(5), 1439–1457 (2015)
27. H.T. Nguyen, E.A. Walker, *A First Course of Fuzzy Logic* (CRC Press, Boca Raton, 1997)
28. D. Ralescu, Y. Ogura, S. Li, Set defuzzification and choquet integrals, International. J. Uncertain. Fuzziness Knowl.-Based Syst. **9**, 1–12 (2001)
29. C.S. Hönig, *Aplicações da topologia à análise*. Projeto Euclides, Edgard Blücher (1976)
30. H.P. Palaro, L.C. Barros, *Comparação entre esperança fuzzy e esperança estocástica*, Anais do XXIII CNMAC – Congresso Nacional de Matemática Aplicada e Computacional (Santos–SP), SBMAC – Sociedade Brasileira de Matemática Aplicada e Computacional (2000)
31. A. Kandel, *Fuzzy Mathematical Techniques with Applications* (Addison-Wesley Publishing Co., Reading, 1986)
32. E. Massad, N.R.S. Ortega, L.C. Barros, C.J. Struchiner, *Fuzzy Logic in Action: Applications in Epidemiology and Beyond* (Springer, Berlin, 2008)
33. J.J. Buckley, *Fuzzy Probability and Statistics*. Studies in Fuzziness and Soft Computing (Springer, Berlin, 2006)
34. J. M. C. Sousa, U. Kaymak, and S. M. Vieira, *Probabilistic fuzzy system tutorial: Part ii - probabilistic fuzzy models.*, Jul 2013, IEEE International Conference on Fuzzy Systems (FUZZ-IEEE 2013), Hyderabad, India
35. M.A. Gil, M. López-Diaz, D.A. Ralescu, Overview on the development of fuzzy random variable. Fuzzy Sets Syst. **157**, 2546–2557 (2006)
36. W.O. Bussab, P.A. Morettin, *Estatística Básica*, 5th edn. (Editora Saraiva, São Paulo, 2002)
37. M.C. Koissi, A.F. Shapiro, Fuzzy formulation of the lee-carter model for mortality forecasting. Insu.: Math. Econ. **39**, 287–309 (2006)
38. M. Missio, *Modelos de edp intregrados a lógica fuzzy e métodos probabilísticos no tratamento de incertezas: uma aplicação em febre aftosa em bovinos*. Tese de Doutorado, IMECC-UNICAMP, Campinas (2008)
39. L.T. Gomes, *Um estudo sobre o espalhamento da dengue usando equações diferenciais parciais e lógica fuzzy*. Dissertação de mestrado, IMECC-UNICAMP, Campinas (2009)

Chapter 8
Fuzzy Dynamical Systems

God evaluates several worlds, but makes exists the best of them.
(Leibniz – 16th Century)

Abstract This chapter presents an introduction to fuzzy dynamical systems both continuous and discrete. To study the dynamical case, the concept of fuzzy derivative and fuzzy integral are presented. Several kinds of derivatives are explored and consequently, several types of fuzzy differential equations are studied. The discrete case is studied by means of an interactive process. Lastly, all cases are illustrated using the Malthusian Model.

Certainly Leibniz considered many facts that lead him to conclude his thought above. In remains for us to resolve if this best world given to us by God is clear (exact, precise, deterministic) or hazy (inexact, imprecise, fuzzy). As we shall see next, our resolution of the "best of all worlds" is that this world in many instances is hazy.

This chapter briefly introduces fuzzy dynamical systems with the intention to illustrate the power of the fuzzy logic for studying evolutionary systems. As usually done in deterministic and stochastic systems we distinguish two cases here: continuous and discrete. In the continuous case, some type of derivative to represent the continuous variation rate will appear. In the discrete case, the system evolution is established in an iterative process.

8.1 Continuous Fuzzy Dynamical Systems

This section presents some approaches used to study continuous fuzzy dynamical systems. The fundamental difference of each one of the methods is the treatment given to the variation rate and/or how it is related to the state variables. The first approach evolves the Hukuhara derivative. Originally developed for functions with values in classical sets [1] and subsequently adapted for functions with values in fuzzy sets [2]. This adaptation to fuzzy functions (functions with values in fuzzy sets) is done using Theorem 1.4 which gives the representation of fuzzy sets (Chap. 1). The

© Springer-Verlag Berlin Heidelberg 2017
L.C. de Barros et al., *A First Course in Fuzzy Logic, Fuzzy
Dynamical Systems, and Biomathematics*, Studies in Fuzziness
and Soft Computing 347, DOI 10.1007/978-3-662-53324-6_8

second approach uses fuzzy differential inclusions [3, 4], while the third is simply given by the fuzzification of the deterministic solution, supposing that the initial condition and/or some parameter of the differential equation is given by a fuzzy set. Finally, the fourth approach differs from the others because the rate is related to the state variables given by some fuzzy rules instead of an equation. We would like to stress that in the last three cases, we did not use any notion of derivatives of fuzzy functions, but just the concept of derivative for deterministic functions.

Before we develop each concept listed above, we want to note that recently, Barros, Gomes and Tonelli [5] and Gomes, Barros and Bede [6] have investigated a "new" type of fuzzy differential equation in which the extension principle is used to fuzzify the derivative operator and not the deterministic solution as cited in the third approach above. From Theorem 1.4 and some other conditions, it is possible to conclude that this methodology yields fuzzy differential equations whose solutions match those of Hüllermeier [4]. We emphasize that in this approach we have, in fact, derivatives for fuzzy functions, which do not exist in Hüllermeier's methodology. Also, the derivative for fuzzy interactive processes have been studied from a "new" view point (see [7, 8]).

We motivate the derivatives for the above approaches using the "Malthusian growth model". We emphasize that Malthus did not originally prescribe any mathematical equation describing population growth, he just enunciated that the population would grow geometrically while the food would grow at an arithmetic rate, once there was no control mechanism (disease, poverty, etc.). The first mathematical interpretation of the Malthus conjecture was through a deterministic model that posits that "the growth of a population is proportional to the population itself". So, the continuous mathematical model, known as the Malthus model, is given by the differential equation

$$\begin{cases} \frac{dx}{dt} = \lambda x \\ x(0) = x_0 \end{cases}, \tag{8.1}$$

where $x(t)$ is the number of individuals at each instant t and x_0 indicates the initial number of individuals of the population.

This model assumes that all involved quantities are given by real numbers. We suppose that both λ and x_0 are well determined, and so, there is no uncertain data. However, if we consider that there are uncertainties in the growth rate λ or in the initial condition x_0, we must rethink the meaning of $\frac{dx}{dt}$ and how this variation is related to the state variable x.

Assuming that the uncertainties are random, the model (8.1) can be treated by stochastic differential equations [9–11]. However, if the uncertainty is modeled by fuzzy subsets, the differential equation can be treated in several forms such as:

- *Fuzzy differential equations* (from the Hukuhara derivative point of view) - in this case the notion of fuzzy derivative is necessary [2, 12–15];
- *Fuzzy differential inclusions* [3, 4, 16, 17];
- *Extension of the deterministic solution* [17, 18];
- *Fuzzy Rule Base* (Sect. 6.4 of Chap. 6 and Chap. 9).

We next present an introduction to the integral and differential calculus for fuzzy functions, that is, functions with domain in the set real numbers and the set of fuzzy number.

8.1.1   Integration and Differentiation of Fuzzy Functions

Here we consider only the one dimensional case, that is, the case in which the function is defined on an interval of the real line with values in the set of fuzzy numbers:

$$u : [a, b] \to \mathcal{F}(\mathbb{R}), \quad a \geq 0,$$

where $\mathcal{F}(\mathbb{R})$ denotes the set of fuzzy numbers. Information of the more general case about integration and differentiation of fuzzy functions can be found in [12–15, 19] or articles on fuzzy mathematics.

For the one dimensional case, we define the derivative of $u(.)$ from its α-levels. We recall (see [14]) that the function $u : [a, b] \to \mathcal{F}(\mathbb{R})$ associating a fuzzy number $u(t)$ to each real number t is well-defined if, and only if, for each $\alpha \in [0, 1]$ there exists real functions

$$u_1^\alpha, u_2^\alpha : [a, b] \to \mathbb{R}$$

such that the α-levels of $u(t)$ are $[u_1^\alpha(t), u_2^\alpha(t)]$, that is,

$$[u(t)]^\alpha = [u_1^\alpha(t), u_2^\alpha(t)]. \tag{8.2}$$

Before we present the concepts of derivative and integral we will use u' to denote the derivative and $\int_a^b u(t)dt$ to denote the integral of fuzzy functions $u : [a, b] \to \mathcal{F}(\mathbb{R})$.

Definition 8.1 (*Hukuhara Derivative*) The fuzzy function $u' : [a, b] \longrightarrow \mathcal{F}(\mathbb{R})$ whose α-levels are given by

$$[u'(t)]^\alpha = [(u_1^\alpha)'(t), (u_2^\alpha)'(t)], \tag{8.3}$$

for all $\alpha \in [0, 1]$, is the derivative of the fuzzy function $u(.)$, which we call the *Hukuhara derivative*. Of course we are supposing the existence of the classical derivatives $(u_1^\alpha)'(t)$ and $(u_2^\alpha)'(t)$.

Thus the α-levels of the fuzzy derivative are the classical derivatives at the endpoints of the α-levels of u. For example, the fuzzy function u that associates for each $t > 0$ the triangular fuzzy number $(0; t; 2t)$, that is, $u(t) = (0; t; 2t)$, has α-levels $[u(t)]^\alpha = [\alpha t, 2t - \alpha t]$ according to (2.6). Therefore, $[u'(t)]^\alpha = [\alpha, 2 - \alpha]$, for all $t > 0$. We observe that the existence of $u'(t)$ necessarily implies that the interval $[u_1^\alpha(t), u_2^\alpha(t)]$ satisfies Theorem 1.4.

Fig. 8.1 Fuzzy function
$u(t) = At$ and its α-levels

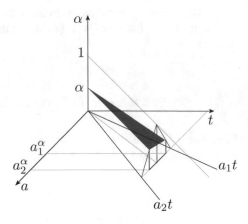

The integral of $u : [a, b] \to \mathcal{F}(\mathbb{R})$ is also defined by its α-levels. The Aumann[1] integral, originally defined for functions that assume values in classical sets (see [12]), is defined next.

Definition 8.2 The integral of u in $[a, b]$, denoted $\int_a^b u(t) \, dt$, is the fuzzy number with α-levels:

$$\left[\int_a^b u(t) \, dt \right]^\alpha = \left[\int_a^b u_1^\alpha(t) \, dt, \quad \int_a^b u_2^\alpha(t) \, dt \right], \tag{8.4}$$

where $\int_a^b u_1^\alpha(t) \, dt$ and $\int_a^b u_2^\alpha(t) \, dt$ are the Riemann integrals of the real functions u_1^α and u_2^α.

Existence of $\int_a^b u(t) dt$ necessarily implies that the intervals

$$\left[\int_a^b u_1^\alpha(t) \, dt, \int_a^b u_2^\alpha(t) \, dt \right]$$

satisfy Theorem 1.4. As observed for derivatives, we also suppose that the functions u_1^α and u_2^α are Riemann integrable in the interval $[a, b]$. Observe that if u is a real function ($u : [a, b] \to \mathbb{R} \subset \mathcal{F}(\mathbb{R})$), then the concepts of derivative and integral above are the same as the classical ones.

Example 8.1 Let us consider the fuzzy function $u(t) = At$, $t \geq 0$, where A is a fuzzy number, such that the α-levels are given by the intervals $[A]^\alpha = [a_1^\alpha, a_2^\alpha]$ (Fig. 8.1).
We have $[u(t)]^\alpha = [u_1^\alpha(t), u_2^\alpha(t)] = [a_1^\alpha t, a_2^\alpha t]$, so that

---

[1]Aumann won the Nobel prize for economics 2005.

$$[u'(t)]^\alpha = [(u_1^\alpha)'(t), (u_2^\alpha)'(t)] = [(a_1^\alpha t)', (a_2^\alpha t)'] = [a_1^\alpha, a_2^\alpha] = [A]^\alpha.$$

Therefore,

$$u'(t) = A.$$

On the other hand,

$$\left[\int_a^b u(t)\,dt\right]^\alpha = \left[\int_a^b u_1^\alpha(t)\,dt, \ \int_a^b u_2^\alpha(t)\,dt\right] = \left[\int_a^b a_1^\alpha t\,dt, \ \int_a^b a_2^\alpha t\,dt\right]$$

$$= \left[a_1^\alpha\left(\frac{b^2}{2} - \frac{a^2}{2}\right), \ a_2^\alpha\left(\frac{b^2}{2} - \frac{a^2}{2}\right)\right] = \left(\frac{b^2}{2} - \frac{a^2}{2}\right)[a_1^\alpha, a_2^\alpha]$$

$$= \left(\int_a^b t\,dt\right)[A]^\alpha.$$

Thus,

$$\int_a^b u(t)\,dt = \int_a^b At\,dt = A\int_a^b t\,dt = \left(\frac{b^2 - a^2}{2}\right)A.$$

We observe that $\int_a^b t\,dt$ is the Riemann integral that, multiplied by a fuzzy number A, gives us the Aumann's integral of $u(t) = At$.

We do not have the aim of making an extended and deep study of differentiability and integrability of fuzzy functions. However, for the study of stability of dynamical systems, we need the basic concepts of integral and derivative as well as that of metric in $\mathcal{F}(\mathbb{R})$.

Definition 8.3 The *metric in the space fuzzy numbers*, $\mathcal{F}(\mathbb{R})$, stems from the Hausdorff–Pompeiu metric, and is given by

$$\mathscr{D}(A, B) = \sup_{0 \le \alpha \le 1} d_H([A]^\alpha, [B]^\alpha), \tag{8.5}$$

where d_H is the Hausdorff–Pompeiu's metric for compact intervals of $\mathbb{R}$, whose definition is

$$d_H(I, J) = \max(\sup_{x \in I} d(x, J), \ \sup_{y \in J} d(y, I)), \tag{8.6}$$

where $d(x, J) = \inf_{j \in J} d(x, j)$ and $d(r, s) = |r - s|$.

Puri and Ralescu [20] proved that, with this metric, the metric space $\mathcal{F}(\mathbb{R})$ is complete, that is, they proved that every convergent sequence of fuzzy numbers converges to a fuzzy number.

The following theorem is important in the study of fuzzy differential equations.

Theorem 8.1 *If $F, G : [a, b] \to \mathcal{F}(\mathbb{R})$ are differentiable functions and $\lambda \in \mathbb{R}$, then*

(a) F and G are continuous under the metric $\mathcal{D}$;
(b) $(F + G)'(t) = F'(t) + G'(t)$;
(c) $(\lambda F)'(t) = \lambda F'(t)$.

Proof See [12, 14].   ∎

The following theorem is a version of the Fundamental Theorem of Calculus for the fuzzy case, using derivative and integral concepts presented above.

Theorem 8.2 *Let $F : [a, b] \longrightarrow \mathcal{F}(\mathbb{R})$ be continuous. Then the function $G(t) = \int_a^t F(s) \, \mathrm{d}s$ is derivable and $G'(t) = F(t)$ for all $t \in [a, b]$.*

Proof See [12, 14].   ∎

Moreover, the following result also holds:

Theorem 8.3 *Let $F : [a, b] \longrightarrow \mathcal{F}(\mathbb{R})$ be integrable. Then for all $c \in [a, b]$ we have*

$$\int_a^c F(t) \, \mathrm{d}t + \int_c^b F(t) \, \mathrm{d}t = \int_a^b F(t) \, \mathrm{d}t. \tag{8.7}$$

These theorems give us the basics needed to study of fuzzy differential equations. From the concepts of derivative and integrals above, we begin the study of *fuzzy differential equations*.

8.1.2   Fuzzy Initial Value Problem (FIVP)

We consider the fuzzy initial value problem to be

$$\begin{cases} u'(t) = F(t, u(t)) \\ u(a) = u_0 \end{cases}, \tag{8.8}$$

where $F : [a, b] \times \mathcal{F}(\mathbb{R}) \to \mathcal{F}(\mathbb{R})$ and $a > 0$.

Lemma 8.4 *Let $F : [a, b] \times \mathcal{F}(\mathbb{R}) \to \mathcal{F}(\mathbb{R})$ be continuous. Then the function*

$$u : [a, b] \longrightarrow \mathcal{F}(\mathbb{R})$$

is a solution of (8.8) if, and only if, it is continuous and satisfies the integral equation

$$u(t) = u(a) + \int_a^t F(s, u(s)) \, \mathrm{d}s. \tag{8.9}$$

Proof See [12, 14].

As an illustration, let us consider $u(t) = At$. We saw in the Example 8.1 that $u'(t) = A$. So,

$$u(t) = Aa + \int_a^t A \, ds = u(a) + \int_a^t u'(s) \, ds.$$

∎

Corollary 8.5 *If $u(t)$ is a solution of (8.8) then, for each $\alpha \in [0, 1]$, the function $d(t) = \operatorname{diam}[u(t)]^\alpha$ is nondecreasing.*

Proof $\operatorname{diam}([u(t)]^\alpha) = u_2^\alpha(t) - u_1^\alpha(t)$. So, according to Lemma 8.4, we have

$$[u(t)]^\alpha = [u_1^\alpha(a), u_2^\alpha(a)] + \left[\int_a^t F_1^\alpha(s, u(s)) \, ds, \int_a^t F_2^\alpha(s, u(s)) \, ds \right]$$

$$= \left[u_1^\alpha(a) + \int_a^t F_1^\alpha(s, u(s)) \, ds, \ u_2^\alpha(a) + \int_a^t F_2^\alpha(s, u(s)) \, ds \right].$$

Thus,

$$\operatorname{diam}([u(t)]^\alpha) = u_2^\alpha(t) - u_1^\alpha(t)$$

$$= (u_2^\alpha(a) - u_1^\alpha(a)) + \int_a^t \left[F_2^\alpha(s, u(s)) - F_1^\alpha(s, u(s)) \right] ds$$

is nondecreasing, since $(F_2^\alpha(s, u(s)) - F_1^\alpha(s, u(s))) \geq 0$ for all $s \in [a, b]$. ∎

Example 8.2 To illustrate some applications of *fuzzy differential equations* we suppose that in the Malthus model, only the initial condition is fuzzy and we consider positive variation rate (**population in expansion**) and negative variation rate (**population in retraction**).

• Let us consider the fuzzy Malthusian model with positive variation rate $\lambda > 0$, population in expansion.

$$\begin{cases} u'(t) = \lambda u(t) \\ u(0) = u_0 \in \mathcal{F}(\mathbb{R}) \end{cases}. \tag{8.10}$$

Suppose that $[u(t)]^\alpha = [u_1^\alpha(t), u_2^\alpha(t)]$ and that the initial condition is fuzzy and is given by the α-levels $[u_0]^\alpha = [u_{01}^\alpha, u_{02}^\alpha]$.

According to Definition 8.1, for each $\alpha \in [0, 1]$, we need to solve the equation

$$\begin{cases} [u'(t)]^\alpha = \lambda[u_1^\alpha(t), u_2^\alpha(t)] \\ u_0 \in \mathcal{F}(\mathbb{R}) \text{ and } \lambda > 0 \end{cases}. \tag{8.11}$$

Multiplying fuzzy numbers by a positive real number λ, we have that the solution to this equation is obtained from the solution of the deterministic α-levels equations:

$$\begin{cases} (u_1^\alpha)'(t) = \lambda u_1^\alpha(t), & \text{with } u_1^\alpha(0) = u_{01}^\alpha \\ (u_2^\alpha)'(t) = \lambda u_2^\alpha(t), & \text{with } u_2^\alpha(0) = u_{02}^\alpha \end{cases}.$$

For each α, the solution of the system (8.11) exists and is given by:

$$\begin{cases} u_1^\alpha(t) = u_{01}^\alpha e^{\lambda t} \\ u_2^\alpha(t) = u_{02}^\alpha e^{\lambda t} \end{cases}. \tag{8.12}$$

Observe that if $[u_0]^1$ is a zero width interval, that is, $u_{01} = u_{02} = x_0$ then $[u(t)]^1$ behaves like the solution of the deterministic Malthusian model, that is, $[u(t)]^1 = x_0 e^{\lambda t}$.

- We now consider the fuzzy Malthusian model with negative variation rate $\lambda < 0$, **population in retraction**.

$$\begin{cases} u'(t) = -\lambda u(t) \\ u_0 \in \mathcal{F}(\mathbb{R}) \text{ and } \lambda > 0 \end{cases}. \tag{8.13}$$

According to Definition 8.1, for each $\alpha \in [0, 1]$ we must solve the equation

$$[u'(t)]^\alpha = -\lambda[u_1^\alpha(t), u_2^\alpha(t)],$$

The multiplication of a negative and an $\alpha - level$ interval yields

$$\begin{cases} (u_1^\alpha)'(t) = -\lambda u_2^\alpha(t), & \text{with } u_1^\alpha(0) = u_{01}^\alpha \\ (u_2^\alpha)'(t) = -\lambda u_1^\alpha(t), & \text{with } u_2^\alpha(0) = u_{02}^\alpha \end{cases}, \tag{8.14}$$

whose solution is

$$u_1^\alpha(t) = \frac{u_{01}^\alpha - u_{02}^\alpha}{2} e^{\lambda t} + \frac{u_{01}^\alpha + u_{02}^\alpha}{2} e^{-\lambda t} \tag{8.15}$$

$$u_2^\alpha(t) = \frac{u_{02}^\alpha - u_{01}^\alpha}{2} e^{\lambda t} + \frac{u_{01}^\alpha + u_{02}^\alpha}{2} e^{-\lambda t}.$$

Thus, the solution of problem (8.14) is the fuzzy function $u(\cdot)$ with α-levels given by the above equations (8.15). Figure 8.3 represents the solution of decay in Malthusian fuzzy model.

Remarks:

1. The diameter of $[u(t)]^\alpha$, given by

$$\text{diam}([u(t)]^\alpha) = u_2^\alpha(t) - u_1^\alpha(t) = (u_{02}^\alpha - u_{01}^\alpha)e^{\lambda t},$$

is always increasing in t, except if $u_{02}^\alpha = u_{01}^\alpha$, that is, $u_0 \in \mathbb{R}$. This is the major criticism of the fuzzy derivative and in particular of Hukuhara derivative. There is a clear difficulty in defining the concept of stability, as well as an attractor, with that type of fuzzy differential equation.

2. Solving $u' = -\lambda u$ is different from solving $u' + \lambda u = 0$ [21].
3. If we have a FIVP whose direction field is an extension of a deterministic field, then every deterministic solution is a *preferred solution*, in sense that it has membership degree equal to one on the set of fuzzy solutions. This result is formalized and proved in [12]. To illustrate this fact, let us restrict ourselves to the FIVP of the Malthusian equation previously studied. Associated with this problem we have the deterministic IVP

$$\begin{cases} x'(t) = -\lambda x(t) \\ \quad x_0 \in \mathbb{R} \end{cases}, \tag{8.16}$$

whose solution is

$$x(t) = x_0 e^{-\lambda t}.$$

Thus, if $x_0 \in [u_0]^1$, then it is easy to see that

$$u_1^\alpha(t) \le x(t) \le u_2^\alpha(t), \quad \forall \alpha \in [0, 1].$$

This means that $x(t) \in [u(t)]^1$ for all t. Then the deterministic solution $x(t)$ has membership degree 1 in the set of fuzzy solutions. Therefore, it is a *preferred* solution (see Figs. 8.2 and 8.3).

According to Remark **1**, there is a difficulty in defining stability for this type of differential equation, since the diameter of the solutions increases with time for all α in the interval $[0, 1]$. Researchers have sought to circumvent this anomaly by using other methods to study continuous fuzzy dynamical systems, that is, with **continuous variation rate** in some sense. Two methods that are able to resolve the problem of increasing diameters in the solution to some FIVP obtained via Hukuhara derivative are fuzzy differential inclusion and the Extension Principle methods (see [17]). Another approach was proposed by Bede and Gal [22] extending the Hukuhara derivative (this method will not be discussed here).

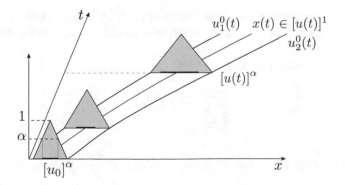

Fig. 8.2 Solution of the fuzzy Malthusian model for population in expansion ($\lambda > 0$)

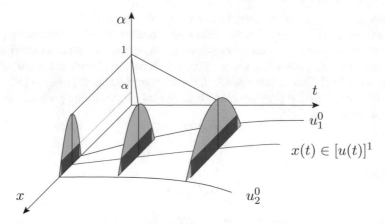

Fig. 8.3 Decay in Malthusian fuzzy model ($\lambda < 0$)

The method of fuzzy differential inclusions requires knowledge of multivalued function analysis and classical differential inclusions. For this reason, we only present the main ideas to introduce and illustrate its potential applications (the reader might consult [16, 17, 23–26], and others texts of multivalued analysis).

The Extension Principle method can be considered to be simpler because it requires only the application of the extension principle on deterministic solutions. More specifically, from the deterministic solution, for every fixed t, it can be seen as a function of the initial condition x_0 to which we apply the Extension Principle of Zadeh. Therefore, this method is applicable only for fuzzy systems that originate from deterministic ones.

8.1.3   Generalized Fuzzy Initial Value Problem (GFIVP)

We continue our study of continuous fuzzy systems by looking at the GFIVP from two distinct approaches, via fuzzy differential inclusions and via the principle of Zadeh's extension.

Let us consider the problem

$$\begin{cases} \dfrac{du}{dt} = F(t, u(t)) \,, \\ u(a) = u_0 \end{cases} \tag{8.17}$$

where $F : [a, b] \times \mathcal{F}(\mathbb{R}) \longrightarrow \mathcal{F}(\mathbb{R})$, $u_0 \in \mathcal{F}(\mathbb{R})$ and $\dfrac{du}{dt}$ represents the continuous variation rate of the function $u(.)$ in some sense. If $\dfrac{du}{dt}$ is the Hukuhara's derivative of the unknown function $u(.)$, the study of *GFIVP* is reduced to what we discussed in Sect. 8.1.2.

A function $u : [a, b] \to \mathcal{F}(\mathbb{R})$ is a solution of (8.17) in the various ways we will analyze it, if, and only if, it satisfies Eq. (8.17) and $u(a) = u_0$. To this generalized problem we define, for each fixed $t \geq 0$, a family of functions given by

$$\psi_t : \mathcal{F}(\mathbb{R}) \to \mathcal{F}(\mathbb{R})$$
$$u_0 \mapsto \psi_t(u_0) := u(t, u_0),$$

where $u(t, u_0)$ is a solution of (8.17) at the instant t, with initial condition $u(a) = u_0$.

The purpose of the following subsections is to suggest two ways to obtain the family ψ_t.

Fuzzy Initial Value Problem via Fuzzy Differential Inclusion

We begin with differential inclusions as an alternative approach to the Hukuhara derivative. To study a fuzzy initial value problem, the concept of derivative of a fuzzy function is not used. The derivative used is the usual one of deterministic functions and the fuzzy solution of (8.17) is "constituted" from deterministic functions. There are several ways of using the differential inclusions to adapt them to the fuzzy context (see [3, 4, 17, 24]).

Here we will follow the suggestion of Hüllermeier [4]. The idea is the following: the field $F : [a, b] \times \mathcal{F}(\mathbb{R}) \to \mathcal{F}(\mathbb{R})$ is such that, for each pair (t, u) we have $F(t, u) \in \mathcal{F}(\mathbb{R})$, and so the fuzzy solution of (8.17) will be made up of all deterministic trajectories that satisfy the classical differential inclusions,

$$\begin{cases} x'(t) \in [F(t, x(t))]^\alpha \\ \quad x(a) \in [u_0]^\alpha \end{cases} . \tag{8.18}$$

A deterministic function $x_\alpha : [a, b] \to \mathbb{R}$ is a solution of (8.17), with membership degree α, if it is absolutely continuous and satisfies (8.18) for almost every $t \geq a$. Then, the fuzzy solution of (8.17) is the fuzzy function $u : [a, b] \to \mathcal{F}(\mathbb{R})$ whose α-levels are

$$[u]^\alpha = \{x_\alpha : [a, b] \to \mathbb{R}, \text{ that are solutions of (18)}\}.$$

Under certain conditions of regularity of F, Diamond [27] proved that the sets $\{x_\alpha : [a, b] \longrightarrow \mathbb{R}, \text{ that are solutions of (8.18)}\}$ satisfy Theorem 1.4 of the representation in the space of functions, and in this case, the function u is well-defined.

Thus, for each t, the functions $\psi_t : \mathcal{F}(\mathbb{R}) \longrightarrow \mathcal{F}(\mathbb{R})$ associated with *GFIVP* (8.17) are given by:

$$\psi_t(u_0) = u(t, u_0),$$

where u is a solution of (8.17) in the Hüllermeier's sense. In this case, the α-levels of $\psi_t(u_0)$ are the intervals $[\psi_t(u_0)]^\alpha$.

Let us illustrate the concepts presented here with the Malthusian model and verify that the diameters of the α-levels of the solutions $[\psi_t(u_0)]^\alpha$ are slowly increasing for populations in expansion and decrescent for populations that are contracting.

Example 8.3 (*Growth rate well determined*) If $\lambda \in \mathbb{R}$ and $u_0 \in \mathcal{F}(\mathbb{R})$, then the Malthus model has the form

$$\begin{cases} x'(t) = \lambda x(t) \\ x_\alpha(0) \in [u_0]^\alpha = [u_{01}^\alpha, u_{02}^\alpha] \end{cases} \tag{8.19}$$

whose fuzzy solution is formed by the deterministic functions

$$x_\alpha(t) = x_\alpha(0)e^{\lambda t}, \text{ with } x_\alpha(0) \in [u_{01}^\alpha, u_{02}^\alpha].$$

Thus,

$$[\psi_t(u_0)]^\alpha = [u_{01}^\alpha e^{\lambda t}, u_{02}^\alpha e^{\lambda t}] = [u_{01}^\alpha, u_{02}^\alpha]e^{\lambda t},$$

so that

$$\psi_t(u_0) = u_0 e^{\lambda t}.$$

The diameters of the α-levels of the fuzzy solution $\psi_t(u_0)$ are

$$\text{diam}([\psi_t(u_0)]^\alpha) = (u_{02}^\alpha - u_{01}^\alpha)e^{\lambda t}.$$

Therefore, for populations in expansion ($\lambda > 0$), we have the diameter increasing with time t, and for contracting populations in retraction ($\lambda < 0$) the diameter is decreasing.

Example 8.4 (*Growth rate and uncertain initial condition*) If the growth rate and the initial condition are uncertain, that is, $\Lambda \in \mathcal{F}(\mathbb{R})$, with $[\Lambda]^\alpha = [\lambda_1^\alpha, \lambda_2^\alpha]$, and $u_0 \in \mathcal{F}(\mathbb{R})$, then the Malthusian model takes the form:

$$\begin{cases} x'(t) \in [\Lambda x(t)]^\alpha = x(t)[\lambda_1^\alpha, \lambda_2^\alpha] \\ x_\alpha(0) \in [u_0]^\alpha = [u_{01}^\alpha, u_{02}^\alpha] \end{cases} \tag{8.20}$$

whose fuzzy solution is given by the deterministic functions:

$$x_\alpha(t) = x_\alpha(0)e^{\lambda t}, \text{ with } \lambda \in [\lambda_1^\alpha, \lambda_2^\alpha] \text{ and } x_\alpha(0) \in [u_{01}^\alpha, u_{02}^\alpha].$$

Therefore, assuming that $\lambda_1^\alpha \geq 0$ (**strong expansion**), we have

$$[\psi_t(u_0)]^\alpha = [u_{01}^\alpha e^{\lambda_1 t}, u_{02}^\alpha e^{\lambda_2 t}],$$

and in this case, diam$[\psi_t(u_0)]^\alpha$ grows with t, since $\lambda_2^\alpha > \lambda_1^\alpha > 0$.

On the other hand, supposing that $\lambda_2^\alpha < 0$ (**strong contraction**),

$$[\psi_t(u_0)]^\alpha = [u_{01}^\alpha e^{\lambda_2^\alpha t}, u_{02}^\alpha e^{\lambda_1^\alpha t}],$$

and in this case, $\text{diam}[\psi_t(u_0)]^\alpha$ decreases with t, since $\lambda_2^\alpha > \lambda_1^\alpha$. We leave to the reader the cases in which λ_1^α and λ_2^α have opposite signs.

Applications of fuzzy differential inclusions to biological phenomena can be found in the literature, but as yet, they are few in number. The reader might consult [16] for models in epidemiology, and [17, 26] in population dynamics. Comparisons between the solutions of Hukuhara and Hüllermeier can be found in [28].

Fuzzy Initial Value Problem Via Zadeh's Extension

Another approach to obtain a fuzzy solution to the *GFIVP* (8.17) is by using the Zadeh extension that was explained in Chap. 2. In this case, if only the initial condition and/or some parameter of the field F are/is fuzzy, then the *GFIVP* solutions are obtained through the fuzzification of the deterministic solutions by the principle of extension.

As we did in the case of fuzzy differential inclusions, we will study two different cases here. In the first case, only the initial condition is given by a fuzzy number. In the second case, we assume that the initial condition and/or some parameter of the initial value problem are/is fuzzy.

Case (a) – Fuzzy Initial Condition

- We consider that only the initial condition is fuzzy. In this case, the initial value problem is given by

$$\begin{cases} \dfrac{dx}{dt} = f(t, x(t)) \\[2mm] x(a) = u_0 \in \mathcal{F}(\mathbb{R}) \end{cases}, \tag{8.21}$$

with $f : [a, b] \to \mathbb{R}$ continuous.
Assuming that for every initial condition $x_0 \in \mathbb{R}$ the deterministic problem

$$\begin{cases} \dfrac{dx}{dt} = f(t, x(t)) \\[2mm] x(a) = x_0 \end{cases}, \tag{8.22}$$

admits unique solution ϕ_t then, for every t, the fuzzy solution ψ_t of (8.21) is defined as the Zadeh's extension of the deterministic solution ϕ_t, namely

$$\text{If } u_0 \in \mathcal{F}(\mathbb{R}) \text{ then } \psi_t(u_0) = \widehat{\phi_t}(u_0).$$

In this case, because ϕ_t is continuous with respect to the initial condition so that, by Theorem 2.1, we have

$$[\psi_t(u_0)]^\alpha = [\widehat{\phi_t}(u_0)]^\alpha = \phi_t([u_0]^\alpha) = \phi_t([u_{01}^\alpha, u_{02}^\alpha]).$$

We notice that the above formula indicates that the membership degree of x_0 to u_0 is the same as that of $\phi_t(x_0)$ to $\widehat{\phi}_t(u_0)$, for all t. With this procedure we find the solution to the Malthusian model.

- If $\lambda \in \mathbb{R}$ and $u_0 \in \mathcal{F}(\mathbb{R})$, we have

$$
\begin{cases}
\dfrac{dx}{dt} = \lambda x(t) \\[2mm]
x(0) = u_0
\end{cases}. \tag{8.23}
$$

The deterministic flow of the Malthusian model (8.1) is given by $\phi_t(x_0) = x_0 e^{\lambda t}$. Therefore, using Definition 2.1, the fuzzy flow is $\widehat{\phi}_t(u_0) = u_0 e^{\lambda t}$, whose α-levels are given by

$$
[\widehat{\phi}_t(u_0)]^\alpha = \phi_t([u_0]^\alpha) = [u_0]^\alpha e^{\lambda t} = [u_{01}^\alpha, u_{02}^\alpha] e^{\lambda t}.
$$

So, for every t, the diameters of the α-levels of the fuzzy solution are given by

$$
\text{diam}([\widehat{\phi}_t(u_0)]^\alpha) = (u_{02}^\alpha - u_{01}^\alpha) e^{\lambda t}
$$

which coincides with those obtained in the previous case of differential inclusions (8.19). This allows us to conclude that such diameters grow for populations in expansion and decrease for contracting populations.

Case (b) – Fuzzy Parameter and Initial Condition

- We suppose now that the *GFIVP* (8.17) is fuzzy because some parameters (Λ) and also the initial condition are fuzzy. Thus, the initial value problem takes the form

$$
\begin{cases}
\dfrac{dx}{dt} = \widehat{f}(t, \Lambda, x(t)) \\[2mm]
x_\alpha(0) = u_0 \in \mathcal{F}(\mathbb{R})
\end{cases}. \tag{8.24}
$$

In this case, we have the previous case and add a new equation ($y = \lambda$, with $y' = 0$). That is, looking at the parameter as a variable and in the original deterministic model (8.22), we add the pair (λ, x_0) to initial condition. For a mathematical formalism of this method the reader may consult [17, 29]. Let us illustrate this case still considering the Malthusian model.

- Suppose we have that the growth rate $\Lambda \in \mathcal{F}(\mathbb{R})$ and the initial condition $u_0 \in \mathcal{F}(\mathbb{R})$. We know that the deterministic solutions of the expanded Malthusian model (8.1)

$$
\begin{cases}
\dfrac{dx}{dt} = \lambda x \\[2mm]
\dfrac{dy}{dt} = 0 \\[2mm]
x(0) = x_0 \text{ and } y(0) = \lambda
\end{cases}
$$

are given by $\phi_t(\lambda, x_0) = x_0 e^{\lambda t}$, where x_0 and λ are real numbers. Now, if

$$[\Lambda]^\alpha = [\lambda_1^\alpha, \lambda_2^\alpha] \quad and \quad [u_0]^\alpha = [u_{01}^\alpha, u_{02}^\alpha]$$

then the solution of (8.24) with $\widehat{f}(t, \Lambda, x(t)) = \Lambda x$ is given by

$$[\psi_t(\Lambda, u_0)]^\alpha = [\widehat{\phi_t}(\Lambda, u_0)]^\alpha = \phi_t([\lambda_1^\alpha, \lambda_2^\alpha], [u_{01}^\alpha, u_{02}^\alpha]). \qquad (8.25)$$

Therefore, assuming that $\lambda_1^\alpha \geq 0$ (**strong expansion**),

$$[\psi_t(\Lambda, u_0)]^\alpha = [u_{01}^\alpha e^{\lambda_1^\alpha t}, u_{02}^\alpha e^{\lambda_2^\alpha t}],$$

and in this case, $\mathrm{diam}[\psi_t(\Lambda, u_0)]^\alpha$ increase with t, since $\lambda_2^\alpha > \lambda_1^\alpha$. On the other hand, supposing that $\lambda_2^\alpha \leq 0$ (**strong contraction**),

$$[\psi_t(\Lambda, u_0)]^\alpha = [u_{01}^\alpha e^{\lambda_2^\alpha t}, u_{02}^\alpha e^{\lambda_1^\alpha t}],$$

and in this case, $\mathrm{diam}[\psi_t(\Lambda, u_0)]^\alpha$ decreases with t, since $\lambda_2^\alpha > \lambda_1^\alpha$. The cases in which λ_1^α and λ_2^α have opposite signs we leave to the reader.

As the reader can see, the solutions to the model of Malthus obtained via differential inclusion and via extension principle are the same. This was not a coincidence just for the model that was chosen. Under certain conditions such methods produce the same solutions (see [17] for details).

The use of this type of variational equations has been accepted by researchers from many areas, in particular with regard to issues related to biological phenomena. Jafelice et al. [30] used this methodology to study the dynamics of HIV with treatment, considering the action of the fuzzy delay in action of the drug.

The study of stability of stationary states (equilibrium) plays a key role in dynamical systems. Therefore, we present next, an introduction to stability of fuzzy dynamical systems formulated via fuzzy differential inclusions and/or via the Extension Principle. We want to emphasize that there is a consolidated theory of stability of fuzzy dynamical systems. We offer some results below. But these are somewhat specific.

Stability of Continuous Fuzzy Dynamical Systems

Let us start this section defining stationary states (or equilibrium) for *GFIVP* (8.17).

Definition 8.4 (*Equilibrium*) A fuzzy number $\bar{u} \in \mathcal{F}(\mathbb{R})$ is a *point of equilibrium* or a *stationary state* of (8.17) if

$$\psi_t(\bar{u}) = \bar{u}, \quad \text{for all } t \geq a,$$

that is, if $\bar{u}$ is a fixed point for all ψ_t.

Remember that for a deterministic initial value problem, equilibrium points are those whose derivative is zero, and these are exactly the fixed points of their solutions, viewed as functions of the initial conditions. Because here we have no notion of derivative to fuzzy functions we define equilibrium as fixed points of the flows generated by *GFIVP'S*.

Now we are only interested in the initial value problems that are *autonomous*, that is, the field F does not depend explicitly on t. Let us consider only the autonomous systems whose **IVP's** has unique solution. The great advantage of autonomous systems, which will be explored here, comes from the fact that their solutions have the property of flow, which we will explain below.

We will present results of stability only for *autonomous generalized fuzzy initial value problems AGFIVP* namely

$$\begin{cases} \dfrac{du}{dt} = F(u(t)) \\ u(a) = u_0 \in \mathcal{F}(\mathbb{R}) \end{cases}. \tag{8.26}$$

It is known that, for this problem, the family of solutions ψ_t has the property of flow:

(1) $\psi_0(u_0) = u_0$ for all $u_0 \in \mathcal{F}(\mathbb{R})$, that is, ψ_0 is the identity function on $\mathcal{F}(\mathbb{R})$;
(2) $\psi_{t+s}(u_0) = \psi_t(\psi_s(u_0)) = (\psi_t o \psi_s)(u_0)$ for all $u_0 \in \mathcal{F}(\mathbb{R})$.

Property (2) above characterizes a flow. It means that, starting from a state u_0, the state reached at time $t + s$, $\psi_{t+s}(u_0)$, is the same as that reached $\psi_t(\psi_s(u_0))$, at time t, starting with $\psi_s(u_0)$.

Examples of such flows are the solutions of deterministic autonomous initial value problems and also those flows generated by differential inclusions (see [4]).

Proposition 8.6 *Given the deterministic autonomous initial value problem*

$$\begin{cases} \dfrac{dx}{dt} = f(x(t)) \\ x(a) = x_0 \end{cases}, \tag{8.27}$$

let us consider the AGFIVP (8.26) associated with IVP (8.27)

$$\begin{cases} \dfrac{dx}{dt} = f(x(t)) \\ x(a) = u_0 \in \mathcal{F}(\mathbb{R}) \end{cases}. \tag{8.28}$$

Under these conditions, any equilibrium point of (8.27) is an equilibrium point of (8.28). Moreover the real numbers that are equilibria of (8.28) are also equilibria of (8.27) if the solution is given by the extension method or by fuzzy differential inclusion.

Proof By Theorem 2.1 we have

$$[\widehat{\phi}_t(\chi_{\{\overline{x}\}})]^\alpha = \phi_t([\chi_{\{\overline{x}\}}]^\alpha) = \phi_t(\overline{x}),$$

where $\chi_{\{\overline{x}\}}$ is the membership function of $\overline{x}$, ϕ_t is the deterministic flow and $\widehat{\phi}_t$ is the fuzzy flow.

Thus,

$$\phi_t(\overline{x}) = \overline{x} \iff [\widehat{\phi}_t(\chi_{\{\overline{x}\}})]^\alpha = [\chi_{\{\overline{x}\}}]^\alpha,$$

that is, $\overline{x}$ is an equilibrium of (8.27) if and only if $\chi_{\{\overline{x}\}}$ is an equilibrium of (8.28). ∎

The stability of continuous dynamical systems will be studied through flows of its solutions. Using the metric $\mathscr{D}$ (Definition 8.3), we define stability of equilibrium points.

Definition 8.5 (*Stability*) Let $\overline{u}$ be an equilibrium point of (8.28). Then it is:

(a) *Stable,* if $\forall \varepsilon > 0$ there exists $\delta > 0$ such that

$$\text{if } \mathscr{D}(\overline{u}, u) \leq \delta, \text{ then } \mathscr{D}(\overline{u}, \psi_t(u)) \leq \varepsilon, \text{ for all } t \geq a,$$

(the equilibrium points that are not stable are said *unstable*);

(b) *Asymptotically stable,* if it is stable and there is $r > 0$ such that

$$\lim_{t \to +\infty} \mathscr{D}(\psi_t(u), \overline{u}) = 0 \text{ whenever } \mathscr{D}(\overline{u}, u) \leq r.$$

It is easily seen that with this notion of stability, it is not possible to have asymptotically stable equilibrium for continuous fuzzy systems, for which the derivative used is the Hukuhara derivative. Recall that for such systems the diameters of α-levels of the solutions are always increasing. The main stability result that we next develop is for continuous fuzzy systems whose solutions are obtained through the Zadeh's extension principle.

We remark that, with the Definition 8.5 of stability, it is easy to verify that the Malthusian population model in contraction, whose solutions are obtained via fuzzy differential inclusions or Zadeh's extension, are asymptotically stable. The following result generalizes this observation.

Theorem 8.7 *Let $\overline{x}$ be an equilibrium of the deterministic initial value problem (8.27). Then,*

(a) *$\overline{x}$ is stable for* IVP *(8.27) if and only if $\chi_{\{\overline{x}\}}$ is stable for* AGFIVP *(8.28);*

(b) *$\overline{x}$ is asymptotically stable for* IVP *(8.27) if and only if $\chi_{\{\overline{x}\}}$ is asymptotically stable for* AGFIVP *(8.28).*

Proof See [17]. ∎

Corollary 8.8 *Let $\overline{x}$ be an equilibrium point of (8.27). Then, the equilibrium point $\chi_{\{\overline{x}\}}$ of (8.28) will be stable if $f'(\overline{x}) < 0$, and unstable if $f'(\overline{x}) > 0$.*

Proof Recall that this hypothesis is sufficient for asymptote stability in the classical case. The conclusion follows from Theorem 8.7.   ∎

To end this section we notice that although Theorem 8.7 is quite intuitive, it reveals something that we consider important. If $\bar{x}$ is asymptotically stable for (8.27) then $\bar{x}$ attracts points of $\mathbb{R}$. Now, to be asymptotically stable in the fuzzy space $(\mathcal{F}(\mathbb{R}), \mathscr{D})$ means that the point attracts fuzzy sets, and therefore attracts their level sets, which are compact subsets of $\mathbb{R}$. From the modeling point of view, this means that the stability of $\bar{x}$ is independent of the uncertainties of the initial conditions. A more general study of stability of fuzzy systems via the Extension Principle can be found in [17]. By using Zadeh's extension, Cecconello [29] studied the flows in fuzzy metric spaces and the existence of periodic orbits from classical autonomous systems.

At the beginning of Sect. 8.1 we promised four approaches for continuous fuzzy dynamical systems, so we introduce the last one, fuzzy systems where the directions field is given by a fuzzy rule base.

P-Fuzzy Initial Value Problem

The nomenclature p-fuzzy means partially fuzzy. These systems are partially fuzzy in the sense that the direction field F of the respective *IVP* is known only partially. However, its solution (trajectory) is crisp, since in each instant t it is a real number obtained after a process of defuzzification. Formally we have,

Definition 8.6 A *p-fuzzy IVP* is given by

$$\begin{cases} \dfrac{du}{dt} = F(t, u(t)) \\ u(a) = u_0 \end{cases}, \qquad (8.29)$$

where F is partly known and described by a fuzzy rule base (see Chap. 5).

Given a fuzzy rule base and a particular defuzzification of the output of fuzzy rule base, we have that the solution $u(t)$ of (8.29) belongs to $\mathbb{R}$. In this case, we have the method of Sect. 6.4 where F is the function given by fuzzy controllers. Following this line of thinking, we will study the IVP

$$\begin{cases} \dfrac{dx}{dt} = f(x) \\ x(a) = x_0 \end{cases}, \qquad (8.30)$$

where f is replaced by a fuzzy rule base consistent with studied phenomenon. For example, in the Malthusian model, the growth rate of a population is directly proportional to the population. The rule base built here is for the rate of change per unit of time, denoted by $\frac{dX}{dt}$, with respect to the population X. Thus x is the value of input variable X, while $\frac{dx}{dt}$ is the value of the output variable $\frac{dX}{dt}$. We will take only four qualifiers for each of these linguistic variables, summarized in Frame 8.1.

R_1 : **If** the population (X) is "very small" (MB) **then** the rate is

"very small" (MB)

R_2 : **If** the population (X) is "small" (B) **then** the rate is "small" (B)

R_3 : **If** the population (X) is "average" (M) **then** the rate is "average" (M)

R_4 : **If** the population (X) is "high" (A) **then** the rate is "high" (A)

Frame 8.1: Rule base for modeling the variation of population based on its density.

The membership functions that correspond to each value of the linguistic variables of the rule base are given in Fig. 8.4.

Fig. 8.4 Membership functions of rule base (Frame 8.1)

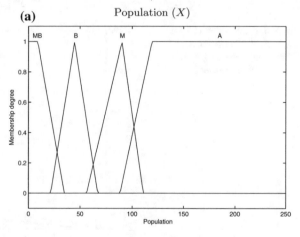

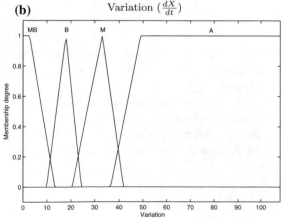

Fig. 8.5 Granules for the
Malthusian model and
possible growth function f

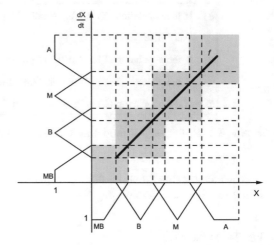

Fig. 8.6 Solutions $x(.)$ for
the Malthusian p-fuzzy and
for deterministic case with
$a = 9.5\%$ and $x_0 = 2$

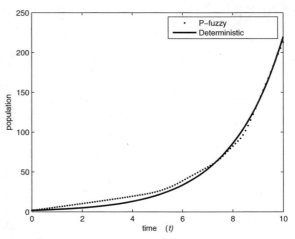

Figure 8.5 illustrates the rules of Frame 8.1 in granular form, supposing that each
of the above quantifiers are given by a triangular fuzzy number and corresponding
to the underlying f.

Adopting the Mamdani fuzzy controller and with center of mass as a defuzzificator, combined with the Euler method (see details in Sect. 6.4 and in Chap. 9),
we obtain the solution of the p-fuzzy Malthusian model whose graph is depicted in
Fig. 8.6. A more detailed study about p-fuzzy systems will be given in Chap. 9.

8.2 Discrete Fuzzy Dynamic System

A discrete dynamical system is given by a recurrence or iterative process. In this section we introduce *discrete fuzzy dynamical systems* as a generalization of the classical ones. To illustrate the process, we use once more the population models - the exponential (Malthus) and logistic (Verhulst) models.

Definition 8.7 A *discrete fuzzy dynamic system* is an iterative process of fuzzy subsets

$$\begin{cases} u_{t+1} = F(u_t) \\ u_0 \in \mathcal{F}(\mathbb{R}) \end{cases}, \tag{8.31}$$

where $F : \mathcal{F}(\mathbb{R}) \to \mathcal{F}(\mathbb{R})$ is a function between spaces of fuzzy subsets.

Definition 8.8 Given $u_0 \in \mathcal{F}(\mathbb{R})$ and F as in Definition 8.7, the iteration sequence $u_0, F(u_0), F(F(u_0)), \ldots$, is called a *solution* or a *positive orbit* of u_0.

According to these definitions, the flow ψ_t for discrete systems is given by successive compositions of field F:

$$\begin{aligned}
\psi_0(u_0) &= F^0(u_0) = & u_0 \\
\psi_1(u_0) &= F^1(u_0) = & F(u_0) \\
\psi_2(u_0) &= F^2(u_0) = & F(F(u_0)) \\
&\vdots \quad = \quad \vdots \quad = & \vdots \\
\psi_t(u_0) &= F^t(u_0) = & F(F^{t-1}(u_0)),
\end{aligned}$$

for $t \in \mathbb{N}$.

Thus, if $u_0 \in \mathcal{F}(\mathbb{R})$, then the iterates defined above and its limit, when limit exists in the metric $\mathscr{D}$), are in $\mathcal{F}(\mathbb{R})$, since the metric space $(\mathcal{F}(\mathbb{R}), \mathscr{D})$ is complete (see [20]). We note that, in a discrete system, the time is proportional to the number of iterations performed. Based on Definition 8.4 we have the following definition.

Definition 8.9 (*Equilibrium*) A fuzzy number $\overline{u} \in \mathcal{F}(\mathbb{R})$ is an equilibrium point of the fuzzy discrete system (8.31) if $\psi_t(\overline{u}) = \overline{u}$, for all $t \geq 0$. That is, $F(\overline{u}) = \overline{u}$, and $\overline{u}$ is a fixed point of F.

Next we will briefly analyze the dynamics of the Malthusian model, assuming that we have the uncertainty in the initial condition, which is reasonable for problems of dynamics of population, especially when starting with a very large or estimated population. A typical example is the initial number of bacteria in a culture.

8.2.1 Discrete Fuzzy Malthusian Model

Let us assume that, as in the continuous case, in each generation t, the number of individuals is proportional to the population in the previous generation. Furthermore, the initial condition is uncertain and is given by $u_0 \in \mathcal{F}(\mathbb{R})$ so that their α-levels are the closed intervals $[u_0]^\alpha = [u_{01}^\alpha, u_{02}^\alpha] \subset \mathbb{R}^+$, for all $\alpha \in [0, 1]$. As we did in the continuous case, we also distinguish two situations:

Case (a) Growth rate is crisp and initial condition is uncertain

- If $\lambda > 0$, the discrete fuzzy Malthusian model is given by:

$$\begin{cases} u_{t+1} = \lambda u_t \\ u_0 \in \mathcal{F}(\mathbb{R}) \end{cases}.$$ (8.32)

The solution of (8.32) is given by

$$u_t = \lambda^t u_0,$$ (8.33)

whose α-levels are $[u_t]^\alpha = \lambda^t [u_0]^\alpha = [\lambda^t u_{01}^\alpha, \lambda^t u_{02}^\alpha]$.

Case (b) Growth rate and initial condition are uncertain

- In this case, besides the initial condition, we also have that the growth rate (Λ) is fuzzy. If $\Lambda \in \mathcal{F}(\mathbb{R})$ with $[\Lambda]^\alpha = [\lambda_1^\alpha, \lambda_2^\alpha]$ and $u_0 \in \mathcal{F}(\mathbb{R})$, the discrete fuzzy Malthusian model is given by:

$$\begin{cases} u_{t+1} = \Lambda u_t \\ u_0 \in \mathcal{F}(\mathbb{R}) \end{cases},$$ (8.34)

with fuzzy solution

$$u_t = \Lambda^t u_0,$$ (8.35)

whose α-levels are $[u_t]^\alpha = [(\lambda_1^\alpha)^t u_{01}^\alpha, (\lambda_2^\alpha)^t u_{02}^\alpha]$.

Equilibrium Points

According to the above solutions (8.33) and (8.35), we conclude that if $\lambda \neq 1$ ($\Lambda \neq \widehat{1}$) then the unique equilibrium of the discrete fuzzy Malthusian system is the fuzzy point $\chi_{\{0\}}$, and if $\lambda = 1$ ($\Lambda = \widehat{1}$) then any initial condition $u_0 \in \mathcal{F}(\mathbb{R})$ is an equilibrium point.

Unlike the continuous case, the fuzzy differential equations, as we saw in Sect. 8.1.2, can have diameters of the solution that decrease, increase or stay the same. For our example above we have, if $\lambda \in \mathbb{R}$,

$$diam[u_t]^\alpha = diam[\lambda^t u_0]^\alpha = \lambda^t diam[u_0]^\alpha$$

and so,

$$\lim_{t \to +\infty} diam[u_t]^\alpha = \begin{cases} 0 & \text{if } 0 < \lambda < 1 \\ +\infty & \text{if } \lambda > 1 \\ diam[u_0]^\alpha & \text{if } \lambda = 1 \end{cases}.$$

Stability of the Equilibrium Point $\chi_{\{0\}}$

We have, for metric $\mathscr{D}$, that

$$\mathscr{D}(\chi_{\{0\}}, u_0) = \sup_{0 \le \alpha \le 1} d_H([\chi_{\{0\}}]^\alpha, [u_0]^\alpha) = u_{02}^0$$

and

$$\mathscr{D}(\chi_{\{0\}}, u_t) = \mathscr{D}(\chi_{\{0\}}, \lambda^t u_0) = \lambda^t u_{02}^0.$$

Thus, for the model (8.32), $\chi_{\{0\}}$ is stable if $0 < \lambda \le 1$, and asymptotically stable if $0 < \lambda < 1$ since at this case $\lim_{n \to +\infty} \mathscr{D}(\chi_{\{0\}}, u_t) = 0$. For $\lambda > 1$, the equilibrium $\chi_{\{0\}}$ is unstable. We leave it to the reader to study the case in which the growth rate Λ is fuzzy.

The conclusions we obtain for the discrete fuzzy Malthusian model with respect to stability, are actually more general as we discuss below. Let the discrete deterministic system be

$$x_{t+1} = f(x_t). \tag{8.36}$$

Associated with this system, we have a fuzzy system (8.31) (it is sufficient to consider in (8.31) the extension $\widehat{f}$ of the function f). Now, if $\bar{x}$ is an equilibrium point of the system (8.36), then $\chi_{\{\bar{x}\}}$ is an equilibrium of system (8.31) obtained by the fuzzification of the deterministic field f, and these equilibria have the same characteristics of stability. The following theorem allows us to characterize the types of stability for the equilibrium of discrete fuzzy dynamical systems which come from deterministic systems. This is the discrete version of Theorem 8.7.

Theorem 8.9 *Let $f : \mathbb{R} \to \mathbb{R}$ be a continuous function and $\widehat{f}$ its Zadeh's extension. Then,*

(a) *$\chi_{\{\bar{x}\}}$ is an equilibrium to the fuzzy system $u_{t+1} = \widehat{f}(u_t)$ if, and only if, $\bar{x}$ is an equilibrium of the deterministic system $x_{t+1} = f(x_t)$;*
(b) *$\chi_{\{\bar{x}\}}$ is stable to the fuzzy system $u_{t+1} = \widehat{f}(u_t)$ if, and only, if $\bar{x}$ is stable of the deterministic system $x_{t+1} = f(x_t)$;*
(c) *$\chi_{\{\bar{x}\}}$ is asymptotically stable to the fuzzy system $u_{t+1} = \widehat{f}(u_t)$ if, and only if, $\bar{x}$ is asymptotically stable of the deterministic system $x_{t+1} = f(x_t)$.*

Proof (see [12, 31, 32]). ∎

Corollary 8.10 *Suppose that f is continuously differentiable. Then the equilibrium $\chi_{\{\bar{x}\}}$ of the discrete fuzzy system $u_{t+1} = \widehat{f}(u_t)$ will be asymptotically stable if $|f'(\bar{x})| < 1$, and unstable if $|f'(\bar{x})| > 1$.*

Proof Remember that the hypotheses of the corollary above are sufficient for stability on the deterministic case (see [33]). The conclusion is a consequence of Theorem 8.9. ∎

These last two results hold in a more general context (see [12, 31]).

Returning to the Malthus model, because $\bar{x} = 0$ is asymptotically stable for the deterministic case, Corollary 8.10 allows us to conclude that $\chi_{\{0\}}$ is asymptotically stable for the discrete fuzzy model of Malthus, if $0 < \lambda < 1$.

For cases of nonlinear systems, such as the *logistic model*, the dynamic changes dramatically for discrete fuzzy systems. Since the fuzzy space $\mathcal{F}(\mathbb{R})$ contains $\mathbb{R}$, it is reasonable that the number of critical points of fuzzy systems is greater than the deterministic case. Furthermore, new periodic orbits appear. Also, the bifurcation diagram is different from the one that appear in the classical case. Let us check these facts for the logistic model (or Verhulst).

8.2.2 Discrete Fuzzy Logistic Model

The deterministic logistic model (or Verhulst model) supposes an inhibition in growth when the population is very high as $t \to +\infty$. Its mathematical formulation is given by

$$\begin{cases} x_{t+1} = ax_t(1 - x_t) \\ x_0 \in \mathbb{R}^+ \end{cases}, \tag{8.37}$$

where x_t denotes the population density in the generation t and a is the rate of intrinsic growth, $1 \leq a \leq 4$.

The equilibria of this equation are $\bar{x} = 0$ and $x_a = 1 - \dfrac{1}{a}$. We also known that $\bar{x} = 0$ is unstable, and $x_a = 1 - \dfrac{1}{a}$ is asymptotically stable if $1 < a < 3$. Furthermore, when $a = a_1 = 3$ (the first bifurcation value), the fixed point $x_a = 1 - \dfrac{1}{a}$ loses stability and thereafter, the population oscillates between two values $[x_1, x_2]$ until the next value of the bifurcation that is $a = a_2 = 1 + \sqrt{6}$. At a_2 this orbit of period 2 loses stability and there appears an orbit of period 4 that is stable until the next value of the bifurcation $a = a_3$. This duplication behavior of the orbit periods (Fig. 8.7) still occurs until the system reaches chaos at $a^* = 3.569\ldots$ (see [33]).

Remember that in the discrete logistic model, we are assuming that the population is homogeneous and that the growth rate a is constant for the entire population. However, in any community there are physical and behavioral differences among the individuals of the population. This heterogeneity is more pronounced when individuals are considered separately and less pronounced when considering the group. However, in this example, we consider the same rate a for the entire population. Unlike the analysis we made on the Malthusian model, here we will study only the case where the initial condition is fuzzy and the parameter a is deterministic. We leave, as a challenge to the reader, the case where the growth rate is also fuzzy (the reader may consult [34]).

So, let us consider the fuzzy case where a is real, with $1 \leq a \leq 4$, and the initial condition being a fuzzy number, that is

Fig. 8.7 Deterministic
bifurcation diagram [31]

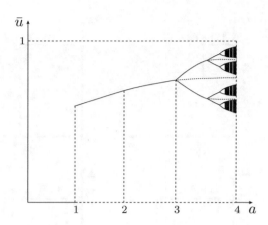

$$\begin{cases} u_{t+1} = \widehat{f}(u_t) \\ u_0 \in \mathcal{F}(\mathbb{R}) \end{cases}, \tag{8.38}$$

where f is the normalized logistic function $f(x) = ax(1 - x)$ and $\widehat{f}$ is its Zadeh's extension.

Equilibrium Points

The equilibrium points of the fuzzy system (8.38) are the fixed points of $\widehat{f}$, that is, the fuzzy numbers u that are solutions of the equation

$$\widehat{f}(u) = u$$

or equivalently, for the level set, since f is continuous (from Theorem 2.1),

$$[\widehat{f}(u)]^\alpha = f([u]^\alpha) = [u]^\alpha = [u_1^\alpha, u_2^\alpha]$$

for all $\alpha \in [0, 1]$, that is,

$$\begin{cases} u_1^\alpha = \min_{u_1^\alpha \le x \le u_2^\alpha} f(x) \\ u_2^\alpha = \max_{u_1^\alpha \le x \le u_2^\alpha} f(x) \end{cases}. \tag{8.39}$$

Denoting by $\hat{0}$ and $\hat{x}_a$ the characteristic functions of the fixed points 0 and $x_a = 1 - \frac{1}{a}$ of the function f and using a direct calculation, we obtain the fixed points of $\widehat{f}$ on $\mathcal{F}(\mathbb{R})$ (see [12, 31]).

- If $1 \le a \le 2$, the fixed points of the fuzzy logistic equation are $\hat{0}$, $\hat{x}_a$ and $\bar{u}_1$, where $\bar{u}_1$ is given by $[\bar{u}_1]^\alpha = [0, x_a]$, $\forall \alpha \in [0, 1]$.
- If $2 < a \le 3$, beyond the fixed points $\hat{0}$ and $\hat{x}_a$, we also have $\bar{u}_2$, given by $[\bar{u}_2]^\alpha = [0, \frac{a}{4}]$, $\forall \alpha \in [0, 1]$.

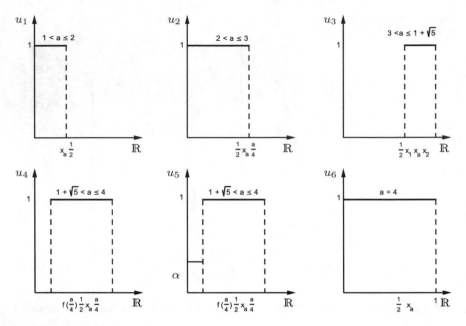

Fig. 8.8 Equilibrium points of the logistic fuzzy system [31]

- If $3 < a \leq 1 + \sqrt{5}$, beyond the fixed points $\hat{0}$, $\hat{x}_a$ and $\overline{u}_2$, we have the fixed point $\overline{u}_3$ with $[\overline{u}_3]^\alpha = [x_1, x_2]$, $\forall \alpha \in [0, 1]$, where x_1 and x_2 are fixed points of $\widehat{f}$, that is $f(x_1) = x_2$ and $f(x_2) = x_1$.
- If $1 + \sqrt{5} < a < 4$, the fixed points are $\hat{0}$, $\hat{x}_a$, $\overline{u}_2$, $\overline{u}_3$, $\overline{u}_4$, where $[\overline{u}_4]^\alpha = [f(\frac{a}{4}), \frac{a}{4}]$ and $\overline{u}_5$ which is given by

$$[\overline{u}_5]^\alpha = \begin{cases} [0, f(\frac{a}{4})] & \text{if } \alpha \leq \overline{\alpha} \\ [f(\frac{a}{4}), \frac{a}{4}] & \text{if } \alpha > \overline{\alpha} \end{cases}$$

  for all $\alpha \in [0, 1]$ and some $\overline{\alpha}$.
- If $a = 4$, the fixed points are: $\hat{0}$, $\hat{x}_a$ and $\overline{u}_6$ with $[\overline{u}_6]^\alpha = [0, 1]$ for all $\alpha \in [0, 1]$.

Figure 8.8 illustrates the fixed points of this example.

Stability of Equilibria

The stability of the equilibrium points $\hat{0}$, $\hat{x}_a$ and cycles of $\widehat{f}$, which are characteristic functions of f cycles, are the same when studying f or $\widehat{f}$, according to Theorem 8.9.

The only new fixed points (fuzzy) of $\widehat{f}$ that are asymptotically stable are $\overline{u}_3$ and $\overline{u}_4$. The others are unstable. Details of this study can be found in [12, 31, 34].

Figure 8.9 represents the bifurcations of equilibrium points and shows the change in magnitude when we vary the parameter a. For the fuzzy model, the deterministic branch is equal to the classical bifurcation diagram (Fig. 8.7) and fuzzy bifurcation

Fig. 8.9 Bifurcation diagram for the fuzzy case [31]

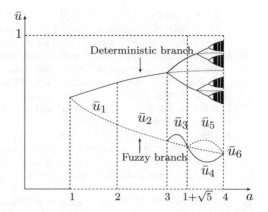

illustrates the new fixed points according to our results. As already pointed out for the deterministic case, $a = 3$ is a bifurcation value, that is, if a is slightly greater than 3, the fixed point x_a ceases to be stable and there appears a new orbit with period 2. For values of a slightly more than $1 + \sqrt{6}$, there appears an orbit of period 4. For values near to 3.89, there is a chaotic behavior in the dynamics of this equation (see [33, 35]). The fuzzy equation also has bifurcation values of $a = 1$, $a = 2$, $a = 3$ and $a = 1 + \sqrt{5}$. The bifurcation diagram below illustrates the dynamics of the logistic model above assuming an initial condition fuzzy.

We stress that the above study deals only with fuzzy equilibrium points. The periodic orbits (cycles) studied are deterministic and as can be shown (see [31, 32]), does not change the type of stability when they are considered in Euclidean or fuzzy spaces. Studies of fuzzy periodic orbits have been developed recently and we already know that every deterministic periodic orbit of period 2^p gives rise to a fuzzy orbit of period 2^{p-1}, $p \geq 2$ (see [34]).

An example of this is the deterministic orbit of period 2 that became the fuzzy equilibrium point $\bar{u}_3$, with α-levels $[\bar{u}_3]^\alpha = [x_1, x_2]$ for all $\alpha \in [0, 1]$. We will not study fuzzy chaos. The interested reader might consult [36, 37].

We want to close this chapter by commenting that, as we saw above, there are several approaches to fuzzy dynamical systems. Besides those presented here, the reader can find others referring, for example, to [38]. The p-fuzzy systems, formally described in Sect. 8.1.5, both for the discrete and continuous cases, will be revisited in greater detail in Chap. 9.

References

1. M. Hukuhara, Integration des applications mesurables donc la valeur est un compact convexe. Funkcialaj Ekvacioj **10**, 205–223 (1967)
2. M.L. Puri, D.A. Ralescu, Differentials of fuzzy functions. J. Math. Anal. Appl. **91**, 552–558 (1983)

3. V.A. Baidosov, Fuzzy differential inclusions. PMM USSR **54**(1), 8–13 (1990)
4. E. Hüllermeier, An approach to modelling and simulation of uncertain dynamical systems. Int. J. Uncertain. Fuzziness Knowl.-Based Syst. **5**, 117–137 (1997)
5. L.C. Barros, L.T. Gomes, P.A. Tonelli, Fuzzy differential equations: an approach via fuzzification of the derivative operator. Fuzzy Sets Syst. **230**, 39–52 (2013)
6. L.T. Gomes, L.C. Barros, B. Bede, *Fuzzy Differential Equations in Various Approaches* (Springer, Berlin, 2015)
7. L.C. Barros, F.S. Pedro, Fuzzy differential equations with interactive derivative, Fuzzy Sets Syst. (2016). (accepted for publication)
8. E. Esmi, F.S. Pedro, L.C. Barros, W.A. Lodwick, *Frèchet Derivative for Linearly Correlated Fuzzy Function* (2016). (submitted for publication)
9. L. Arnold, *Random Dynamical Systems*, 2nd edn. (Springer, Berlin, 2003)
10. D. Maki, M. Thompson, *Mathematical Models and Applications* (Prentice-Hall, Englewood Cliffs, 1973)
11. L. San Martin, M.S.F. Marques, *Cálculo estocástico*, 18o. Colóquio da SBM, IMPA, Rio de Janeiro (1991)
12. L.C. Barros, Sobre sistemas dinâmicos fuzzy - teoria e aplicação, Tese de Doutorado, IMECC-UNICAMP, Campinas (1997)
13. B. Bede, Mathematics of fuzzy sets and fuzzy logic, *Studies in Fuzziness and Soft Computing*, vol. 295 (Springer, Berlin, 2013)
14. O. Kaleva, Fuzzy differential equations. Fuzzy Sets Syst. **24**(3), 301–318 (1987)
15. S. Seikkala, On the fuzzy initial value problem. Fuzzy Sets Syst. **24**(3), 319–330 (1987)
16. L.C. Barros, R.C. Bassanezi, R.Z.G. Oliveira, Fuzzy differential inclusion: An application to epidemiology, in *Soft Methodology and Random Information Systems*, vol. I, ed. by M. Lopez-Diaz, M.A. Gil, P. Grzegorzewski, O. Hyrniewicz, J. Lawry (Springer, Warsaw, 2004), pp. 631–637
17. M.T. Mizukoshi, Estabilidade de sistemas dinâmicos fuzzy, Tese de Doutorado, IMECC-UNICAMP, Campinas (2004)
18. Y. Chalco-Cano, H. Román-Flores, Comparison between some approaches to solve fuzzy differential equations. Fuzzy Sets Syst. **160**(11), 1517–1527 (2009)
19. P. Diamond, P.E. Kloeden, *Metric Spaces of Fuzzy Sets: Theory and Applications* (World Scientific Publishing Company, Singapore, 1994)
20. M.L. Puri, D.A. Ralescu, Fuzzy random variables. J. Math. Anal. Appl. **91**, 409–422 (1986)
21. T.G. Bhasker, V. Lakshmikantham, V. Devi, Revisiting fuzzy differential equations. Nonlinear Anal. **58**, 351–358 (2004)
22. B. Bede, S.G. Gal, Generalizations of the differentiability of fuzzy-number-valued functions with applications to fuzzy differential equations. Fuzzy Sets Syst. **151**, 581–599 (2005)
23. J.P. Aubin, A. Cellina, *Differential inclusions - set-value maps and a viability theory* (Springer, Berlin, 1984)
24. Y. Chalco-Cano, Algumas contribuições na teoria fuzzy multívoca, Tese de Doutorado, IMECC-UNICAMP, Campinas (2004)
25. Y. Chalco-Cano, R.C. Bassanezi, M.T. Mizukoshi, M. Rojas-Medar, Population dynamics by fuzzy differential inclusion, Kybernetes (2004)
26. V. Krivan, G. Colombo, A non-stochastic approach for modeling uncertainty in population dynamics. Bull. Math. Biol. **60**, 721–751 (1998)
27. P. Diamond, Time-dependent differential inclusions, cocycle attractors and fuzzy differential equation. IEEE Trans. Fuzzy Sets Syst. **7**, 734–740 (1999)
28. L.C. Barros, P.A. Tonelli, Fuzzy pertubation of vector fields, in *Proceedings of Joint 9th IFSA World Congress and 20th NAFIPS International Conference (Vancouver, Canada)*, NAFIPS, North American Fuzzy Information Processing Society and IFSA, the International Fuzzy Systems Association, ed. by M.H. Smith, W.A. Gruver, L. O'Higgins Hall (IEEE, 2001), pp. 3000–3002
29. M.S. Ceconello, Sistemas Dinâmicos em Espaços Métricos Fuzzy - Aplicações em Biomatemática, Tese de Doutorado, IMECC-UNICAMP, Campinas (2010)

30. R.M. Jafelice, L.C. Barros, R.C. Bassanezi, A fuzzy delay differential equation model for hiv dynamics, IFSA-EUSFLAT (2009), pp. 265–270
31. L.C. Barros, R.C. Bassanezi, P.A. Tonelli, Fuzzy modelling in population dynamics. Ecol. Model. **128**, 27–33 (2000)
32. R.C. Bassanezi, L.C. Barros, P.A. Tonelli, Attractors and asymptotic stability for fuzzy dynamical systems. Fuzzy Sets Syst. **113**(3), 473–483 (2000)
33. L. Edelstein-Keshet, *Mathematical Models in Biology* (McGraw-Hill, México, 1988)
34. K.F. Magnago, Abordagem fuzzy em modelos populacionais discretos, Tese de Doutorado, IMECC-UNICAMP, Campinas (2005)
35. R.L. Devaney, *An Introduction to Chaotic Dynamical Systems* (Bejamin/Cummings, Menlo Park, Califórnia, 1989)
36. P.E. Kloeden, Chaotic iterations of fuzzy sets. Fuzzy Sets Syst. **42**(1), 37–42 (1991)
37. H. Roman-Flores, A note on transitivity in set-valued discrete systems. Chaos Solitons Fractals **17**, 99–104 (2003)
38. D.D. Majumder, K.K. Majumdar, Complexity analysis, uncertainty management and fuzzy dynamical systems. Kybernetes **33**, 1143–1184 (2004)

Chapter 9
Modeling in Biomathematics: Demographic Fuzziness

The word is the golden thread of thought.

(Socrates – 5th Century)

Abstract This chapter explores the notion of demographic fuzziness in modeling of bio-mathematical phenomena. The concept of demographic fuzziness is illustrated by looking at both continuous and discrete models. The relatively new idea of p-fuzzy systems, which combines dynamical systems with fuzzy logic, is illustrated via the dynamical models.

This chapter and the next use the concepts of demographic and environmental fuzziness. These terms come from the stochastic literature (see [1–3]) and our use is an adaptation for fuzzy biomathematical models presented in this chapter and Chap. 10.

The essential feature of mathematical modelling of variational processes using deterministic equations is the "exactness" obtained in the prediction of the studied phenomenon. Such predictions are definitely dependent on the hypotheses about the precision of the state variables and about the parameters inserted in the models via "mean values" of a data set.

The classical biomathematical models, in particular population dynamics and epidemiology models, are mostly based on physical-chemical hypotheses, in which the reaction between two substances (state variables) is modeled by the product of their concentration - the *law of mass action*. The same law is used in the Lotka–Volterra models of interactions between two species and in the Kermack–MacKendrick epidemiology models (see [4]). The parameter representing predation rate of the predator-prey model or the force of infection in the epidemiology models are "mean" values simulated or obtained empirically.

In the models that deal with uncertainty, for instance the stochastic models, the solutions are stochastic processes whose mean values can be obtained a posteriori, when the variable's distribution density and/or the parameters related to the analyzed phenomenon are available. However, if in addition to quantifying the elements of a population, we also want to take into account certain qualities of the individuals, the variables should "capture" such uncertainties. For instance, in the prey population

© Springer-Verlag Berlin Heidelberg 2017
L.C. de Barros et al., *A First Course in Fuzzy Logic, Fuzzy Dynamical Systems, and Biomathematics*, Studies in Fuzziness and Soft Computing 347, DOI 10.1007/978-3-662-53324-6_9

of some species, we can consider the difficulty of preying each specific prey, such as age, health, habitat, etc.

The various types of uncertainty arising from biomathematical phenomena may generate distinct models. When we choose a stochastic model, we are implicitly assuming knowledge of the parameter's probability distribution. Nevertheless, if in the given phenomenon we intend to take into account the heterogeneity as being gradual, that is, fuzzy and not originating from randomness, how do we model these characteristics mathematically?

For example, if we have a "*smoker*" population at instant t_0, subject to some mortality rate, we may want to know how this population will be composed in the future. If we consider that each individual is simply a smoker or non-smoker, the problem can be solved through a deterministic model, considering each population individually. On the other hand, if we initially have the probability distribution of the smokers, we can use a stochastic model to study the evolution of this initial distribution. However, if the characteristic of *being a smoker* depends on how many cigarettes a person smokes a day, the potency of such cigarettes, smoking intervals, etc., we should also characterize smoking as *degree*. In this case, each individual belongs to the smoker population with a specific degree of belonging. If the individual does not smoke, the degree of belonging is zero. If s/he smokes 3 packs a day we can say that s/he is a smoker of degree 1. Now, if s/he smokes 10 cigarettes a day, how much of a "smoker" will s/he be? This subjectivity may be expressed by a function φ_A, where $\varphi_A(x)$ indicates the degree which a person who smokes x cigarettes is in agreement with the definition of "smoker". A study about the life expectancy of a group, considering the quantity of cigarettes smoked a day, was done by A. Kandel [5].

The variational fuzzy models may admit many types of uncertainties (*fuzziness*), described in coefficients, initial conditions or by the state variables themselves. If the subjectivity comes from the state variable or from the parameters, we have *demographic fuzziness* or *environmental fuzziness*, respectively. Thus, when the state variables are modeled by fuzzy set theory, we have demographic fuzziness, and when only the parameters are fuzzy we have environmental fuzziness. In general, both types of fuzziness are present in the biological phenomena.

The observation above suggest that adopting environmental fuzziness allows us to use classical concepts of variation rate, since the state variables are deterministic. This approach will be explored in Chap. 10. For demographic fuzziness, we should employ some variation concept that is compatible with the notion of uncertain variables.

There are many possibilities for modeling demographic fuzziness. Given that, in this case, the state variation is uncertain, any of the processes seen in the Sects. 8.1.2 and 8.1.3 could be used for continuous models. The chosen process is related to the most suitable phenomenon in question. On the other hand, if the model is discrete, we have the methodology of Sect. 8.2 as an option. However, due to the richness of **p-fuzzy** systems (see below), we will use this methodology to study the evolution of dynamical systems in which the state variables are uncertain.

The systems considered here are autonomous, i.e., the variations (or variation rates) do not depend explicitly on time. Furthermore, the state variables and their variations are considered linguistic. This way, the state variables are correlated to their variations, not by means of equations - which is the most common case in the literature - but by means of fuzzy rules whose main characteristic is having the *state variables as input, while the variations are outputs.* As noted in Sect. 8.1.5, the systems studied here are referred to as **p-fuzzy**, because the direction field, partially known a priori, is obtained from fuzzy controllers. Recall that p-fuzzy is an abbreviation for partially fuzzy. Since in such methodologies, processes of defuzzification are expected, the final solution of a p-fuzzy system is crisp, this is, a precise value $x(t)$ that represents the state variable in each instant t. The p-fuzzy systems may be discrete or continuous. For clarity, we first study the discrete case and then the continuous case.

9.1 Demographic Fuzziness: Discrete Modeling

Many concepts in this section the reader can find in [6, 7]. The mathematical modelling of the phenomena analysed here are fundamentally provided by fuzzy controllers. For this reason, we will not adopt the index "r", that indicates the number of rules in the direction field, to distinguish it from the deterministic model.

The discrete p-fuzzy systems have the form:

$$\begin{cases} x_{t+1} = F(x_t) \\ \quad x_0 = x(t_0) \end{cases}, \tag{9.1}$$

where $F : \mathbb{R}^n \to \mathbb{R}^n$ is the function $F(x) = x + \Delta x$, and Δx is the defuzzified output, given by a fuzzy controller for the input x. A discrete p-fuzzy system is nothing but a sequence of differences $x_{t+1} - x_t = f(x_t)$, in which the variation function $f(x) = \Delta x$ is the output of the fuzzy controller. Figure 9.1 represents a discrete p-fuzzy system schematically. Ortega et al. [8] applied this method in association with Zadeh's Extension Principle to study the evolution the rabies in dogs for the sate of São Paulo in Brazil.

We are modeling with linguistic variables. What we wish to convey is not only how obtain meaningful qualitative models compatible with words but also show how some linguistic variables already exhibit a quantitative character suggesting its

Fig. 9.1 Architecture in a discrete p-fuzzy model [7]

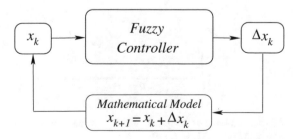

relation in the model itself. For example, we might have a linguistic variable "tall". Linguistically, tall already suggests short as well as positively tall and negatively tall. That is, some words suggest opposites.

For a better understanding of the stability of equilibrium points of p-fuzzy systems, some remarks about the fuzzy rule-base with semantic opposition are necessary.

9.1.1   Fuzzy Rules with Opposite Semantics

The Malthusian principle for population growth is

"the population's variation is proportional to the population at each instant".

The first attempt to model this principal could generate Frame 8.1, whose antecedents and consequents are represented in Fig. 8.4a, b, respectively. Based on these rules, the Mamdani controller and the defuzzification given by the center of mass, the p-fuzzy system (9.1) leads us to the trajectory illustrated in Fig. 9.2.

According to Fig. 9.2, the discrete p-fuzzy system produces a trajectory compatible with the Malthusian exponential model, in which the number of deaths is smaller than the number of births. However, this exponential unbounded growth is not observed in reality. There are factors in nature such as food, competition with other individuals, competition for space, light, etc, that limit the population to a certain threshold carrying capacity, providing stability in a given environment. Factors

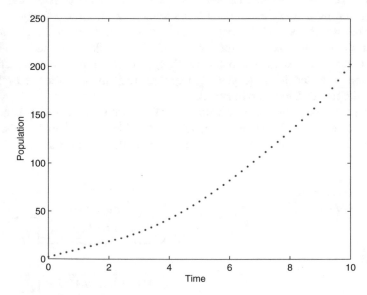

Fig. 9.2 Number of fuzzy individuals as a function of time from the discrete p-fuzzy system and rule base Frame 8.1, with $x(0) = 2$

such as these result in a process of population "inhibition" in such a way that, for very large populations, the variation is small or even negative.

R_1 : **If** (X) is "low" (A_1) **then** the variation is "low positive" (B_1)

R_2 : **If** (X) is "average low" (A_2) **then** the variation is "average positive" (B_2)

R_3 : **If** (X) is average (A_3) **then** the variation is "high positive" (B_3)

R_4 : **If** (X) is "average high" (A_4) **then** the variation is "average positive" $(B_4 = B_2)$

R_5 : **If** (X) is "high" (A_5) **then** the variation is "low positive" $(B_5 = B_1)$

R_6 : **If** (X) is "very high" (A_6) **then** a variation is "low negative" (B_6)

Frame 9.1: Fuzzy rule-base to model population variation based on its density, with semantic opposition

In order to improve the Malthusian model, information such as those that limit growth, should be included in the rule base. If we expect stability of equilibrium, the rule base should contain rules with **semantic opposition** in the consequents. Semantic opposition is characterized here by the alternating signs in the variations. A theoretical study of this subject can be found in [9]. For instance, we could refine the rule-base of Frame 8.1 in order to obtain the rule-base of Frame 9.1 with semantic opposition in the successive rules R_5 and R_6, in which the fuzzy sets of antecedents and consequents are illustrated in Fig. 9.3a, b, respectively. This rule base using Mamdani's controller and the defuzzification of the center of mass, the p-fuzzy system produces the trajectory shown in Fig. 9.4.

The trajectory presented in Fig. 9.4 has qualitative behavior compatible with the models that present inhibition, such as the logistic models of Gompertz, Montroll, etc [4, 10, 11].

To simplify the study of equilibrium of p-fuzzy systems, we will make some requirements of the rule base. One of them is regarding its monotonicity, i.e., the rules must be displayed using an **ordinal scaling**. For example, the rules of Frame 9.1 exhibit such an order: the antecedents are monotonically displayed from the "smallest" to the "largest". This facilitates the search for possible equilibria of the model. Clearly, not ordering does not eliminate equilibrium points. The existence of such points depend, among other factors, of the existence of semantic opposition in the rules. Rules without semantic opposition imply the non-existence of hyperbolic equilibria (see [12]), which are the ones of our interest. On the other hand, rules with semantic opposition imply the possibility of such equilibria. The existence of such points depends on the "continuity" in the rule base. In the classic case, such a guarantee comes from Bolzano's Theorem [13, 14].

It is worth noting that we are not interested in the study of dynamics around non-hyperbolic equilibrium points. Intuitively, non-hyperbolic equilibrium means that the variation around it does not change in sign (see [12]).

(a)   Antecedent fuzzy sets for population (*X*).

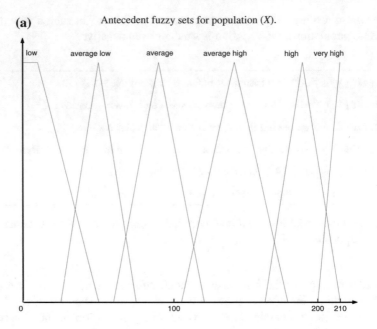

(b)   Consequent fuzzy sets for variations (Δ*X*).

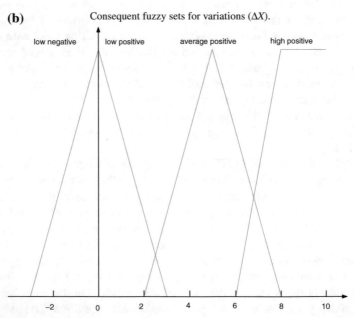

Fig. 9.3 Membership function for Frame 9.1

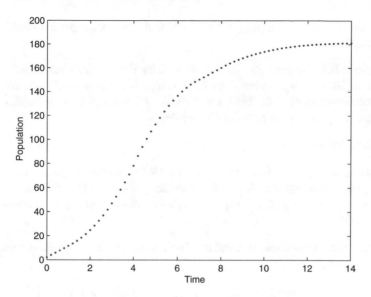

Fig. 9.4 Solution of the discrete p-fuzzy system for the rule-base of Frame 9.1 and $x_0 = 2$

9.1.2 Equilibrium and Stability of One-Dimensional Discrete p-Fuzzy Systems

The fuzzy rule base we use for this chapter will satisfy some properties, enumerated below, in such a way that facilitates the search for possible equilibrium points of the system.

(i) The universes must be bounded interval sets of real numbers.
(ii) The fuzzy sets of the rule base must be **fuzzy numbers**.
(iii) The rule base must cover its associated universe, in the sense that each element of the universe has a **non-zero** degree of belonging to at least one of the fuzzy numbers of the rule base.
(iv) At most two rules can be activated at once, i.e., each element of the universe must have non-zero belonging to at most two antecedents.
(v) Any element whose membership value is 1 can belong to only one fuzzy set, that is, this element has a zero degree of belonging to any other fuzzy member of the rule-base.
(vi) The rule base must be **monotonically ordered** (increasing or decreasing), i.e., the qualifiers of the antecedents must be "ordered": *small, medium, large*, for example. Formally, this means that the largest element of the support of the antecedent of rule R_i should be smaller than the one that follows, rule R_{i+1}.

We next study equilibrium and stability for dynamical system given by field $F(x) = x + \Delta x$ of p-fuzzy system (9.1).

Definition 9.1 (*Rule ordering*) A rule base with the six properties above will be called well-ordered.

Proposition 9.1 *Suppose the the rule base with the p-fuzzy system (9.1) is well-ordered and that the p-fuzzy numbers A_i and A_{i+1}, of consecutive rules, have continuous membership functions. Then, for each $x \in I^* = \mathrm{supp}\{A_i\} \bigcap \mathrm{supp}\{A_{i+1}\} \neq \emptyset$, the output Δx is continuous and differentiable.*

Proof See [6, 7]   ∎

Corollary 9.2 *Suppose that the rule base for (9.1) is well-ordered and is composed of triangular, trapezoidal and/or bell-shaped fuzzy numbers. Under these conditions, for all $x \in I^* = \mathrm{supp}\{A_i\} \bigcap \mathrm{supp}\{A_{i+1}\} \neq \emptyset$, the output Δx is continuous and differentiable.*

Definition 9.2 (*Equilibrium*) A real number $\overline{x}$ is an *equilibrium point* of the discrete p-fuzzy system (9.1) if

$$F(\overline{x}) = \overline{x} \iff \overline{x} + \Delta\overline{x} = \overline{x} \iff \Delta\overline{x} = 0.$$

Theorem 9.3 (Existence of Equilibrium) *Suppose that a rule base satisfies conditions of Proposition 9.1 and that the rules R_i and R_{i+1}, with antecedents A_i and A_{i+1}, exhibit semantic opposition in the consequents B_i and B_{i+1}. Under these conditions, the interval*

$$I^* = \mathrm{supp}\{A_i\} \bigcap \mathrm{supp}\{A_{i+1}\} \neq \emptyset$$

contains at least one equilibrium of the system (9.1).

Proof The proof is based on the fact that the semantic opposition implies a change of sign of Δx in the interval I^*. We know that Δx is continuous (Proposition 9.1) therefore from Bolzano's Theorem, the proof is complete.   ∎

Figure 9.5 illustrates Theorem 9.3.

The study of uniqueness of equilibrium of p-fuzzy systems is large and the interested reader can consult [7]. In what follows we will only mention some results.

For p-fuzzy systems in which the rule base satisfies Proposition 9.1, the output Δx has an explicit expression with respect to the membership functions of the antecedents and consequents of the rules that exhibit semantic opposition. Given this, it is possible to study properties regarding uniqueness of equilibrium in the interval I^*.

A first general result is the following. If Δx vanishes in I^* and is monotone, then the p-fuzzy system (9.1) has an unique equilibrium point in I^*. A sufficient condition for Δx to be monotone is that its derivative does not change its sign. In what follows, we will only state the result for determining the equilibrium for consequents that are symmetric.

Theorem 9.4 (Uniqueness of equilibrium for symmetric outputs) *Suppose that a rule base satisfies the conditions of Proposition 9.1, and that the rules R_i and R_{i+1},*

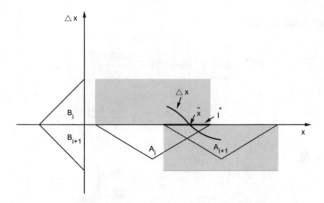

Fig. 9.5 Existence of equilibrium for the rule base with semantic opposition: "$B_i > 0$ and $B_{i+1} < 0$"

with antecedents A_i and A_{i+1}, exhibit semantic opposition and the membership functions of the consequentes B_i and B_{i+1} are symmetric, i.e., $\varphi_{B_i}(s) = \varphi_{B_{i+1}}(-s)$ for all s in the universe. Under these conditions, the interval $I^* = \text{supp}\{A_i\} \cap \text{supp}\{A_{i+1}\}$ has an unique equilibrium $\overline{x}$ of the p-fuzzy system (9.1), given by

$$\overline{x} = \max_{x \in I^*}[\min(\varphi_{A_i}(x), \varphi_{A_{i+1}(x)})],$$

or as the solution of the equation

$$\varphi_{A_i}(x) = \varphi_{A_{i+1}}(x),$$

provided it exists.

  Moreover, the following useful formula for the stability study holds:

$$\frac{d(\Delta x)}{dx}\Big|_{x=\overline{x}} = \frac{[\varphi_{B_{i+1}^+}^{-1}(\varphi_{A_i}(\overline{x}))]^2[\varphi'_{A_i}(\overline{x}) - \varphi'_{A_{i+1}}(\overline{x})]}{4\displaystyle\int_0^{\varphi_{A_i}(\overline{x})} \varphi_{B_{i+1}^+}^{-1}(s)\,ds}. \tag{9.2}$$

where $\varphi_{B_{i+1}^+}$ is the membership function of B_{i+1} restricted to the right side of this set.

Proof See [6, 7]. An illustration of the existence of $\overline{x}$ is given in Fig. 9.5 ∎

The study we will present next on the stability of equilibrium of discrete p-fuzzy systems is developed using Corollary 8.10 for classic discrete systems.

Theorem 9.5 (Stability of equilibrium of discrete p-fuzzy systems) *Suppose that $\overline{x}$ is an equilibrium of the p-fuzzy system (9.1). Under this condition, the following statements hold:*

(a) $\bar{x}$ is asymptotically stable if

$$|F'(\bar{x})| < 1 \iff \left|1 + \frac{d(\Delta x)}{dx}\bigg|_{x=\bar{x}}\right| < 1$$

$$\iff -2 < \frac{d(\Delta x)}{dx}\bigg|_{x=\bar{x}} < 0.$$

(b) $\bar{x}$ is unstable if

$$\frac{d(\Delta x)}{dx}\bigg|_{x=\bar{x}} < -2 \ or \ \frac{d(\Delta x)}{dx}\bigg|_{x=\bar{x}} > 0.$$

It is worth observing that, depending on the sign of $\frac{d(\Delta x)}{dx}|_{x=\bar{x}}$, we will have a variety of forms for the behavior of the stability of discrete systems:

(i) If $-1 < \frac{d(\Delta x)}{dx}|_{x=\bar{x}} < 0$, $\bar{x}$ is asymptotically stable with monotone convergence;
(ii) If $-2 < \frac{d(\Delta x)}{dx}|_{x=\bar{x}} < -1$, $\bar{x}$ is asymptotically stable with oscillant convergence;
(iii) If $\frac{d(\Delta x)}{dx}|_{x=\bar{x}} < -2$, $\bar{x}$ is an unstable oscillant.

The following example illustrates the concepts seen above.

Example 9.1 Consider the discrete p-fuzzy system whose rule base exhibits self-inhibition and is given by the rules of Frame 9.1, and whose antecedents and consequents are given in Fig. 9.3. We can observe semantic opposition in the consequents B_5 and B_6 of the rule base. Therefore, we have only one equilibrium region, the interval

$$I^* = \text{supp}\{A_5\} \bigcap \text{supp}\{A_6\} = [200, 210].$$

Since in this region the consequents B_5 and B_6 are symmetric and

$$\varphi_{A_5}(x) = \frac{210 - x}{20} \text{ and } \varphi_{A_6}(x) = \frac{x - 200}{20},$$

then, from Theorem 9.4, the only equilibrium point is the solution of the equation

$$\varphi_{A_5}(x) = \varphi_{A_6}(x) \iff \frac{210 - x}{20} = \frac{x - 200}{20} \iff \bar{x} = 205.$$

The stability of this equilibrium is determined from formula (9.2) for $\frac{d(\Delta x)}{dx}|_{x=\bar{x}}$, in Theorem 9.4. Since

$\varphi_{B_6^+}(x) = 1 - x \implies \varphi_{B_6^+}^{-1}(x) = 1 - x \implies \varphi_{B_6^+}^{-1}(\varphi_{A_5}(\bar{x})) = \frac{3}{4}$. Moreover,

$$\varphi_{A_5}(\bar{x}) = \frac{1}{4}, \ \varphi_{A_5}'(\bar{x}) = -\frac{1}{20}, \ \varphi_{A_6}'(\bar{x}) = \frac{1}{20}$$

and

$$\int_0^{\varphi_{A_5}(\overline{x})} \varphi_{B_6^+}^{-1}(s)\,\mathrm{d}s = \int_0^{\frac{1}{4}} (1-s)\,\mathrm{d}s = \frac{7}{32}.$$

Hence,

$$\frac{\mathrm{d}(\Delta x)}{\mathrm{d}x}\Big|_{x=205} = \frac{(\frac{3}{4})^2[(-\frac{1}{20}) - \frac{1}{20}]}{4\cdot(\frac{7}{32})} = -\frac{9}{240}.$$

In this way,

$$-1 < \frac{\mathrm{d}(\Delta x)}{\mathrm{d}x}\Big|_{x=205} < 0.$$

Therefore, according to Theorem 9.5(a), $\overline{x} = 205$ is asymptotically stable.

It is possible to verify that small perturbations in the rule base sets cause qualitative changes in the type of stability of the system's equilibrium (see [6, 7, Sect. 4.1.1] and Exercise 9.1). This means that the p-fuzzy system considered is structurally unstable. This fact is in complete agreement with the discrete model of Verhulst studied in Sect. 8.2.2.

An interesting aspect of the discrete p-fuzzy systems that may be explored, from a practical point of view, is its use in adjusting parameters from theoretical models. Supposing that the system of Example 9.1 represents the dynamics of a population with inhibition, a deterministic model should have the same properties as the p-fuzzy model. For example, if we wanted to adjust a discrete Verhulst model to the p-fuzzy model studied above, the carrying capacity K and the intrinsic growth rate a should satisfy $205 = K - \frac{1}{a}$, since the equilibrium of the discrete Verhults model is given by $\overline{x} = K - \frac{1}{a}$. The adjustment itself would be done from the values generated by the p-fuzzy system. Clearly this methodology should be applied more carefully if we wanted to adjust the discrete p-fuzzy model to a classic continuous model, for the previously observed reasons regarding structural stability. However, if the equilibrium of the discrete p-fuzzy system has the same qualitative properties as the continuous one, that is if the p-fuzzy equilibrium is stable, then it is possible to use the data generated by the discrete p-fuzzy model for the parameter adjustment of the continuous theoretical model.

Exercise 9.1 Change the support of the antecedents A_5 and A_6 of Frame 9.1 that contains equilibrium, in order to obtain a stable oscillatory equilibrium, and study it from the point of view of the previously obtained results. After that, make changes to obtain unstable non-zero equilibrium. (Suggestion: Combine Formula (9.2) with the results of Theorem 9.5).

We will conclude this section by presenting an introduction to bi-dimensional p-fuzzy systems.

9.1.3 Discrete p-Fuzzy Predator-Prey Model

Our approach deals with a specific predator-prey type model, in which we simulate the population of prey and predators and calculate its phase plane. In order to study this dynamical system by means of a discrete p-fuzzy system, we consider that the input variables are the number of prey (X) and the number of predators (Y), where the qualitative properties are that the prey favors the predators and are disfavored by them. The outputs ΔX and ΔY represent, respectively, the variation of prey and predator populations. All the variables are linguistic and each one of them can be described by terms such as low (B), average (M) and high (A) for the state variables while high positive (A^+), average positive (M^+), low positive(B^+), low negative (B^-), and high negative (A^-) are terms for the respective variations. Suppose that such terms are modeled by fuzzy sets whose membership functions are obtained from a specialist. Such functions are represented in Fig. 9.6.

The membership functions of the consequents for the population variations are illustrated in Fig. 9.7.

The correlation of the linguistic variables is given by a rule base, which should be consistent with the characteristics of an iterative predator-prey type system, as mentioned above.

The rule base, presented in Frame 9.2 can be represented graphically in Fig. 9.8, where the arrows indicate the magnitudes and directions of the variations. As in the one dimensional case, here we also adopt Mamdani's inference method with defuzzification given by the center of mass.

The dynamics of the bi-dimensional discrete p-fuzzy system consists of obtaining the populations from the iterative system:

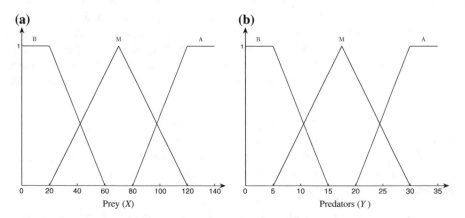

Fig. 9.6 Antecedent membership functions of populations of Frame 9.2

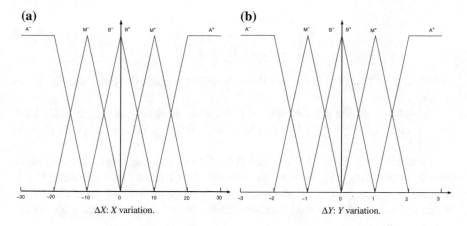

Fig. 9.7 Consequent membership functions of the population variation of Frame 9.2

1. If X is B and Y is B then ΔX is M^+ and ΔY is M^-

2. If X is B and Y is M then ΔX is B^+ and ΔY is A^-

3. If X is B and Y is A then ΔX is M^- and ΔY is M^-

4. If X is M and Y is B then ΔX is A^+ and ΔY is B^+

5. If X is M and Y is A then ΔX is A^- and ΔY is B^-

6. If X is A and Y is B then ΔX is M^+ and ΔY is M^+

7. If X is A and Y is M then ΔX is B^- and ΔY is A^+

8. If X is A and Y is A then ΔX is M^- and ΔY is M^+

Frame 9.2: Rule base for a discrete p-fuzzy prey-predator system

Fig. 9.8 Representation of
the rule base of (9.3)

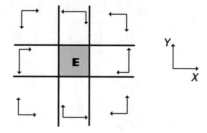

$$\begin{cases} x_{n+1} = x_n + \Delta_1 [x_n, y_n] \\ y_{n+1} = y_n + \Delta_2 [x_n, y_n] \\ \quad x_0, \ y_0 \in \mathbb{R} \text{ are given} \end{cases} \tag{9.3}$$

where $\Delta_1 [x, y]$ and $\Delta_2 [x, y]$ are the defuzzified outputs for the input $(X, Y) = (x, y)$.

The solution of the p-fuzzy system (9.3), with the fuzzy sets given in Figs. 9.6 and 9.7, and $(x_0, y_0) = (70, 14)$, can be visualized in Fig. 9.9, and its phase plane in Fig. 9.10.

We observe that there exists a region **E** not "covered" by any rule. However, since there is semantic opposition in the consequents of the rules 4 and 5, related to **E**, it is expected that the equilibria of the system lies in this region. If we wanted to fill the whole region **E** "continuously", we should have rules relating to average populations.

For example:

"If X is M and Y is M then ΔX is B and ΔY is B".

We stress the fact that when we use the term "Average Population" for the linguistic variable, we are in fact, a priori, considering the existence of an equilibrium fuzzy value for the real system. It is like saying that we have some information of the type, "the prey favor the predators and are disfavored by them", i.e. *the equilibrium is always around the average*.

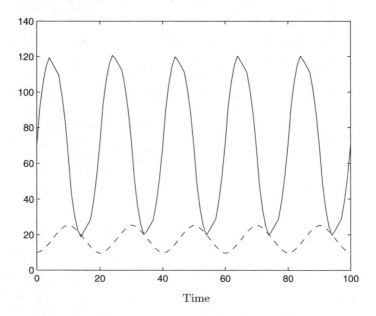

Fig. 9.9 The *dashed* and *solid lines* represent the predators and prey, respectively

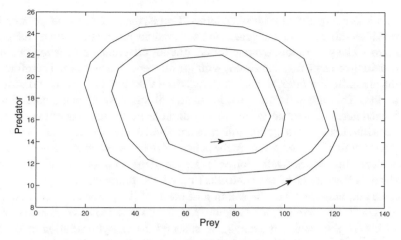

Fig. 9.10 Phase-plane of the system, with initial condition (70, 14)

9.2 Demographic Fuzziness: Continuous Modeling

There are many approaches to continuous fuzzy dynamical systems (see Chap. 8).
Here our interest in the p-fuzzy approach. Such systems play an important role when
one wants to model some continuous dynamical system where the direction field is
only partially known, as discussed in Sect. 6.4 of Chap. 6. We observed there that
such systems are good approximators of theoretic systems. As in the discrete case,
here we are not interested in this property, therefore we will omit the index "r" of
the field "f_r". Here the mathematical model for the studied phenomenon is given by
the IVP

$$\begin{cases} \dfrac{dx}{dt} = f(x) \, , \\ x(t_0) = x_0 \end{cases} \tag{9.4}$$

where the direction field is given by a fuzzy controller. The following section has the
objective of emphasizing the differences between the discrete and continuous p-fuzzy
systems, since in both cases we essentially use the outputs of a fuzzy controller.

9.2.1 Characteristics of a Continuous p-Fuzzy Systems

Recall that we are studying autonomous systems (the direction fields do not depend
explicitly on the time). This means that the rules correlate the inputs, which are state
variables, with the variation rates which are the output variables. Formally, the rule
base of a continuous p-fuzzy systems is similar to the one of a discrete system. The
difference lies essentially on the formulation of each rule. In the discrete systems,

the variations are qualified in absolute terms. That is, the qualifications are stated for
the time intervals in which the generation successions occur (successive changes in
the inputs). The generations overlap for continuous case and the variation rate must
have qualitative properties consistent with the concept of derivative. Therefore, the
qualifications for the outputs must be compatible with the concept of variation per
unit of time. This unit of time has nothing to do with successive generations, which is
not defined here. As we said before, in a continuous model the generations overlap.

The methodology of fuzzy controllers that we will use here is Mamdani's methodology with defuzzification given by the center of mass. Moreover, we will consider
well-ordered rule bases (Definition 9.1). Hence, depending on the rules, the field
f (which is the output of the controller) may have properties that guarantee the
existence and uniqueness of the solution of the IVP (9.4). For instance, under the
hypotheses of Theorem 9.3, the function f may be known to be continuous or differentiable. If f is explicitly known, we can find the analytic solution of the IVP
(9.4) by traditional methods. However, depending on the complexity of f, one has
to employ numerical methods in order to obtain numerical estimates for the solution
of the given IVP. Since, by fuzzy controller methods, f is implicitly known, it is
always possible, under mild assumptions to use numerical methods.

9.2.2   Numerical Methods for the Solution of the Continuous p-Fuzzy System IVP

The estimates x_n will be obtained by means of numerical methods for the ordinary
differential equations (ODE) such as Euler and Runge–Kutta methods, or by means
of numerical methods for integration (see [15–17]).

(a) (**Euler Method for ODE**) This method generates the estimates x_n as follows:

$$x_{n+1} = x_n + hf(t_n, x_n),$$

where h is the step size and f is the mapping produced by the fuzzy controller.

(b) (**Second Order Runge–Kutta Methods for ODE**) The second-order Runge–
Kutta method we adopt here, also known as Improved Euler's Method, generate the
estimates

$$x_{n+1} = x_n + \frac{h}{2}[f(t_n, x_n) + f(t_n + h, x_n + hf(t_n, x_n))].$$

Higher order methods can also be used.

(c) (**Numerical Integration Methods**) The estimates x_n can also be obtained by
some integration numerical method such as Trapezoidal or Simpson's Rule, modify-
ing the IVP (9.4) in such a way that the ODE is transformed into an integral equation
(see [18]).

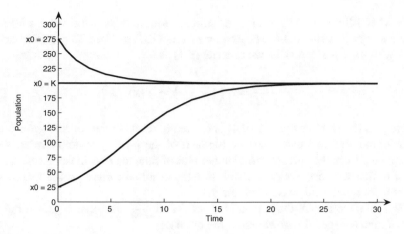

Fig. 9.11 Trajectories of Verhults model with $K - 200$, $x_0 - 25$; 200 and 270

We illustrate, in what follows, the methodology proposed here for the model of population growth with inhibition, as Verhulst's model. The traditional Verhulst model for population growth is governed by the IVP

$$\begin{cases} \dfrac{1}{x}\dfrac{dx}{dt} = a\left(1 - \dfrac{x}{K}\right), \\ x(t_0) = x_0 \end{cases} \tag{9.5}$$

where a is the intrinsic growth rate and K is the carrying capacity. The classical solution of (9.5), that represent the populations $x(t)$ at each instant t, is given by

$$x(t) = \frac{K}{(\frac{K}{x_0} - 1)e^{-at} + 1}. \tag{9.6}$$

Hence,

$$\begin{cases} x \text{ is increasing if } x_0 < K \\ x \text{ is constant if } x_0 = K \\ x \text{ is decreasing if } x_0 > K \end{cases},$$

which is illustrated in Fig. 9.11.

Recall that in this example, the function that models the direction field is given explicitly by

$$g(x) = \frac{dx}{dt} = ax\left(1 - \frac{x}{K}\right). \tag{9.7}$$

However, to adopt our methodology we do not need to know explicitly such an expression. Here it is presented for the sake of comparison with the qualitative properties of the classic trajectories and those produced by the continuous p-fuzzy system.

In what follows we will obtain the estimates for the logistic trajectories from the methodology described at the beginning of this ODE section. To compare the the rules with the classic models, we re-write (9.7) as

$$\frac{1}{x}\frac{dx}{dt} = a\left(1 - \frac{x}{K}\right) = f(x), \tag{9.8}$$

where f is linear. Note that Eq. (9.8) is written in terms of the specific growth rate. This formulation facilitates the development of the p-fuzzy system's rules. Rules constructed from the percent variation per unit of time may be, in some cases, more intuitive than the formulation derived from the absolute variations. For this reason, we will not use the rule base in Frame 9.1.

We will denote by X the population (input) and $\frac{1}{X}\frac{dX}{dt}$ the relative growth rate per unit of time (or specific growth rate - the output).

R_1 : **If** X is "very low" (A_1) then $\frac{1}{X}\frac{dX}{dt}$ is "high positive" (B_1)

R_2 : **If** X is "low" (A_2) then $\frac{1}{X}\frac{dX}{dt}$ is "high positive" ($B_2 = B_1$)

R_3 : **If** X is "average" (A_3) then $\frac{1}{X}\frac{dX}{dt}$ is "average positive" (B_3)

R_4 : **If** X is "average high" (A_4) then $\frac{1}{X}\frac{dX}{dt}$ is "average positive" ($B_4 = B_3$)

R_5 : **If** X is "high" (A_5) then $\frac{1}{X}\frac{dX}{dt}$ is "low positive" (B_5)

R_6 : **If** X is "very high" (A_6) then $\frac{1}{X}\frac{dX}{dt}$ is "baixa negativa" (B_6)

Frame 9.3: Rules for the continuous fuzzy model

Rule Base

In this rule base, the fuzzy numbers A_i and B_i are the same as the rules of the Frame 9.1, except that the support of B_i, should be between -1 and 1 for modelling opposite semantics, which now must admit positive and negative values. Thus, using the rules of Frame 9.3, we obtain values for f, and with one of the previous numerical methods (see Sect. 9.2.2) we calculate the estimates for Verhulst's model.

To illustrate, we choose Euler's method (for the function $xf(x)$, since the rate for rules of the Frame 9.3 is the specific one) and we obtained the estimates x_n:

$$x_{n+1} = x_n + hx_n f(x_n),$$

whose representation can be seen in Fig. 9.12.

The rules of Frame 9.3 are in agreement with the main characteristics of a general model with inhibited growth that is regulated by a carrying capacity. Verhulst's model, considered above, is a particular case. Besides this model, with small modifications, the same rule base can be made suitable for the inhibition models of Gompertz, Montroll, von Bertalanffy, and others (see [4, 11, 19]).

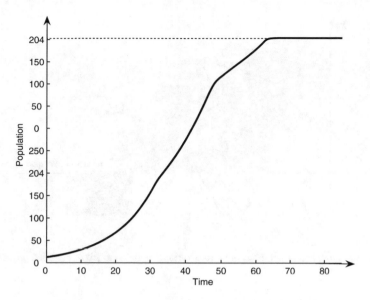

Fig. 9.12 Trajectory of the continuous p-fuzzy model, with $x_0 = 5$, of Frame 9.3

We next briefly study Montroll's general model, and, supposing that the rule base (Frame 9.3) corresponds to Verhulst's model, we will illustrate a method for "adjusting" such rules in order to take into account the particularities of Montroll's model.

9.2.3 A Study of Montroll's p-Fuzzy Model

Most of the continuous autonomous models of population growth, formalized in terms of differential equations, have the form

$$\frac{dx}{dt} = xf(x).$$

The function f, given by $\dfrac{1}{x}\dfrac{dx}{dt}$, is called specific growth of the population, x. We present below some functions extensively used in the literature (see [4, 11, 12]).

Verhulst's Model f is linear and given by

$$f(x) = a\left(1 - \frac{x}{K}\right).$$

Montroll's Model

$$f(x) = a\left(1 - \left(\frac{x}{K}\right)^{s}\right), \text{ with } s > 0.$$

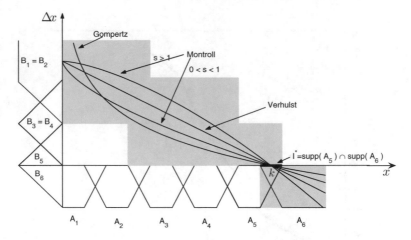

Fig. 9.13 Granules and possibilities of various variational field models of inhibited growth; $\Delta x = \frac{1}{x}\frac{dx}{dt}$

Gompertz's Model

$$f(x) = -a\ln\frac{x}{K}, x > 0.$$

Figure 9.13 below illustrates a rule base in granular form, as well as possibilities for various specific growth functions (f) with inhibition.

Although the models described above have a general form for their rule-base, each of them has a particularity. Here we are only interested in the "adjustment" of the rules in Frame 9.3 for Montroll's model. Depending on the parameter s in Montroll's model, the specific growth is smaller or greater than the one in Verhult's Model (see Fig. 9.13).

- If $s > 1$, the specific growth of Montroll's model is greater than Verhulst's model up to the carrying capacity. After the carrying capacity, Montroll's model grows slower.
- If $0 < s < 1$, we have an inverse situation from the case $s > 1$.

These particularities suggest the changes to be made in Frame 9.3, supposing that it represents Verhulst's model, in order to obtain rules consistent with Montroll's model.

Example 9.2 In what follows we make changes in order to incorporate the particularities of Montroll's models, supposing $0 < s < 1$:

Rule base for Montroll's model with $0 < s < 1$

R_1 : **If** X is "very low" (A_1) then $\frac{1}{X}\frac{dX}{dt}$ is "high positive" (pB_1)

R_2 : **If** X is "low" (A_2) then $\frac{1}{X}\frac{dX}{dt}$ is "high positive" $(pB_2 = pB_1)$

R_3 : **If** X is "average" (A_3) then $\frac{1}{X}\frac{dX}{dt}$ is "average positive" (pB_3)

R_4 : **If** X is "average high" (A_4) then $\frac{1}{X}\frac{dX}{dt}$ is "average positive" $(pB_4 = pB_3)$

R_5 : **If** X is "high" (A_5) then $\frac{1}{X}\frac{dX}{dt}$ is "low positive" (mB_5)

R_6 : **If** X is "very high" (A_6) then $\frac{1}{X}\frac{dX}{dt}$ is "low negative" (mB_6)

Frame 9.4: Rules for the continuous Montroll fuzzy model

The antecedents of the rules of Frame 9.4 are the same as those of Frame 9.3. To model the changes specified in the rules of Frame 9.4, we will use the concept of fuzzy modifier, seen in Sect. 4.5 of Chap. 4.

We will use power modifiers for the specific case considered above, where the power is a parameter $0 < \gamma < 1$, or its inverse $\frac{1}{\gamma}$. We will apply the following modifiers in the consequentes of the rules of Frame 9.3 to obtain the rules of Frame 9.4

$$
\begin{cases}
pB_i = (B_i)^\gamma \iff \varphi_{pB_i}(x) = (\varphi_{B_i}(x))^\gamma, \ i = 1, 2. \\[2mm]
pB_i = \begin{cases} (B_i^-)^\gamma \iff \varphi_{pB_i^-}(x) = (\varphi_{B_i^-}(x))^\gamma \\[1mm] (B_i^+)^{\frac{1}{\gamma}} \iff \varphi_{pB_i^+}(x) = (\varphi_{B_i^+}(x))^{\frac{1}{\gamma}} \end{cases}, \ i = 3, 4. \\[4mm]
mB_i = (B_i)^{\frac{1}{\gamma}} \iff \varphi_{mB_i}(x) = (\varphi_{B_i}(x))^{\frac{1}{\gamma}}, \ i = 5, 6.
\end{cases}
$$

where B_i^- and B_i^+ are respectively the right-hand side and left-hand side of the fuzzy set B_i. Figure 9.14 illustrates the consequents of the rules of Frames 9.3 and 9.4.

With this new rule base we obtain a trajectory for Montroll's p-fuzzy model, that may be visualized in Fig. 9.15.

Exercise 9.2 Redo the example above assuming $s > 1$.

We conclude this section with remarks about the parameter estimates of the p-fuzzy model. For example, as in Verhulst's model, the equilibrium in the Montroll's p-fuzzy model belongs of the interval

$$ I^* = \text{supp}\,(A_5) \bigcap \text{supp}\,(A_6) = [200, 210], $$

since there is semantic opposition in the consequents mB_5 and mB_6. This value will be the carrying capacity (K) of Montroll's theoretic model, in which the direction field is given by $f(x) = a(1 - (\frac{x}{K})^s)$. Since the antecedents A_5 and A_6 are the same as in Example 9.1, the equilibrium is the solution to the equation

$$ \varphi_{A_5}(x) = \varphi_{A_6}(x) \implies \bar{x} = 205. $$

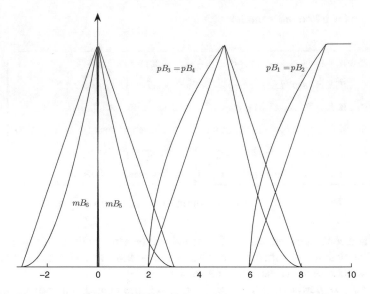

Fig. 9.14 Consequents of rule base of Frame 9.3 and their respective modifications

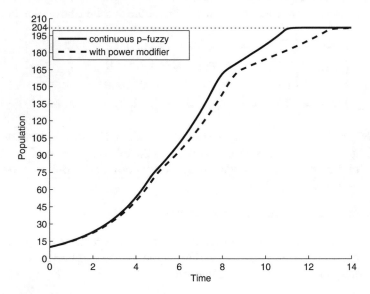

Fig. 9.15 Trajectory of the continuous p-fuzzy models for the base rules of Frame 9.3 and modified rules ($\gamma = 0.05$), according to Frame 9.4

Therefore, the carrying capacity K must be equal to 205. The parameter a can be obtained from a least squares type adjustment. Clearly both a and K may be obtained by adjusting the direction field or the classic solution of the model.

A study on how to obtain the parameters for continuous p-fuzzy models can be found in [7, 20]. The stability of such systems are obtained through similar results to the ones we employed in the discrete p-fuzzy systems.

The suggestion above to approach Montroll's model from Verhulst's model is not unique. It is only one among many other possibilities, such as translating the consequents of the rule base or apply the extension principle to the function $f(x) = 1 - x^s$.

The following section concludes this chapter and deals with p-fuzzy continuous systems for two-dimensional models.

9.3 Bi-Dimensional Models: Predator-Prey and p-Fuzzy Lotka–Volterra

We will briefly review the classical Lotka–Volterra model and develop the corresponding p-fuzzy model. We want to point out that our formulation of the p-fuzzy Lotka–Volterra model does not use the solution given by classical model. The hypothesis (see below) of classical model are re-interpreted by fuzzy rules for p-fuzzy model. The objective of describing this model is to compare both approaches, classic and p-fuzzy.

Lotka–Volterra Predator-Prey Model
About the year 1925, Lotka and Volterra developed one of the most widely used biomathematical models that tracks remarkably well the interactions between prey and predators and is of great importance to the field of biomathematics. The model is known as the Lotka–Volterra Predator-Prey Model.

The model created by Volterra explained the changes observed in the weakfish and shark populations in the Adriatic Sea, given the downtime in the fishing activities during World War I and resumed after the end of the war.

The classic Lotka–Volterra Predator-Prey Model assumes that:

1. The prey and the predators are distributed uniformly in the same habitat, i.e., all the predators have the same chance of finding each prey;
2. An encounter between the elements of the two species is random, and has rate proportional to the size of both populations, the higher the number of prey, the easier it is to find them, and the greater number of predators, the more the attacks;
3. The prey population grows exponentially in the absence of predators (unlimited growth in the presence of lack of predators);
4. The predator population decreases exponentially in the absence of prey (decreasing by lack of food);
5. The predator population is favored by the excess of food;
6. The prey population is disfavored by the increase of predators.

These six hypothesis (see [4, 10, 19])) are summarized in the next equations, which is called the Lotka–Volterra Model:

$$\begin{cases} \dfrac{dx}{dt} = ax - \alpha xy \\ \dfrac{dy}{dt} = -by + \beta xy \end{cases}. \tag{9.9}$$

The state variables x and y are, respectively, the number of prey and predators at each instant t. The parameters represent:

- a: population growth rate in the absence of predators;
- $\frac{\alpha}{\beta}$: predator efficiency, i.e., the efficiency of conversion of a unit of mass of prey in a unit of mass of predators, since α represents the success of the attacks and β represents the conversion rate of prey biomass into predators;
- b: mortality rate of predators in the absence of prey.

The equilibrium points of the system (9.9) are $(0, 0)$, that is an unstable saddle point, and $\left(\frac{b}{\beta}, \frac{a}{\alpha}\right)$, that is a stable center (see [4, 19]). The cyclic nature of the solutions explains the variations observer empirically found in a population of prey and predators.

9.3.1   Predator-Prey p-Fuzzy Model

The previous subsection presented Lotka–Volterra's hypotheses that characterize a predator-prey model whose population oscillate in time. This is consistent with empirical observations in such an ecosystems [4, 10, 11]. The results, consistent with the studied phenomenon, made Lotka–Volterra theoretic model a paradigm for the predator-prey type models. In Sect. 9.1.3 we modeled the main property of a predator-prey system, which was that the prey favors the growth of the predators and are disfavored by the them. As a consequence, the phase plane results in oscillating trajectories. In this section we want to go beyond this. We intend to reproduce, by means of a two-dimensional continuous p-fuzzy system, a phase plane similar to the Lotka–Volterra continuous model, in which the trajectories are cycles (see Fig. 9.16). To do so, it is necessary to re-interpret the six hypotheses above as follows:

1'. No individual in either species has an advantage coming from the environment, so that there does not exist individual "quality" involved, and it is natural that the state variables just represent quantities;
2'. There is interaction between the species;
3'. There is no self-inhibition in the prey, so that for a given number of predators, the specific growth of the prey is a negative or a positive constant;
4'. For a given number of prey, the specific growth of the predators is a negative or a positive constant;

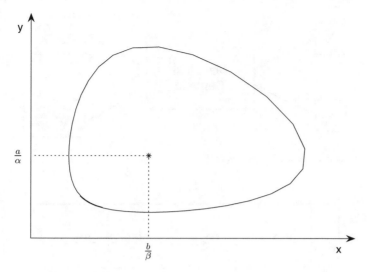

Fig. 9.16 Phase plane of the Lotka–Volterra model (9.9)

5'. The specific growth of the predators increases with the number of prey;
6'. The specific growth of the prey decreases with the number of predators.

The hypotheses 3'–6' indicate that interaction is typical of prey-predator and that, if one species is maintained constant, the other one will have Malthusian increase/decrease that is, its specific growth will be constant.

Note that if the rules of Malthusian p fuzzy model (Frame 8.1) had been stated in terms of the specific growth,the rules should have been qualified with the same adjective, that is, the consequent would be the same for all rules. Considering the above observations, our objective is to obtain a fuzzy rule base that "replaces" Eq. (9.9) in order to model the dynamics between prey and predators by means of a continuous Lotka–Volterra p-fuzzy model.

We have all the linguistic input variables, the number of prey (X) and the number of predators (Y), and we have two output variables, the relative variation of the number of prey per unit of time, denoted by $\frac{1}{X}\frac{dX}{dt}$, which is the specific growth of the prey, and the relative variation of the number of predators per unit of time, denoted by $\frac{1}{Y}\frac{dY}{dt}$, the specific growth of the predators. Figure 9.17 represents a scheme of the model.

The values assumed by the variable X are: low (A_1), average low (A_2), average high (A_3), and high (A_4). The values assumed by the variable Y are: low (B_1), average low (B_2), average high (B_3), and high (B_4).

Both specific growths, $\frac{1}{X}\frac{dX}{dt}$ and $\frac{1}{Y}\frac{dY}{dt}$, will assume the values: high positive (P_2), low positive (P_1), low negative (N_1) and high negative (N_2). In the above scheme (Fig. 9.17), the knowledge base is translated into a set of fuzzy rules that play the role of a direction field. From the six re-interpretations for Lotka–Volterra's hypotheses above, specially observation 6', we propose the fuzzy rule base of Frame 9.5.

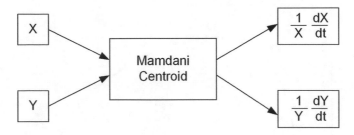

Fig. 9.17 System based on fuzzy rules for (9.9)

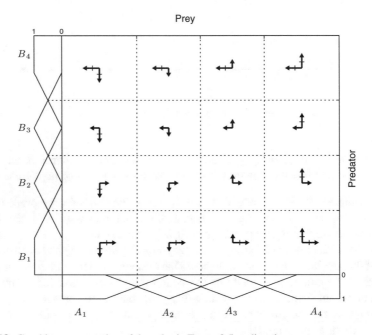

Fig. 9.18 Graphic representation of the rules in Frame 9.5 as direction vectors

We can represent the rule base graphically considering that there is no variation in the specific growths, with respect to the magnitudes and direction of each species when we maintain the quantity of the other one constant (Malthusian growth for each species, given by the other). For example, for a fixed quantity of predators, the specific variation of prey must be constant (see horizontal arrows in Fig. 9.18). Of course, other rule bases could have been adopted. Note that the related magnitudes are uncertain, both for the variables and for the specific growths.

Figure 9.18 illustrates the rule base of Frame 9.5. The horizontal and vertical arrows represent the magnitudes and direction of $\frac{1}{X}\frac{dX}{dt}$ and $\frac{1}{Y}\frac{dY}{dt}$, respectively. Figure 9.18 is exhibited in order to make a comparison with the representation of the classic differential equations direction field. For the sake of curiosity, and to convince

If X is A_1 and Y is B_1 then $\frac{1}{X}\frac{dX}{dt}$ is P_2 and $\frac{1}{Y}\frac{dY}{dt}$ is N_2
If X is A_2 and Y is B_1 then $\frac{1}{X}\frac{dX}{dt}$ is P_2 and $\frac{1}{Y}\frac{dY}{dt}$ is N_1
If X is A_3 and Y is B_1 then $\frac{1}{X}\frac{dX}{dt}$ is P_2 and $\frac{1}{Y}\frac{dY}{dt}$ is P_1
If X is A_4 and Y is B_1 then $\frac{1}{X}\frac{dX}{dt}$ is P_2 and $\frac{1}{Y}\frac{dY}{dt}$ is P_2
If X is A_1 and Y is B_2 then $\frac{1}{X}\frac{dX}{dt}$ is P_1 and $\frac{1}{Y}\frac{dY}{dt}$ is N_2
If X is A_2 and Y is B_2 then $\frac{1}{X}\frac{dX}{dt}$ is P_1 and $\frac{1}{Y}\frac{dY}{dt}$ is N_1
If X is A_3 and Y is B_2 then $\frac{1}{X}\frac{dX}{dt}$ is P_1 and $\frac{1}{Y}\frac{dY}{dt}$ is P_1
If X is A_4 and Y is B_2 then $\frac{1}{X}\frac{dX}{dt}$ is P_1 and $\frac{1}{Y}\frac{dY}{dt}$ is P_2
If X is A_1 and Y is B_3 then $\frac{1}{X}\frac{dX}{dt}$ is N_1 and $\frac{1}{Y}\frac{dY}{dt}$ is N_2
If X is A_2 and Y is B_3 then $\frac{1}{X}\frac{dX}{dt}$ is N_1 and $\frac{1}{Y}\frac{dY}{dt}$ is N_1
If X is A_3 and Y is B_3 then $\frac{1}{X}\frac{dX}{dt}$ is N_1 and $\frac{1}{Y}\frac{dY}{dt}$ is P_1
If X is A_4 and Y is B_3 then $\frac{1}{X}\frac{dX}{dt}$ is N_1 and $\frac{1}{Y}\frac{dY}{dt}$ is P_2
If X is A_1 and Y is B_4 then $\frac{1}{X}\frac{dX}{dt}$ is N_2 and $\frac{1}{Y}\frac{dY}{dt}$ is N_2
If X is A_2 and Y is B_4 then $\frac{1}{X}\frac{dX}{dt}$ is N_2 and $\frac{1}{Y}\frac{dY}{dt}$ is N_1
If X is A_3 and Y is B_4 then $\frac{1}{X}\frac{dX}{dt}$ is N_2 and $\frac{1}{Y}\frac{dY}{dt}$ is P_1
If X is A_4 and Y is B_4 then $\frac{1}{X}\frac{dX}{dt}$ is N_2 and $\frac{1}{Y}\frac{dY}{dt}$ is P_2

Frame 9.5: Fuzzy rules for the predator-prey p-fuzzy model

ourselves of the power of the p-fuzzy methodology, the rule base in fact "generates" a classic direction field for an ODE. Figure 9.19 below illustrates the direction field produced by the rule base of Frame 9.5.

Let us go back to our example. Figure 9.19 is very useful in the study of the system dynamics. For example, from this figure, one can locate the region of the plane that contains the possible non-zero equilibrium points of the system. In our case, this region is

$$E = [\text{supp}\,(A_2) \bigcap \text{supp}\,(A_3)] \times [\text{supp}\,(B_2) \bigcap \text{supp}\,(B_3)] = I_x \times I_y.$$

Fig. 9.19 Graphic
representation of the
direction field generated by
the rules of Frame 9.5

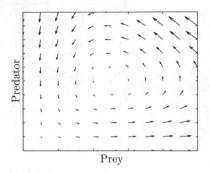

We observe that the semantic opposition occurs in this region. It is also possible to suggest that the interactions of φ_{A_2} with φ_{A_3} and of φ_{B_2} with φ_{B_3} are strong candidates for being the equilibrium of this system. We can adopt such values for the equilibrium of a classic Lotka–Volterra model (9.9) and, together with the adjustments, obtain the value of a, b, α, and β. However, we will study next methods for obtaining the parameters of the classic models from p-fuzzy models. We refer the reader interested in this topic to some recent work on p-fuzzy systems [7, 18, 20, 21].

Our interest here is to illustrate the proposed method in order to produce a trajectory that represents the evolution of the p-fuzzy system. Figures 9.20 and 9.21 represent the membership functions of each of the fuzzy values used for antecedents/consequents in our example. Using Mamdani's Inference Method and the defuzzification of the center of mass we obtain the values for $\frac{1}{x}\frac{dx}{dt}$ and $\frac{1}{y}\frac{dy}{dt}$.

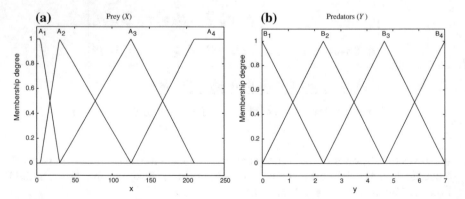

Fig. 9.20 Membership function of the antecedents

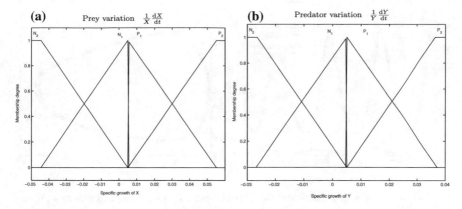

Fig. 9.21 Membership function of the consequents

At each instant t, the number of prey and predators is given by the formulas

$$
\begin{cases}
x(t) = x(t_0) + \displaystyle\int_{t_0}^{t} \dfrac{dx}{dt}(s)\,ds \\[4mm]
y(t) = y(t_0) + \displaystyle\int_{t_0}^{t} \dfrac{dy}{dt}(s)\,ds
\end{cases}
\tag{9.10}
$$

Since the outputs are $\frac{1}{x}\frac{dx}{dt}$ and $\frac{1}{y}\frac{dy}{dt}$, we should multiply them by the input values x and y, respectively, in order to obtain the derivatives $\frac{dx}{dt}$ and $\frac{dy}{dt}$. However, the analytic expressions for each of these derivatives are not known. To estimate the trajectories given by (9.10), in each interval $[t_{i-1}, t_i]$, we approximate $\frac{dx}{dt}(t)$ by $\frac{dx}{dt}(t_{i-1})$, in such a way that the integral $\int_{t_{i-1}}^{t_i} \frac{dx}{dt}(s)\,ds$ is approximated by $(t_i - t_{i-1})\frac{dx}{dt}(t_{i-1})$.

The values of $x(t)$ and $y(t)$ are thus given by the equations,

$$
\begin{cases}
x(t_i) = x(t_{i-1}) + hx'_{i-1} \\
y(t_i) = y(t_{i-1}) + hy'_{i-1}
\end{cases},
\tag{9.11}
$$

where $t_i = t_0 + ih$ and x', y' are the outputs of the controller corresponding to the input values $x_{i-1} \approx x(t_{i-1})$ and $y_{i-1} \approx y(t_{i-1})$, respectively.

Simulations of the trajectories produced by the p-fuzzy system above follow the steps:

- To start the process, we use the values $x_0 = 100$, $y_0 = 3$, $h = 0.1$ and $t_0 = 0$;
- Initial data for the fuzzy controller are prey population x_0 and predator population y_0;

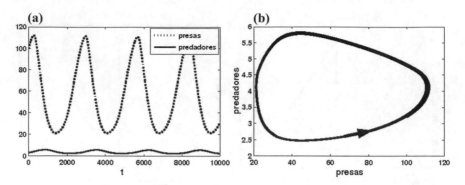

Fig. 9.22 a Evolution of population in time; **b** Phase plane for p-fuzzy system with $x_0 = 100$ and $y_0 = 3$ [22]

- The outputs provided by the fuzzy controller, multiplied by the inputs, give us the values x_0' and y_0';
- From (9.11), we find x_1 and y_1;
- x_1 and y_1 are the new input values of the controller, and so on.

Using Eq. (9.11), we obtain the phase plane and the trajectories illustrated in Fig. 9.22.

Moreover, using the initial data above and the p-fuzzy system given by the rule base of Frame 9.5, combined with the system (9.11), it is possible to conclude that the equilibrium point is $P_e = (77.5; 3.5)$.

We could compare the coordinates of P_e with the classical theoretical equilibrium $P = \left(\frac{b}{\beta}, \frac{a}{\alpha}\right)$, to obtain relations between $a, b, \alpha\beta$, if we were interested in finding the parameters of a classic Lotka–Volterra model to produce the trajectories represented in Fig. 9.16. From this, we could use adjustments to finally find each of these parameters.

The first published work that uses continuous p-fuzzy models to the interaction between species can be found in [18]. If uses the methodology given above to model the relation between plant lice and lady-bugs in the biological control of a disease called "Sudden Death of the Citrus". The plant louse is supposedly the host of the virus that causes sudden death and is the prey. The lady-bug, that eats the plant louse, is the predator. In this predator-prey system the p-fuzzy model assumes inhibition in both species. Therefore, the rules should take this into account in such a way that the trajectories no longer exhibit a cyclic nature, but have cyclic limits. Such p-fuzzy model exhibits qualitative properties that coincide with the classic Holling–Tanner model. From this, a study of the stability and parameters adjustments of this model was done.

An important aspect of the p-fuzzy systems explored by the authors of [18, 22] is how easy it deals with possible heterogeneities in the populations. For instance, for the specific case of the sudden death, the predators show many levels of predation, depending on its stage, larval or adult. In this case, the authors chose, as the state variables the number of plant lice and the predation potential. This takes into account not only the number of predators, but also their qualities.

References

1. K.B. Athreya, S. Karlin, On branching processes with random environments: I: extinction probabilities. Ann. Math. Stat. **42**(5), 1499–1520 (1971)
2. R.M. May, *Stability and Complexity in Model Ecosystems*, vol. 6 (Princeton University Press, Princeton, 1973)
3. M. Turelli, Stochastic community theory: a partially guided tour. Biomathematics **17**, 321–339 (1986)
4. L. Edelstein-Keshet, *Mathematical Models in Biology* (McGraw-Hill, México, 1988)
5. A. Kandel, *Fuzzy Mathematical Techniques with Applications* (Addison-Wesley Publishing Co., Reading, 1986)
6. J.D.M. Silva, *Análise de estabilidade de sistemas dinâmicos p-fuzzy com aplicações em biomatemática* (Tese de Doutorado, IMECC-UNICAMP, Campinas, 2005)
7. J.D.M. Silva, J. Leite, R.C. Bassanezi, M.S. Cecconello, Stationary points—i: one-dimensional p-fuzzy dynamical systems. J. Appl. Math. **2013**, 1–11 (2013)
8. N.R.S. Ortega, L.C. Barros, E. Massad, Fuzzy gradual rules in epidemiology. Kybernetes **32**, 460–477 (2003)
9. J.C.R. Pereira, *Análise de dados qualitativos - estratégias metodológicas para as ciências da saúde, humanas e sociais*, 3rd edn. (Edusp-Fapesp, São Paulo, 2003)
10. A.G. Gomes, M.C. Varriale, *Modelagem de ecossistemas: Uma introdução*, vol. 1 (Editora UFSM, Santa Maria-RS, 2001)
11. J. Murray, *Mathematical Biology* (Springer, New York, 1990)
12. J. Hale, H. Koçak, *Dynamics and Bifurcations* (Springer, New York, 1991)
13. T.M. Apostol, *Calculus*, vol. 2, 2nd edn. (Editorial Reverté, Mexico, 1975)
14. H.L. Guidorizzi, *Um curso de cálculo*, vol. 1, 5th edn. (Livros Técnicos e Científicos Editora S. A., Rio de Janeiro, 2001)
15. M.C.C. Cunha, *Métodos numéricos*, 2nd edn. (Editora da UNICAMP, Campinas, 2000)
16. W.E. Milne, *Numerical Calculus* (Princeton University Press, Princeton, 2015)
17. M.A.G. Ruggiero, V.L.R. Lopes, *Cálculo numérico, aspectos teóricos e computacionais*, 2nd edn. (Makron Books, São Paulo, 1997)
18. M.S. Peixoto, *Sistemas dinâmicos e controladores fuzzy: Um estudo da dispersão da morte súbita dos cítros em São Paulo* (Tese de Doutorado, IMECC-UNICAMP, Campinas, 2005)
19. R.C. Bassanezi, W.C. Ferreira Jr., *Equações diferenciais com aplicações* (Edit. HARBRA, São Paulo, 1998)
20. M.R.B. Dias, L.C. Barros, Differential equations based on fuzzy rules, in IFSA/EUSFLAT Conference, pp. 240–246 (2009)
21. L.C. Barros, R.Z.G. Oliveira, M.B.F. Leite, R.C. Bassanezi, Epidemiological models of directly transmitted diseases: an approach via fuzzy sets theory. Int. J. Uncertain. Fuzziness Knowl.-Based Syst. **22**(05), 769–781 (2014)
22. M.S. Peixoto, L.C. Barros, R.C. Bassanezi, Predator-prey fuzzy model. Ecol. Model. **214**(1), 39–44 (2008)

Chapter 10
Biomathematical Modeling in a Fuzzy Environment

> *As far as the laws of mathematics refer to reality, they are not certain; as far as they are certain, they do not refer to reality.*
> (Albert Einstein)

Abstract This chapter looks at the influence of the environment in a population as a whole, that is, it looks at processes in which the environment affects all individuals equally. We illustrate this phenomenon via four models.

Chapter 9 stated that the methods of incorporating uncertainties in mathematical models are quite varied and mentioned that there two such ways of incorporating fuzzy uncertainty, environmental fuzziness and demographic fuzziness. Whereas the aim of Chap. 9 was the incorporation of demographic fuzziness in models, this chapter focuses on environmental fuzziness. Thus, for pedagogical and didactic purposes and for clarity, we have distinguished these two types of fuzziness inherent in modeling biomathematical systems: *demographic fuzziness* (Chap. 9) and *environmental fuzziness*, this chapter. These terms, demographic and environmental fuzziness, have their origin in dynamic population modeling (see [1–3]). "Demographic stochasticity (or 'within-individual variability', - ... individuals who are apparently identical have different life spans and produce different numbers of offspring. ... Environmental stochasticity - Environments vary unpredictably through time in ways that affect all individuals equally" (Turelli [3], p. 321).

The estimation of the entity such as the future "number of descendents" in a population, already inherently exhibits stochastic or fuzzy uncertainty properties because of the existence of perturbations in the conditions surrounding any population as a whole. Examples of this nature are abundant - how the cost of living in a particular locality influences the life expectancy in a group of people, how, in a predator-prey model, the natural surroundings favor either the predator or the prey, how in a survival of the fittest model nature is favorable to one or another of the competitors at various periods of time. Through translation of rules, environmental fuzziness may be changed into a parameters or demographic fuzziness in biomathematical models. In this chapter we study how to model with environmental fuzziness and compare

© Springer-Verlag Berlin Heidelberg 2017

L.C. de Barros et al., *A First Course in Fuzzy Logic, Fuzzy Dynamical Systems, and Biomathematics*, Studies in Fuzziness and Soft Computing 347, DOI 10.1007/978-3-662-53324-6_10

237

this type of fuzzy model with the deterministic and stochastic ones. Details of similar types of models can be found in [4, 5]. Recall that what we have called environmental fuziness is fuzziness in the parameters of model.

The models we treat next can, from the mathematical point of view, be treated by classical methods without the necessity of new concepts of mathematics to model the evolution of uncertainty in them. For example, if the phenomenon were modeled with differential equations and the rate of change in the differential equation were uncertain, the differential equation may be understood as a family of classical differential equations dependent on the parameters governing the uncertain rates of change (the derivatives) so that the theory of stochastic differential equations may be used. These types of equations are called *random dynamical equations* (see [6]).

Most of the models with uncertainty of interest to us have both types of uncertainties present (demographic and environmental fuzziness) and, in these cases, the modeling is not very different than what has been developed in the previous chapters of this book. However, depending on the purpose of the model, environmental fuzziness can be treated as demographic fuzziness. For this, however, we need to transform all the uncertainty of the variables into the parameters of the mathematical model assuming that such a process makes sense. Let us begin with an example in which environmental fuzziness appears in the model.

10.1 Life Expectancy and Poverty

We can use various indicators to model *poverty,* for example, caloric intake, vitamin intake, basic sanitation, and so on. For this presentation, we will use income of the relevant group we are studying [5].

10.1.1 The Model

Suppose that A is a closed group (no in-migration or out-migration) with $n(t)$ individuals at instant t. Assuming that poverty, here evaluated as the income level, is one factor in the reduction of the number of years of life of all the individuals in A, we can consider that

$$
\begin{cases}
\dfrac{dn}{dt} = -[\lambda_1 + \beta(r)\lambda_2] n \\
n_0 = n(0)
\end{cases},
\tag{10.1}
$$

where:

- λ_1 is the natural death rate (obtained from a group who is under favorable survival conditions);
- $\beta(r)\lambda_2$ indicates the influence of poverty on the increase on the natural death rate λ_1;

- $\beta(r)$ indicates the level to which an individual with income r belongs to the fuzzy set *poverty*, that is, β is a membership function.

We note that the maximum mortality rate is $\lambda_1 + \lambda_2$ which is obtained when $\beta(r) = 1$. The solution to the differential equation (10.1) is

$$n(t) = n_0 e^{-[\lambda_1 + \beta(r)\lambda_2]t}.$$

The membership function β can be represented by a function that is decreasing in r and, here, we think it convenient to adopt a family of curves (see Example 1.5)

$$\beta_k(r) = \begin{cases} [1 - (\frac{r}{r_0})^2]^k & \text{if } 0 < r < r_0 \\ 0 & \text{if } r \geq r_0 \end{cases}, \tag{10.2}$$

where k is a parameter that supplies some characteristics of the group *poverty*.

Recall, from our previous models, the larger the value of k, the smaller the dependence of the individual has in relation to income, that is, the smaller the influence that income has on *poverty*. In this way, intuitively, k reveals if the environment in which the group lives is more or is less favorable to life expectancy.

Observe that (10.1) is a family of ordinary differential equations. Thus, $n(.)$ is a family of solutions of the differential equation indexed by r, that is, for each fixed r, $n(.)$ is a solution of the differential equation corresponding to this r. This set forms the solution of the fuzzy problem (10.1). In this way, suppose that r has a statistical distribution, then $n(t)$ is a random variable for each fixed t. If we wish to select precisely one curve to represent the evolution of the number of individuals over time, a strong candidate is the one that gives us numbers at the midpoint of $n(t)$ for each t. This "mid-curve" is obtained calculating the expectation in the same way as it is done in stochastics/statistics.

Our object in what follows is to obtain an expectation of life expectancy of the group by means of classical mathematical and fuzzy expectation according to the concepts we have seen in Chap. 7.

10.1.2 Statistical Expectation: $E[n(t)]$

Statistical expectation is given by

$$E[n(t)] = \int_{-\infty}^{\infty} n(t)h(r)dr, \tag{10.3}$$

where $h(r)$ is the probability density function of income.

Fig. 10.1 Probability
density function of income -
Pareto distribution

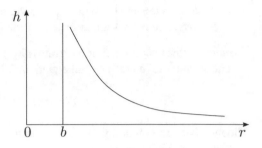

The Pareto distribution for developing countries (see [7]) with parameters a
and b,

$$h(r) = \begin{cases} ab^a r^{-(a+1)} & \text{if } r \geq b \\ 0 & \text{if } r < b \end{cases}.$$

is used for our specific case (Fig. 10.1).
    Therefore,

$$E[n(t)] = n(0)e^{-\lambda_1 t} ab^a \int_b^\infty e^{-\beta_k(r)\lambda_2 t} r^{-(a+1)} dr$$

or

$$E\left[\frac{n(t)}{n(0)}\right] = e^{-\lambda_1 t} ab^a \int_b^\infty e^{-\beta_k(r)\lambda_2 t} r^{-(a+1)} dr. \tag{10.4}$$

- If $r_0 \leq b$, then $\beta_k(r) = 0$ for $r \geq b$ and

$$E[n(t)] = n(0)e^{-\lambda_1 t} ab^a \int_b^\infty r^{-(a+1)} dr = n(0)e^{-\lambda_1 t}.$$

This means that $E[\frac{n(t)}{n(0)}] = e^{-\lambda_1 t}$ for all $a > 0$, that is, in this case the value of b is
sufficiently large so that there is no affect of poverty on the life expectancy of the
group.

- If $r_0 > b$, we have that $ab^a \int_b^\infty e^{-\beta_k(r)\lambda_2 t} r^{-(a+1)} dr < 1$, so that $E[n(t)]$
$< n(0)e^{-\lambda_1 t}$. This means that we can interpret the number

$$ab^a \int_b^\infty e^{-\beta_k(r)\lambda_2 t} r^{-(a+1)} dr$$

as a factor of reduction in the life expectancy due to poverty.

    What follows is the calculation of fuzzy expectation in order for us to compare it
with the statistical expectation given above.

10.1.3   Fuzzy Expectation Value: $FEV\left[\frac{n(t)}{n(0)}\right]$

Let us consider $Y_t(r) = \frac{n(t)}{n_0}$ a membership function of a fuzzy set since we have $\frac{n(t)}{n_0} \in [0, 1]$. Let us next obtain $FEV\left[\frac{n(t)}{n(0)}\right]$ using Theorem 7.1 applying the function

$$H(\alpha) = P\{r : Y_t(r) = \frac{n(t)}{n(0)} \geq \alpha\} = P\{r : e^{-(\lambda_1 + \lambda_2 \beta_k(r))t} \geq \alpha\}$$

$$= P\{r : e^{-\lambda_2 \beta_k(r)t} \geq \alpha e^{\lambda_1 t}\}, \tag{10.5}$$

where P is a probability defined by the density function for income $h(r)$. Thus, $H(\alpha) = 0$ if $\alpha > e^{-\lambda_1 t}$. On the other hand, if $\alpha \leq e^{-\lambda_1 t}$,

$$H(\alpha) = P\{r : \alpha \leq e^{-(\lambda_1 + \lambda_2 \beta_k(r))t} < e^{-\lambda_1 t}\} + P\{r : r \geq r_0\}$$

which, with a little algebraic manipulation, we arrive at

$$H(\alpha) = \begin{cases} 1 & \text{if } 0 \leq \alpha \leq e^{-(\lambda_1 + \lambda_2 \beta_k(b))t} \\ \left[\dfrac{b}{r_0 \sqrt{1 - (-(\frac{\ln \alpha}{\lambda_2 t} + \frac{\lambda_1}{\lambda_2}))^{\frac{1}{k}}}} \right]^a & \text{if } e^{-(\lambda_1 + \lambda_2 \beta_k(b))t} < \alpha \leq e^{-\lambda_1 t} \\ 0 & \text{if } e^{-\lambda_1 t} < \alpha \leq 1 \end{cases} \tag{10.6}$$

It is easy to see that $H(\alpha)$ is continuous over $[0, 1]$, except when $\alpha = e^{-\lambda_1 t}$ and H has a fixed point between $Y_t(b)$ and $e^{-\lambda_1 t}$, that is,

$$Y_t(b) = e^{-(\lambda_1 + \lambda_2 \beta_k(b))t} \leq FEV\left[\frac{n(t)}{n(0)}\right] \leq e^{-\lambda_1 t} (Fig.\ 10.2).$$

Some conclusions can quickly be made which are different than that of statistical expectation. Specifically, if

$$\left(\frac{b}{r_0}\right)^a \geq e^{-\lambda_1 t},$$

then

$$FEV\left[\frac{n(t)}{n(0)}\right] = e^{-\lambda_1 t} = FEV[e^{-\lambda_1 t}].$$

In particular, we have if $b \geq r_0$, then poverty does not affect life expectancy. This was the case with the results that were obtained using statistic expectation. However, fuzzy expectation indicates more. In order for poverty to have no effect on life expectancy, what is of interest is the relationship $\left[\left(\frac{b}{r_0}\right)^a \geq e^{-\lambda_1 t}\right]$ between individual income and the minimal group income. For example, an individual can

Fig. 10.2 $H(\alpha)$ and Fuzzy
Expectation (FEV)

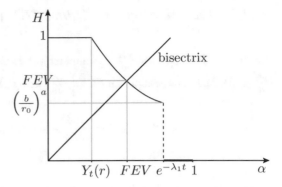

have a relatively small income ($b < r_0$) and even so, not have it interfere with his/her
life expectancy. For this to occur, we just need that $\left(\frac{b}{r_0}\right)^a \geq e^{-\lambda_1 t}$. This is the typical
case of a single person who has all the infrastructure to survive.

We want to emphasize that, from a technical point of view, it is harder to obtain
$E(n(t))$, since it is not integrable in closed form, whereas $FEV\left[\frac{n(t)}{n(0)}\right]$ whose value
is the fixed point of H, can be obtained by the Banach Fixed Point Theorem
(see [8, 9]). If $\left(\frac{b}{r_0}\right)^a < e^{-\lambda_1 t}$, we can compute the value of $FEV\left[\frac{n(t)}{n(0)}\right]$ determined
by the fixed point of H once this function is continuous and decreasing for $\alpha < e^{-\lambda_1 t}$.
We observe that H has the same fixed point as its inverse, that is, as

$$H^{-1}(\alpha) = \exp\left\{-\left[\lambda_1 + \lambda_2 \beta_k(\frac{b}{\alpha^{1/a}})\right]\right\} t, \text{ if } \left(\frac{b}{r_0}\right)^a < \alpha < 1.$$

This model of poverty was used to evaluate the life expectancy of a group of metal
workers in the city of Recife (see Tables 10.1 and 10.2), the capital of the state of
the northeast state of Pernambuco in Brazil. For this group we had some information
about the income and the calculation of life expectancy using classical statistical
methods thus permitting us to compare the statistical methods to the fuzzy methods.

10.1.4 Application: Life Expectancy of a Group of Metal Workers in Recife, Pernambuco - Brazil

We can determine the values of the parameter a and b of the income variable from
Table 10.1 for a Pareto distribution $h(r)$. Now consider the cumulative distribution
of income

$$F(r) = \int_b^r h(x)dx = \int_b^r ab^a x^{-a-1}dx = 1 - b^a r^{-a} = R.$$

Table 10.1 Workers' distribution by minimum wage ranges. Recife, 1988 Source: DIEESE

Minimal salary range	Populational distribution		% of total of payment
	n^0	%	
0 to 2	4003	45.0	21.1
2 to 3	2099	23.6	18.8
3 to 4	933	10.5	12.0
4 to 5	670	7.5	11.0
5 to 6	300	3.4	6.0
6 to 7	264	303.0	6.2
7 to 10	367	4.1	11.1
10 to 15	171	1.9	7.8
over 15	81	0.9	6.1

Table 10.2 Source: Carvalho and Wood (1977)

Income class	Income Cr$	Life expectance(years)
1	1 to 150	40.0
2	151 to 300	45.9
3	301 to 500	50.8
4	over 500	54.4

This means that,

$$\ln(1 - R) = a \ln b - a \ln r.$$

Linearizing the data from Table 10.1, we obtain an approximation of $a \approx 2.031$ and $b \approx 1.726$. Thus,

$$h(r) = \begin{cases} 6.15r^{-3031} & \text{if } r \geq 1.726 \\ 0 & \text{if } r < 1.726 \end{cases}.$$

The table for life expectancy in the northeast of Brazil in 1977, in urban areas, where the minimum salary (which we denote S) was Cr$ 156.00 per month, is given in Table 10.2.

Suppose that income r is proportional to a power of the minimum salary S of the group we are studying, $r = S^m$, where m is a constant. Then, we have

$$\beta_k(S^m) = \begin{cases} [1 - \left(\frac{S}{S_0}\right)^{2m}]^k & \text{if } 0 < S < S_0 \\ 0 & \text{if } S \geq S_0 \end{cases}.$$

Fig. 10.3 Membership
function of poor for $k = 1.51$

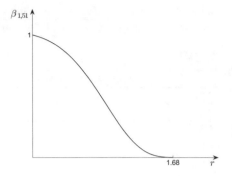

Life expectancy, independent of family income was 54.4 years. From this, the
natural mortality rate is $\lambda_1 = \frac{1}{54.4}$. On the other hand, $\lambda_1 + \lambda_2$ is the highest rate of
mortality of the group which is 40, that is,

$$\lambda_1 + \lambda_2 = \frac{1}{40} \implies \lambda_2 = \frac{1}{40} - \frac{1}{54.4} = 6.618 \times 10^{-3}.$$

Let us consider that the minimum livable wage in 1977 was Cr\$ 500.00 per month
which is equivalent to $S_0 = \frac{500}{156} = 3.2$ minimum salaries. From Table 10.2 we have
two values for life expectancy

$$\text{If } S = 1 \implies \frac{1}{\lambda_1 + \lambda_2 \beta_k(1)} = 45.9$$
$$\text{If } S = 2 \implies \frac{1}{\lambda_1 + \lambda_2 \beta_k(2^m)} = 50.8 \implies$$

$$\lambda_2 \beta_k(1) = \frac{1}{45.9} - \frac{1}{54.4} = 3.404 \times 10^{-3}$$
$$\lambda_2 \beta_k(2^m) = \frac{1}{50.8} - \frac{1}{54.4} = 1.303 \times 10^{-3}.$$

Since $\lambda_2 = 6.618 \times 10^{-3}$, we have

$$\beta_k(1) = 0.514 \implies \left[1 - (\tfrac{1}{S_0})^{2m} \right]^k = 0.514$$
$$\beta_k(2^m) = 0.197 \implies \left[1 - (\tfrac{2}{S_0})^{2m} \right]^k = 0.197.$$

Then, $m = 0.4435$ and $k = 1.51$. Since $S_0 = 3.2$, it must be that $r_0 = (3.2)^{0.4435} \simeq$
1.68 which means the membership function of the fuzzy set $\beta_k(r)$ (Fig. 10.3) is given
by

$$\beta_k(r) = \begin{cases} \left[1 - \left(\frac{r}{3.2}\right)^{0.887} \right]^{1.51} & \text{if } 0 < r < 1.68 \\ 0 & \text{if } r \geq 1.68 \end{cases}. \tag{10.7}$$

Table 10.3 Statistical expectation and fuzzy of number of workers and difference between two methodology

t	$E\left[\frac{n(t)}{n(0)}\right]$	$EF\left[\frac{n(t)}{n(0)}\right]$	$\left\|E\left[\frac{n(t)}{n(0)}\right] - EF\left[\frac{n(t)}{n(0)}\right]\right\| \times 10^3$
1	0.9810872	0.9800555	1.0317
2	0.9625352	0.9605718	1.9634
3	0.9443294	0.941537	2.7924
4	0.9264697	0.9229397	3.5300
5	0.908949	0.9047686	4.1804
10	0.8261962	0.8199376	6.2486
20	0.682632	0.6766003	6.0317
40	0.4660586	0.4687494	2.6908

10.1.5 Comparisons of the Statistical Expected Value and the Fuzzy Expected Value

We have, in hand, the membership function of the set *poverty* ($\beta_{1.51}$), so that we can calculate the average for the metal workers that we have been studying in Sect. 10.1.4, year by year, utilizing the results obtained in Sects. 10.1.2 and 10.1.3. Table 10.3 illustrate these values.

The fourth column of Table 10.3 shows us the various differences between the two methods to calculate life expectancy. In a general manner, Corollary 7.3 guarantees us that the differences are no greater than 0.25. For the values of the table, the largest difference in life expectancy is on the order of 0.63 %.

Moreover, for this specific example, it is easy to see that $FEV\left[\frac{n(t)}{n(0)}\right]$ is in fact between $Y(cb^m)$ and $e^{-\lambda_1 t}$. Thus,

$$\lim_{t \to \infty}\left|E\left[\frac{n(t)}{n(0)}\right] - FEV\left[\frac{n(t)}{n(0)}\right]\right| = 0,$$

that is, $E\left[\frac{n(t)}{n(0)}\right] \simeq FEV\left[\frac{n(t)}{n(0)}\right]$ for t sufficiently large.

Now, as an example, let us suppose that income are given as fixed and let us use Theorem 7.5. Moreover, suppose that the group of workers A have 150 individuals, that is, $\#A = 150 = n_0$ and income is distributed in the following manner:

1. $n_1 = 100$ individuals receive an income of about $r = 2.0$ minimum salaries $\rightarrow$ $Y(2) = e^{-0.0013t}e^{-\lambda_1 t}$;

2. $n_2 = 40$ individuals receive an income of about $r = 2.5$ minimum salaries $\rightarrow$ $Y(2.5) = e^{-0.00057t}e^{-\lambda_1 t}$;

3. $n_3 = 10$ individuals receive an income of about $r = 3.5$ minimum salaries $\rightarrow$ $Y(3.5) = e^{-\lambda_1 t}$.

We can consider that

$$P\{n \mid Y > \alpha\} = \frac{\#\{n \mid Y > \alpha\}}{\#A}.$$

Then,

$$\text{if } Y(2.5) < \alpha \leq Y(3.5) \implies \frac{n_2}{\#A} = \frac{10}{150} = 0.0667;$$

$$\text{if } Y(2.0) < \alpha \leq Y(2.5) \implies \frac{n_2 + n_1}{\#A} = \frac{50}{150} = 0.333.$$

If we now use the fuzzy expected value at time t of $Y(r)$, we have,

$$FEV[Y_t(r)] = \sup_{0 \leq \alpha \leq 1} \inf [\alpha, P\{n \mid Y > \alpha\}]$$

$$= \text{median } \{0.0667; 0.333; e^{-0.0013t - \lambda_1 t}; e^{-0.00057t - \lambda_1 t}; e^{-\lambda_1 t}\}$$

$$= e^{-0.0013t} e^{-\lambda_1 t}.$$

Observe that for $t = 1$ we have $FEF(Y_1(r)) \approx 0.9987 e^{-\lambda_1}$.

On the other hand, if we take the classical average for these same data we obtain

$$E[Y_t] = \frac{100Y_1 + 40Y_2 + 10Y_3}{150} = \frac{e^{-\lambda_1 t}}{150}(100 e^{-0.0013t} + 40 e^{-0.00057t} + 10)$$

so that for $t = 1$

$$E[Y_1] \approx 0.9998 e^{-\lambda_1}.$$

That is, the values $FEF(Y_1(r))$ and $E(Y_1)$ are similar. This corroborates that, in general, $FEV[Y]$ and $E[Y]$ are similar for normalized random variable.

The two following examples have similar characteristics in mathematical models and as such are treated as analogous mathematical tools in terms of building blocks in general biomathematical models. The principal similarity between the two examples as we shall see, is the fact that their uncertainties have their origin in the state variables and so we treat the uncertainty as environmental fuzziness. However, we will "transform" this uncertainty into uncertainty in the parameters. This procedure results in the reduction of complexity in the associated solution methods. To be specific, to treat demographic fuzziness, we will need to use rule-based systems which is generally more complex than if the uncertainty is all in the parameters - environmental fuzziness. However, it is clear that we cannot always use this process of transforming demographic fuzziness to environmental fuzziness. It depends on the situation being modeled.

10.2 The SI Epidemiological Model

The simplest mathematical model to describe the dynamics of directly transmitted illnesses where there is interaction between susceptible individuals and infected individuals is the *SI* model type and it can be represented by the compartmental model depicted by Fig. 10.4.

The classical differential equations that describe the dynamics are given by:

$$\begin{cases} \dfrac{dS}{dt} = -\beta SI \\ \dfrac{dI}{dt} = \beta SI \end{cases}, \tag{10.8}$$

where S is the proportion of susceptible individuals, I is the proportion of infected individuals and β is the coefficient of transmission of the disease. Taking into account that the model is normalized, that is, $S + I = 1$, the number of infected individuals is obtained by the solution to the logistic equation

$$\frac{dI}{dt} = \beta(1 - I)I.$$

whose solution is given by:

$$I = \frac{I_0 e^{\beta t}}{S_0 + I_0 e^{\beta t}}, \tag{10.9}$$

where S_0 and I_0 are the initial proportions of susceptible and infected individuals respectively.

The *SI* model (10.8) is a part of a group of direct disease transmission models. These models are formulated as differential equations and are based on the *law of mass action* whose origin is in kinematic chemistry. The law of mass action postulates that the rate of formation of composites is proportional to the concentration of the reactants. The acceptance of this law is based on the fact that each particle of the reactants are moving independently with respect to all the other particles which means that the mixture is homogeneous so that each particle has the same chance of encountering the other particles. The translation of this law to biomathematical models is made considering that the *encounter* between the variables of the model is their product. Lotka and Volterra, in the same epoch also used this formulation to model the interaction between animal species.

Fig. 10.4 Compartimental diagram of *SI* model

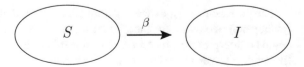

The incorporation of this law into epidemiological models was first made by Kermack-Mackendric (see [10, 11]) based on the hypothesis that infected individuals are homogeneously distributed in the entire population and each infected individual has the same potential to transmit the illness. This is a rather considerable assumption for epidemiological models since there are heterogeneous sources that interfere or accelerate the propagation of an illness, for example, age and/or social class, health habits (washing hands or quarantine, for example).

The model that we are going to propose uses the law of mass action, that is, each infected individual has the same chance of encountering a susceptible individual. This notwithstanding, let us also consider that the chance of new cases of the illness varies from individual to individual. In particular let us consider that a new infection can only occur if a minimal number of viruses (or another pathogenetic agent) is transmitted by the host. In this way, we will take as a factor, the viral (or other pathogen) load as a factor in the propagation of an illness where our assumption is that individuals with a large viral load have a greater chance of transmitting an illness than an individual with a lower viral load (see [12]). Thus, the *SI* model that we present next takes into consideration viral load as a relevant property of an infected individual.

10.2.1 The Fuzzy SI Model

With the heterogeneity in the population described above in mind as we build SI model, we will consider that the higher the viral load, the higher the chance of transmitting the disease. In other words, we will assume that $\beta = \beta(v)$, where v denotes the viral load which will be a non-decreasing function in v. On the other hand, we expect that when the viral load is very low, there is no chance of transmission occurring. That is, we assume that there is a minimum viral load, v_{min}, necessary for there to be the possibility of transmission of the illness. Moreover, after a viral load of v_M, the chance chance of infection is maximum. Lastly, we suppose the there is an upper bound to the viral load which we denote as v_{max}.

We choose, keeping the above in mind, for β the following membership function,

$$\beta(v) = \begin{cases} 0 & \text{if } v \leq v_{min} \\ \dfrac{v - v_{min}}{v_M - v_{min}} & \text{if } v_{min} < v \leq v_M \\ 1 & \text{if } v_M < v \leq v_{max} \\ 0 & \text{if } v > v_{max} \end{cases}. \tag{10.10}$$

The parameter v_{min}, as was mentioned, represents the minimal quantity of virus (pathogens) necessary for there to be a transmission of the illness. This parameter could be interpreted as the threshold value of susceptibility of the group in question. In fact, the larger the value of v_{min}, the larger the quantity of virus necessary for a transmission of the disease to occur and this means that the group in question has

Fig. 10.5 Fuzzy
transmission coefficient β [4]

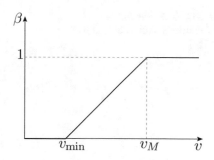

low susceptibility to the illness. In other words, the larger that v_{min} is, the larger the
resistance of the susceptible individuals. Whereas the parameter v_M represents the
viral load above which the chance of transmission is maximum, that is, $\beta(v) = 1$.
Obviously, this does not mean that a transmission of the disease will occur in fact
when $\beta(v) = 1$, just that the chance of transmission is the greatest at this value.

Since $\beta(v) \in [0, 1]$, we can interpret β as a membership function of some fuzzy
set whose domain is the viral load (see Example 7.6) (Fig. 10.5).

Fuzzy Solution

System (10.8), incorporating viral lood, can be seen as a family of ordinary differential equations that has as a solution the functions

$$I(v, t) = \frac{I_0 e^{\beta(v)t}}{S_o + I_0 e^{\beta(v)t}} \tag{10.11}$$

for each fixed v. Now, for each fixed $t > 0$, $I(v, t)$ is a set of real numbers and this
means that for each instant t, a solution (10.11) of the fuzzy problem (10.8) is a
distribution of possible values for the number of infected individuals whose range
lies in the interval $[0, 1]$. Thus,

$$I(v, t) = I_t(v) \in [0, 1]$$

may be interpreted as a membership function of a fuzzy set. If for some reason it is
necessary to adopt a single real-value to represent the number in infected individuals,
we should choose some defuzzification. We could use, for example, the average at
every instant of time t by way of the fuzzy expected value $FEV[I(V, t)]$ using as our
defuzzier of the fuzzy set $I(v, t)$. To make a comparison between the classical and
fuzzy SI models we are calculating the statistic expected value $E[I(V, t)]$ and the
fuzzy expected value $FEV[I(V, t)]$. To do this, let us consider that the viral load V is
a linguistic variable that can be considered *weak* (V_-), *medium* (V_-^+) or *strong* (V_+),
where each of these classifications is a fuzzy set whose membership function is a
triangular fuzzy number dependent on actual viral load associated with the disease
being studied,

Fig. 10.6 Possibility
distribution of viral load ρ
[4]

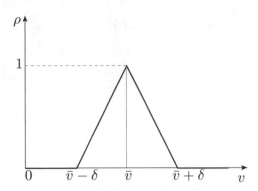

$$\rho(v) = \begin{cases} 1 - \frac{|v - \bar{v}|}{\delta} & \text{if } v \in [\bar{v} - \delta, \bar{v} + \delta] \\ 0 & \text{if } v \notin [\bar{v} - \delta, \bar{v} + \delta] \end{cases}. \tag{10.12}$$

Note that $\rho(v)$ may be viewed as a possibility of occurrence $V = v$ and, in this case ρ becomes a possibility distribution for the variable V. For a fuller interpretation of possibility (say of a fuzzy set like ρ) see Example 7.6 of Chap. 7 (Fig. 10.6).

The parameter $\bar{v}$ is an average value around which each one of the fuzzy sets generated by V distributes itself, whereas δ is half of the distance of the base of the triangles. This triangular fuzzy number may be considered as an ideal dispersion around the average $\bar{v}$. The fuzzy sets generated by the linguistic variable V are classified based on the parameters $v_{\min}$ and v_M that appear in the definition of β.

10.2.2   Expected Value of the Number of Infected Individuals

This section calculates the average number of infected individuals in the distinct cases corresponding to the distributions of the viral load of the group. Since in Chap. 7 we have already defined the fuzzy expected value *FEV*, we now use this definition to define the expected value of the fuzzy set $I(V, t)$ as follows

$$FEV[I(V, t)] = \sup_{0 \le \alpha \le 1} \min[\alpha, \mu\{I(v, t) \ge \alpha\}],$$

where $\mu\{v : I(v, t) \ge \alpha\}$ is the classical measure of the $\alpha - level \ [I(V, t)]^{\alpha}$, which is a classical set. In this way, for each t, the function $H(\alpha)$, whose fixed point is the value of $FEV[I(V, t)]$ according to Theorem 7.1 is given by

$$H(\alpha) = \mu\{v : I(v, t) \ge \alpha\} = \int_{[I(v,t)]^{\alpha}} \rho(v) \mathrm{d}v = 1 - \mu\{v : I(v, t) < \alpha\}.$$

First, observe that $H(0) = 1$ and $H(1) = 0$. For $0 < \alpha < 1$, and setting $k = \frac{S_0}{I_0}$ we have

$$H(\alpha) = 1 - \mu\{v : I(v, t) < \alpha\} = 1 - \mu\{v : \beta(v) < \ln\left(\frac{\alpha k}{1 - \alpha}\right)^{\frac{1}{t}}\} =$$

$$= \begin{cases} 1 & \text{if } \ln(\frac{\alpha k}{1-\alpha})^{\frac{1}{t}} \leq 0 \\ \mu\{v \in [0, B)\} & \text{if } 0 < \ln(\frac{\alpha k}{1-\alpha})^{\frac{1}{t}} < 1 \\ 0 & \text{if } \ln(\frac{\alpha k}{1-\alpha})^{\frac{1}{t}} \geq 1 \end{cases} =$$

$$= \begin{cases} 1 & \text{if } 0 \leq \alpha \leq I_0 \\ \mu\{v \in [0, B)\} & \text{if } I_0 < \alpha < \frac{I_0 e^t}{S_0 + I_0 e^t} \\ 0 & \text{if } \frac{I_0 e^t}{S_0 + I_0 e^t} \leq \alpha \leq 1 \end{cases},$$

where $B = v_{\min} + (v_M - v_{\min}) \ln(\frac{\alpha k}{1-\alpha})^{\frac{1}{t}}$. Note that $v_{\min} < B \leq v_M$.

To calculate the fuzzy expectation, any measure can be used not necessarily a σ-additive one. To this end, in our case, let us adopt a fuzzy measure

$$\mu(A) = \frac{1}{\delta} \int_A \rho(v) dv = \int_A \frac{\rho(v)}{\delta} dv,$$

which is also a probability measure where in that case, $\frac{\rho(v)}{\delta}$ is the probability density function and we note that $\int_A \frac{\rho(v)}{\delta} dv = 1$. With the aim of giving the example of the cases where the viral load is *weak, medium,* or *strong,* let us calculate the fuzzy expectation $FEV[I(V, t)]$ for the three distinct cases according to Fig. 10.7.

- **Weak viral load (V_-).**

This case $B > v_{\min} > \bar{v} + \delta$ and we have $\mu\{v \in [0, B]\} = 1$ and thus,

$$H(\alpha) = \begin{cases} 1 & \text{if } 0 \leq \alpha < I_0 \\ 0 & \text{if } I_0 < \alpha \leq 1 \end{cases}.$$

Fig. 10.7 Classification of viral load [4]

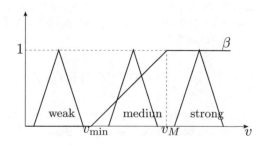

Therefore,

$$FEV[I(V, t)] = I_0.$$

The number if infected at each instant of time t remains the same as at the initial state and so the disease does not propagate. This result is concordant with the fact that in this interval, $\beta(v) = 0$.

- **Strong viral load** (V^+).
  This case $B \leq v_M \leq \bar{v} - \delta$ and we obtain $\mu\{v \in [0, B]\} = 0$. As a result

$$H(\alpha) = \begin{cases} 1 & \text{if } 0 \leq \alpha \leq \frac{I_0 e^t}{S_0 + I_0 e^t} \\ 0 & \text{if } \frac{I_0 e^t}{S_0 + I_0 e^t} < \alpha \leq 1 \end{cases}$$

and therefore,

$$FEV[I(V, t)] = \frac{I_0 e^t}{S_0 + I_0 e^t}.$$

In addition, we obtain the classical solution when $\beta = 1$.

- **Medium viral load** (V_-^+). This case has $v_{\min} < \bar{v} - \delta < \bar{v} + \delta < v_M$ and a direct calculation, though it requires quite a bit of work, gives us the following,

$$H(\alpha) = \begin{cases} 1 & \text{if } 0 \leq \alpha \leq I(\bar{v} - \delta, t) \\ 1 - \frac{1}{2}\left(\frac{B - \bar{v}}{\delta} + 1\right)^2 & \text{if } I(\bar{v} - \delta, t) < \alpha \leq I(\bar{v}, t) \\ \frac{1}{2}\left(\frac{\bar{v} - B}{\delta} + 1\right)^2 & \text{if } I(\bar{v}, t) < \alpha \leq I(\bar{v} + \delta, t) \\ 0 & \text{if } I(\bar{v} + \delta, t) < \alpha \leq 1 \end{cases} \tag{10.13}$$

In accordance with expression (10.13) and the above figure, we can conclude that $H(\alpha)$ is continuous and decreasing with $H(0) = 1$ and $H(1) = 0$. Consequently, H has one and only one fixed point that coincides with $FEV[I(V, t)]$ (Theorem 7.1). Once give the values of the parameters δ, $\bar{v}$, $v_{\min}$ and v_M are used to obtain $FEV[I(V, t)]$ (Fig. 10.8).

It is not hard to see that for each $t > 0$, if $v \in [v - \delta, v + \delta]$ then $I(\bar{v} - \delta, t)$ and $I(\bar{v} + \delta, t)$ are, respectively, the left and right endpoints of a real-valued interval. We also have that if $v_2 \geq v_1$, then $I(v_2, t) \geq I(v_1, t)$. In this way, by the Intermediate-Value Theorem (see [13, 14]), for each $t > 0$ there exists a unique $v = v(t) \in [v - \delta, v + \delta]$ such that

$$FEV[I(V, t)] = I(v(t), t) = \frac{I_0 e^{\beta(v(t))t}}{S_0 + I_0 e^{\beta(v(t))t}}.$$

Therefore, the expectation of the solutions $FEV[I(V, t)]$ does not coincide with any of the solution curves (10.11) of the model. What we have is that for each t, the

Fig. 10.8 Level function $H(\alpha)$ for the medium viral load [4]

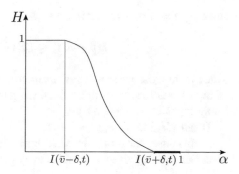

value of $FEV[I(V, t)]$ coincides with $I(v, t)$ for some v. Consequently, changing the instant t, also will change the curve $I(v, t)$, since $FEV[I(V, t)] = I(v(t), t)$ and $v = v(t)$ varies with time. In other words, a curve $FEV[I(V, t)] = I(v(t), t)$ is not a solution of the original autonomous differential equation

$$\frac{dI}{dt} = \beta(1 - I)I.$$

We make several observations based on what we presented above.

• While there are susceptible individuals and $\bar{v} - \delta - v_{min} > 0$, the expectation of the infected $FEV[I(V, t)]$ grow with respect to t, because

$$\lim_{t \to \infty} FEV[I(V, t)] \geq \lim_{t \to \infty} I(\bar{v} - \delta, t) = 1.$$

• The disease can be controlled by $I(\bar{v} + \delta, t)$, that is, making $\bar{v} + \delta - v_{min} \leq 0$, the average number of infected cannot grow since

$$\lim_{t \to \infty} FEV[I(V, t)] \leq \lim_{t \to \infty} I(\bar{v} + \delta, t) = I_0.$$

10.2.3 Statistical Expected Values of the Number in Infected

The way we have considered the parameter $\beta = \beta(v)$, the classical statistical expected value of the number of infected individuals, $E[I(V, t)]$, is given by

$$E[I(V, t)] = \int_{-\infty}^{+\infty} I(v, t) \frac{\rho(v)}{\delta} dv = \frac{1}{\delta} \int_{\bar{v}-\delta}^{\bar{v}+\delta} I(v, t)\rho(v)dv, \tag{10.14}$$

since $\rho(v) = 0$ outside the interval $[\bar{v} - \delta, \bar{v} + \delta]$. So, we have

$$I(\bar{v} - \delta, t) \leq E[I(v, t)] \leq I(\bar{v} + \delta, t).$$

Since there exist various ways for us to calculate the expected value as a function of the parameters, we choose the three particular cases already analyzed using the fuzzy expected value (*FEV*).

Weak viral load: $v_{\min} > \bar{v} + \delta$.

In this case, for all the infected individuals, the transmission coefficient $\beta(v)$ is zero. Substituting $\beta(v) = 0$ and $I(V, t)$ given by (10.11) in (10.14), we obtain:

$$E[I(V, t)] = \frac{1}{\delta} \int\limits_{\bar{v}-\delta}^{\bar{v}+\delta} I(v, t)\rho(v)dv = I_0.$$

Therefore, since all the infected individuals exhibit a viral load less than $v_{\min}$, that is, no individual possesses a minimal viral load necessary for transmission, there occurs no propagation of the disease. We may interpret this situation as one in which the group of individuals is highly resistant ($v_{\min}$ is high), that in turn makes the susceptibility to the disease low. In this case the number of infected remains unaltered from I_0.

Strong viral load: $v_M < \bar{v} - \delta$.

In this case, the coefficient of transmission is maximum for all the infected individuals, that is, $\beta(v) = 1$. After some calculations we obtain

$$E[I(V, t)] = \frac{1}{\delta} \int\limits_{\bar{v}-\delta}^{\bar{v}+\delta} I(v, t)\rho(v)dv = \frac{I_0 e^t}{S_0 + I_0 e^t}. \tag{10.15}$$

Observe that (10.15) coincides with the classical model when we consider the transmission coefficient as constant, that is, $\beta = 1$.

Medium viral load: $\bar{v} - \delta > v_{\min}$ and $\bar{v} + \delta < v_M$.

In this case, similar to we saw for the fuzzy expectation, here also the coefficient of transmission is variable for all infected individuals. All the distribution, the support of the distribution of V is in the region where $\beta(v) = \frac{v - v_{\min}}{v_M - v_{\min}}$. So, to obtain $E[I(V, t)]$ it is necessary to know the values of all the parameters: $\delta, \bar{v}, v_{\min}, v_M$ and $v_{\max}$.

Analogous observations that were made about the propagation of the disease made for the fuzzy expected value also apply here remembering that

$$I(\bar{v} - \delta, t) \leq E[I(v, t)] \leq I(\bar{v} + \delta, t),$$

$$\lim_{t \to \infty} E[I(V, t)] \geq \lim_{t \to \infty} I(\bar{v} - \delta, t) = 1$$

and

$$\lim_{t \to \infty} E[I(V, t)] \leq \lim_{t \to \infty} I(\bar{v} + \delta, t) = I_0.$$

For the statistic expectation, we also have

$$E[I(V, t)] = I(v(t), t)),$$

for some function $v = v(t)$.

To conclude this section we would like to emphasize that unlike the statistic expectation, we could have utilized other fuzzy measures to obtain the fuzzy expectation. This possibility to choose different measures, according to the phenomenon being studied, is what makes the fuzzy expectation a powerful tool in applications. For example, instead of using the measure

$$\mu(A) = \frac{1}{\delta} \int \rho(v) dv,$$

we could have used the **possibilistic measure** (see Chap. 7)

$$\mu(A) = \sup_{v \in A} \rho(v).$$

In our view, this is a very reasonable measure to use for our example if we want to be very conservative in the following sense. It may be that for a particular disease, a group A of infected individuals is evaluated by the one person with the greatest viral load. The expectation of the number of infected individuals, $FEV[I(V, t)]$, could be evaluated with this more conservative measure and from this, mechanisms applied to control the disease could be made according to this figure. To be specific, for the possibility measure, we arrive at a very similar conclusion for the three cases previously analyzed where in the possibilistic measure case the function H becomes

$$H(\alpha) = \begin{cases} 1 & \text{if } 0 \leq \alpha \leq I_0 \\ \sup_{v \in [a, v_{\max}]} \rho(v) & \text{if } I_0 < \alpha \leq \frac{I_0 e^t}{S_0 + I_0 e^t} \\ 0 & \text{if } \frac{I_0 e^t}{S_0 + I_0 e^t} < \alpha \leq 1 \end{cases} \tag{10.16}$$

and $FEV[I(V, t)]$ is the fixed point of the function H.

Let us do a comparative study between the approaches taken above and the deterministic method with the aim of exploring a little more this example.

10.2.4 $I(FEV[V], t)$ Versus $FEV[I(V, t)]$

This section will compare the trajectories of the three cases we have been studying previously above of the curve $FEV[I(V, t)]$, that is, $I(FEV[V], t) = I(\bar{v}, t)$. From the expression of H (10.16), we can conclude that $H(I(\bar{v}, t)) = \frac{1}{2}$ for all t. Thus $FEV[I(V, t)] = I(\bar{v}, t)$ only when $I(\bar{v}, t) = \frac{1}{2}$.

On the other hand, once $FEV[I(V, t)]$ is a fixed point of H we have

$$FEV[I(V, t)] > I(\bar{v}, t) \text{ if } I(\bar{v}, t) < \frac{1}{2}$$
$$FEV[I(V, t)] < I(\bar{v}, t) \text{ if } I(\bar{v}, t) > \frac{1}{2}.$$

In this way, a trajectory due to a medium viral load ($\bar{v}$), does not produce the medium number of infected individuals, as given by $FEV[I(V, t)]$, at every instant. Therefore, from our point of view, it is not correct to adopt an average or modal viral load, $\bar{v}$, to study the evolution of the disease in a population as a whole since $FEV[I(V, t)] = I(\bar{v}, t)$ only at the instant $\bar{t} = \frac{v_M - v_{min}}{\bar{v} - v_{min}} \ln(\frac{S_0}{I_0})$, $S_0 \geq I_0$. We observe that $\bar{t}$ is the inflection point of $I(\bar{v}, t)$ and that $I(\bar{v}, \bar{t}) = \frac{1}{2}$, that is, at the instant $\bar{t}$, the increment of the rate of increase of $I(\bar{v}, t)$ is larger than $I(\bar{v}, \bar{t}) = \frac{1}{2}$ (see Fig. 10.9). Starting with Jensen's inequality [15], we obtain similar results as those commented upon above for the classical expectation, $E(I(V, t))$, by only changing the time $\bar{t}$ at which the curve $I(\bar{v}, t)$ lies above $E(I(V, t))$.

These facts reveal that, for heterogeneous systems, two distinct instants of time can appear in which the uncertainties of the model can induce different values for the system as a whole. If we adopt a **deterministic model** to study the system above, it leads us to adopt $I(\bar{v}, t)$ as a solution since in this case, all the uncertainty should be extracted right at the beginning of the mathematical model which in our case is, $V = \bar{v}$. On the other hand, the **fuzzy model** allows the uncertainties, in this case inherent in the phenomenon, to be extracted in a desired (future) moment resulting in the solution $FEV[I(V, t)]$ or $E[I(V, t)]$ which is more representative of the system as a whole.

Fig. 10.9 Deterministic solution $I(\bar{v}, t)$ with $\bar{v}$ and the fuzzy expected value $FEV[I(V, t)]$ [4]

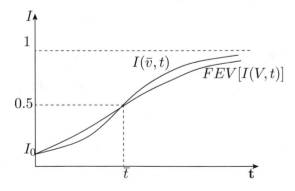

Mathematical models of epidemics are studied, in large part, with the aim of the implementation of policies or strategies to control the disease. We further illustrate this by studying a fuzzy *SI* model.

10.2.5 Control of Epidemics and the Basic Reproductive Number

The discussion in this section is based on the properties of the fuzzy *SI* model, keeping in mind the curve given by the fuzzy expectation $FEV[I(V, t)]$. In our previous development, we obtained conclusions based on the curve $E[I(V, t)]$ [4, 16]. In our previous discussions we saw the following facts.

- If $S_0 > I_0$, while $t < \bar{t} = \frac{v_M - v_{\min}}{\bar{v} - v_{\min}} \ln(\frac{S_0}{I_0})$, then $FEV[I(V, t)] > I(\bar{v}, t)$. Beginning with $t = \bar{t}$ we have that $FEV[I(V, t)] < I(\bar{v}, t)$. In this way we can say that the deterministic model underestimates the number of infected individuals at the beginning of the illness and overestimates the number of infected individuals beginning with $\bar{t}$ (see Fig. 10.9).
- If $S_0 \leq I_0$ then $FEV[I(V, t)] \leq I(\bar{v}, t)$ for all $t > 0$ and in this case, the deterministic model overestimates the number of infected individuals.

Therefore, at the beginning of the illness when $t < \bar{t} = \frac{v_M - v_{\min}}{\bar{v} - v_{\min}} \ln(\frac{S_0}{I_0})$ and $S_0 >> I_0$, we have

$$I(\bar{v}, t) \leq FEV[I(V, t)] \leq I(\bar{v} + \delta, t)$$

and thus, $v(t) \in [\bar{v}, \bar{v} + \delta]$.

Once $FEV[I(V, t)] = I(v(t), t)$ increases with the increase in $v(t)$, we can say that the larger the medium viral load the larger the average number of infected individuals $FEV[I(V, t)]$. Also, the larger the dispersal δ, the larger will be $FEV[I(V, t)]$ and the larger $v_{\min}$ is, the smaller $FEV[I(V, t)]$ will be.

An essential parameter, for epidemiological classical models, is the *basic reproductive number* R_0, which gives the number of secondary cases caused by an infected individual introduced in a population that is totally susceptible [10, 17]. In this way, this parameter indicates under what conditions the disease is propagated in a population. If an infected individual causes more than one new case, that is, if $R_0 > 1$ then the disease will propagate. On the other hand, when $R_0 < 1$ the disease will be extinguished.

The expression for the parameter R_0, for the more simple epidemiological models can be obtained beginning with the condition $dI/dt > 0$, that is, the condition that there occurs an increase in the number of infected. In this case, for the classical normalized *SI* model where $I + S = 1$, we will have

$$\frac{dI}{dt} > 0 \iff \beta SI = \beta(1 - I)I > 0,$$

which holds as long as there exist susceptible individuals in the populations since $\beta >$ 0. In other words we will always have $R_0 > 1$ when $\beta > 0$ and $I < 1$. However, when we use a fuzzy set to describe the parameter β this cannot occur. In our case, according to the analysis we made above, it is easy to verify that a sufficient condition for there to be no transmission of the disease is that no infected individual possesses the minimum or higher viral load. That is, the condition $\bar{v} + \delta < v_{\min}$ should be satisfied. We can therefore define the *fuzzy basic reproductive number* as being the value

$$R_0^{\text{fuzzy}} = \frac{\bar{v} + \delta}{v_{\min}}. \tag{10.17}$$

Classical epidemiological models use, as a prevention control mechanism, the policy of reducing the value of the parameter R_0 in such a way that $R_0 < 1$ so that the disease will not propagate. But for the classical SI model this is not possible since the number of susceptible individuals is always positive as we have seen above.

However, if we consider the number of susceptible individuals was a fuzzy set, that is, $\beta = \beta(v)$ in (10.8), even in this simple model, we will garner additional information about the dynamics of the disease. For example, it is possible to interfere in the illness' transmission by reducing the value of the fuzzy parameter R_0^{fuzzy}. This can be done in two ways: (1) Increasing the value of $v_{\min}$, which means that we increase the resistance of the susceptible individuals (decrease the susceptibility); Increasing the value of $v_{\min}$ could be done through, for example, vaccination, basic sanitation, etc. In this sense, by the fact that the parameter $v_{\min}$ is related to the susceptible individuals, the way to reduce the value of R_0 is referred to as methods of control; (2) the second way to reduce R_0 would be to diminish the value of $\bar{v} + \delta$, by reducing the value of $\bar{v}$ and/or δ. The reduction of the value of δ could be done by means of control of the infected population as in, for example, quarantine or **isolation**. The reduction in $\bar{v}$ is related to measures of **treatment** of the infected individuals.

We finish our discussion of this application by emphasizing that unlike the classical SI model that is quite simple as we presented it, and inadequate for most diseases, even the simple fuzzy SI model is more inclusive whose results are more closely associated with more complex models in which the class of infected are divided into subclasses in accordance with the intensity of the infected (see [18]). A more detailed study of the fuzzy SI models can be found in [4] and fuzzy SIS models in [11, 16, 19].

10.3   A Fuzzy Model of the Transference from Asymptomatic to Symptomatic in HIV$^+$ Patients

The model that we present next can be found in [20, 21]. When we analyze the evolution of a population of individuals from asymptomatic HIV^+ to a class of symptomatic ones, many factors are involved in the process since the rate at which the transference occurs is subject to the factors responsible for the change in the stages of HIV^+. Some of these factors are more crucial and influential than others. For example, the viral load of an individual and the level of $CD4^+$ are fundamental to the determining the next state in a HIV^+ the patient. What we exhibit with this example is to show how we can study a phenomenon, that is typically modeled deterministically, as a fuzzy model that explicitly and effectively uses inexact variables and parameters as they occur in the data and model statement. We demonstrate the transformation of the subjective, uncertain, and inexact variables and parameters into a fuzzy model via environmental fuzziness. To this end, the demographic fuzziness (fuzzy variables) are transformed into environmental (parameters) fuzziness. This being the case, we will consider the rate of transference, from asymptomatic to symptomatic, subjectively dependent on the viral load and the level $CD4^+$. In this way, we can express the rate of transference by a fuzzy set, that is, we express the transference rate via a linguistic variable as developed and studied in Chap. 5. However, to begin, we review the classical deterministic case.

10.3.1   The Classical Model

In 1986 Anderson et al. [22] proposed the following model for the transference of asymptomatic individuals to symptomatic HIV^+ ones,

$$
\begin{cases}
\dfrac{dx}{dt} = -\lambda(t)x \text{ with } x(0) = 1 \\[2mm]
\dfrac{dy}{dt} = \lambda(t)x \text{ with } y(0) = 0
\end{cases}
, \qquad (10.18)
$$

where the function $\lambda(.)$ represents the rate of transference of infected asymptomatic individuals with HIV^+ into symptomatic ones. The state variable x is the proportion of the infected individuals who still do not have symptoms indicative of $AIDS$ and y is the proportion of the individuals that possess clear symptoms of $AIDS$. As a first approximation, Anderson proposes that this rate be given as a linear function

$$
\lambda(t) = at, \text{ with } a > 0,
$$

which means that the solution of the deterministic system (10.18) is

$$
x(t) = e^{-\frac{at^2}{2}} \text{ and } y(t) = 1 - e^{-\frac{at^2}{2}}.
$$

10.3.2 The Fuzzy Model

Let us now consider the rate of transference to be dependent on *viral load* v and the *level of CD4$^+$* c, that is,

$$\lambda = \lambda(v, c).$$

Using the analogous deterministic model given by Anderson, we can write the model as:

$$\begin{cases} \dfrac{dx}{dt} = -\lambda(v, c)x \\ x(0) = 1 \end{cases} \tag{10.19}$$

or as its complementary/dual equation in terms of the variable y,

$$\frac{dy}{dt} = \lambda(v, c)x = k\lambda(v, c)(1 - y) \text{ with } y(0) = 0.$$

The difference in the fuzzy model and the deterministic one is that now the rate of transference λ has a clear biological and linguistical meaning whereas with the deterministic case, this rate was a adjustable parameter. The fuzzy model solution is

$$x(t) = e^{-\lambda(v,c)t} \text{ or } y(t) = 1 - e^{-\lambda(v,c)t}.$$

Each solution can be understood as an element of a family of curves which has initial value equal to 1,

$$x(t) = e^{-\lambda(v,c)t}, \text{ with } t > 0,$$

where λ assumes values dependent on the viral load and the level of $CD4^+$ present in the blood. The values v and c of variables, are characteristic properties of the infected population. The analytic definition of the parameter λ is obtained through a combination of the linguistic meaning of the variables V and $CD4^+$ and a rule base as developed in Chap. 5.

Medical knowledge and research seems to indicate that the parameter most used to control the transference from asymptomatic HIV^+ to symptomatic ones is the value of $CD4^+$. In this way we can simply use $\lambda = \lambda(c)$ as the transference rate in the fuzzy model (10.19). If for every viral load v we have $\lambda = \lambda(c)$, then its graph is approximately the decreasing curve depicted by Fig. 10.10. The equation that defines $\lambda = \lambda(c)$ given next and depicted in Fig. 10.10, was chosen taking in consideration arguments similar to those of the models previously presented (see Chap. 5, Subsect. 5.6.2 for more technical justification) is,

$$\lambda(c) = \begin{cases} 1 & \text{if } c < c_{\min} \\ \dfrac{c_M - c}{c_M - c_{\min}} & \text{if } c_{\min} \leq c \leq c_M, \\ 0 & \text{if } c > c_M \end{cases} \tag{10.20}$$

Fig. 10.10 Transference rate
$\lambda = \lambda(c)$ [21]

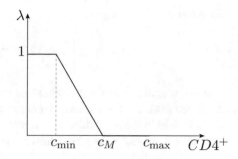

where $c_{\min}$ represents the minimal level of $CD4^+$ required for an individual to become symptomatic and c_M represents the level of $CD4^+$ after which the chance of an infected individual becoming symptomatic is minimal or none.

10.3.3 The Fuzzy Expectation of the Asymptomatic Individuals

The fuzzy expected value provides a type of average value for the values of $x(t, c)$ at each instant of time, since it is a type of defuzzification of the fuzzy set of asymptomatic individuals

$$x(t, c) = e^{-\lambda(c)t}.$$

As we have seen in Chap. 7, to define fuzzy expectation we initially need to choose a fuzzy measure μ. Once this is done, the value of the fuzzy expectation of the asymptomatic individuals $x(t, c)$ is given by

$$FEV[x] = \sup_{0 \le \alpha \le 1} \inf[\alpha, \mu\{x \ge \alpha\}],$$

where $\{x \ge \alpha\} = \{c : x(c) \ge \alpha\}$ and μ is a fuzzy measure. Here, we have, recalling Theorem 7.1, $H(\alpha) = \mu\{c : x(c) \ge \alpha\}$ for each $t > 0$. For this case, a direct calculation results in the following expression of the function H:

$$H(\alpha) = \begin{cases} \mu[c_M, c_{\max}] & \text{if } \alpha = 1 \\ \mu[B, c_{\max}] & \text{if } e^{-t} \le \alpha < 1, \\ 1 & \text{if } \alpha \le e^{-t} \end{cases} \tag{10.21}$$

where $B = c_M - (c_M - c_{\min})(\frac{\ln \alpha}{t}) \implies c_{\min} < B \le c_M$.

The fuzzy measure that we choose is a distribution of levels of $CD4^+$ with different associated possibilities of occurrence. We will assume that the levels of $CD4^+$ has a triangular distribution given by,

$$\rho(c) = \begin{cases} 1 - \frac{|c - \bar{c}|}{\delta} & \text{if } c \in [\bar{c} - \delta, \bar{c} + \delta] \\ 0 & \text{if } c \notin [\bar{c} - \delta, \bar{c} + \delta] \end{cases}. \tag{10.22}$$

Here, we take $\bar{c}$ to be the modal or median value in $[0, c_{\max}]$, with $c_{\max}$ as a maximum limit of viral load in an individual and δ being the dispersion of the levels of $CD4^+$ within the population of interest (those infected with HIV). Thus, with this in mind, we suggest to use the following fuzzy measure μ

$$\mu(A) = \begin{cases} \sup_{c \in A} \rho(c) & \text{if } A \neq \emptyset \\ 0 & \text{if } A = \emptyset \end{cases},$$

where A is a subset of real numbers, containing the domain of possible values of $CD4^+$ (Fig. 10.11).

The subsets A of real numbers of interest are the intervals $A = [B, c_{\max}]$, where $B = c_M - (c_M - c_{\min})(\frac{-\ln \alpha}{t}) \Longrightarrow c_{\min} < B \leq c_M$. Observe that μ is an optimistic measure in the sense that the level of $CD4^+$ of a group is evaluated as being the best level of the individuals of this group.

Consider the level of $CD4^+$ as a linguistic variable with values *low*, *medium* and *high*, each one of these being characterized by a triangular fuzzy set according to the membership function ρ (see Fig. 10.12).

Fig. 10.11 Possibility distribution of $CD4^+$ [21]

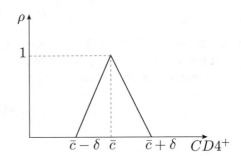

Fig. 10.12 Values of the linguistic variable "level of $CD4^+$" [21]

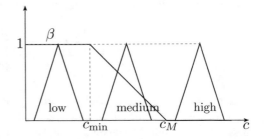

Case 1: The level of $CD4^+$ *low* (C_-).

In this case, we take $c_{\min} > \bar{c} + \delta$. Since $B > c_{\min}$ we have that $\mu[c_M, c_{\max}] = 0$ and $\mu[B, c_{\max}] = 0$. Thus,

$$H(\alpha) = \begin{cases} 1 & \text{if } \alpha \le e^{-t} \\ 0 & \text{if } e^{-t} < \alpha \le 1 \end{cases}$$

so that we obtain $FEV[x] = e^{-t}$ which means that the average number of transferences from asymptomatic to symptomatic has an exponential decay since the expected value of individuals with no HIV symptoms, x, goes to zero exponentially and the transference to symptomatic is an exponential decay.

Case 2: The level of $CD4^+$ *high* $(C+)$.

In this case, we take $c_M \le \bar{c} - \delta$ and $\bar{c} + \delta \le c_{\max}$. Thus, we have $B \le c_M$ and therefore $\mu[c_M, c_{\min}] = 1$ and $\mu[B, c_{\max}] = 1$ which yields

$$H(\alpha) = \begin{cases} 1 & \text{if } \alpha = 0 \\ 0 & \text{if } \alpha > 0 \end{cases}.$$

This means that $FEV[x] = 1$, so that if in the group, the level of $CD4^+$ is high, then there is no transference of asymptomatic individuals to symptomatic ones.

Case 3: The level of CD4$^+$ *medium* (C_-^+).

In this case, we take $\bar{c} - \delta > c_{\min}$ and $\bar{c} + \delta < c_M$ which implies that $\mu[c_M, c_{\max}] = 1$. After a few calculations we have that

$$H(\alpha) = \begin{cases} 1 & \text{if } 0 \le \alpha \le e^{-\lambda(\bar{c})t} \\ \rho(B) & \text{if } e^{-\lambda(\bar{c})t} < \alpha < e^{-\lambda(\bar{c}+\delta)t} \\ 0 & \text{if } e^{-\lambda(\bar{c}+\delta)t} \le \alpha \le 1 \end{cases},$$

where $\rho(B) = \frac{1}{\delta}[-c_M - (c_M - c_{\min})(\frac{\ln\alpha}{t}) + \bar{c} + \delta]$. Since $H(\alpha)$ is a continuous decreasing function with $H(0) = 1$ and $H(1) = 0$, H has a unique fixed point that coincides with $FEV[x]$ (see Chap. 7). Figure 10.13 illustrates this fact.
Thus,

$$e^{-\lambda(\bar{c})t} < FEV[x] < e^{-\lambda(\bar{c}+\delta)t}.$$

We observe that for the three cases of low/medium/high, we always have the inequality

$$e^{-EF[\lambda]t} \le e^{-\lambda(\bar{c})t} \le FEV[x].$$

Fig. 10.13 Representation
of $FEV[x]$ [21]

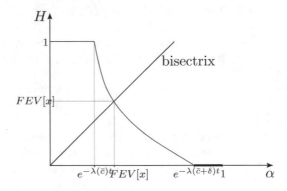

This means that the expected value of the asymptomatic population, at each instant, is larger than the deterministic model which considers the rate of transference (from asymptomatic to symptomatic) as a constant $\lambda(\bar{c}) = \bar{\lambda}$.

10.4   Population Dynamics and Migration of Blow Flies

We close this chapter with the presentation of a two-dimensional model that represents a competition and migration of flies. This model was developed by Castanho et al. [23]. The model comes from a discrete two-dimensional system where the parameters were determined by means of a rule base. This is a environmental fuzziness case because in the model, the uncertainties are all in the parameters. The uncertainties in the parameters are treated by means of fuzzy set theory and the values obtained are via fuzzy controllers.

A deterministic model used by Godoy [24] to analyze the establishment of colonies of blow flies has its foundation based on the incorporation of deterministic models of Prout and McCheney [25] and the stochastic model of Roughgarden [26]. The Godoy model is,

$$
\begin{cases}
N_{1,t+1} = \dfrac{(1 - m_{12})}{2} F_1 S_1 e^{-(f+s)N_{1,t}} N_{1,t} + \dfrac{m_{21}}{2} F_2 S_2 e^{-(f+s)N_{2,t}} N_{2,t} \\[3mm]
N_{2,t+1} = \dfrac{m_{12}}{2} F_1 S_1 e^{-(f+s)N_{1,t}} N_{1,t} + \dfrac{(1 - m_{21})}{2} F_2 S_2 e^{-(f+s)N_{2,t}} N_{2,t}
\end{cases}
. \tag{10.23}
$$

This model relates the dynamics of a population of blow flies with a process of migration between two colonies of blow flies. The variables and parameters are:

1. $N_{i,t}$: the population of blow flies of colony i at time t;
2. F_i: maximal fecundity of the blow flies when these are encountered in colony i;
3. S_i: maximal survival of the blow flies in colony i;

4. m_{ij}: rate of migration from colony i to colony j;

5. f and s represent the variation in fecundity and the survival respectively.

The parameters m_{ij}, F_i and S_i are dependent on a series of factors usually hard to evaluate quantitatively. In this case, it seems that the approach of fuzzy set theory can be useful. So, to obtain the solution of our model, we get the parameters via fuzzy method and substituting them on the deterministic equation (10.23).

Let's consider that the parameters m_{ij}, F_i and S_i are uncertainty and modeled by linguitic variable. Also, consider that these parameters are dependent on two input variables, the *Population* ($N_{i,t}$) and its *Environment* (E_i) which is the habitat of each colony. So, we have based rule fuzzy system (if - then) with two input and three output, according to Frame 10.1. For the input variable *Population*, using the experimental data found in Godoy [24], the linguistic terms adolted were, *Small, Medium* and *Large* according to Fig. 10.14. For the input variable *Environment* the linguistic terms considered were *Hostile, Slightly Unfavourable and Favorable* whose membership functions are given in Fig. 10.15. To model the fuzzy parameter *rate of Migration, m*, as an output variable, dependent on *Population* and on *Environment*, we adopt a rule base given by Frame 10.1. The linguistic terms *Small, Medium* and *Large* representing the rate of migration are given by Fig. 10.16. The memberships values of the output linguistic variables *Fecundity F* (Fig. 10.17) and fuzzy *Survival S* (Fig. 10.18) are intuitively derived considering an interpolation between the experimental values for maxima and minima of these variables.

The result of the equation of Godoy (10.23) with the parameters obtained from fuzzy controller with inference of Mamdani (see Chap. 5) are showed in the Figs. 10.19 and 10.20.

A study of metapopulations of blow flies using a fuzzy dynamic population model was developed in [23, 27].

Fig. 10.14 Fuzzy values of the populations [23]

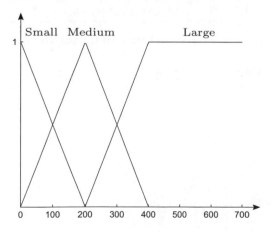

Fig. 10.15 Fuzzy values of the environment [23]

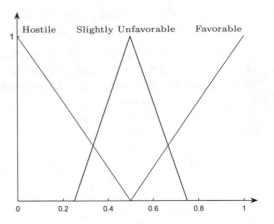

1. **If** Population is Small **and** the Environment is Favorable **then** the Fecundity and Survival are High and Migration is Low;
2. **If** Population is Small **and** the Environment is Slightly Unfavorable **then** the Fecundity is High, the Survival is Medium and Migration is Low;
3. **If** Population is Small **and** the Environment is Hostile **then** the Fecundity is Medium, the Survival is Low and Migration is High;
4. **If** Population is Medium **and** the Environment is Favorable **then** the Fecundity is High, the Survival is Medium and Migration is Low;
5. **If** Population is Medium **and** the Environment is Slightly Unfavorable **then** the Fecundity is Medium, Survival is Low and Migration is High;
6. **If** Population is Medium **and** the Environment is Hostile **then** the Fecundity and Survival are Low and Migration is High;
7. **If** Population is Large **and** the Environment is Favorable **then** the Fecundity is Medium, the Survival is Low and Migration is Moderate;
8. **If** Population is Large **and** the Environment is Slightly Unfavorable **then** the Fecundity and Survival are Low and Migration is High;
9. **If** Population is Large **and** the Environment is Hostile **then** the Fecundity and Survival are Low and Migration is High;

Frame 10.1: Rule base for Blow flies [23].

Fig. 10.16 Fuzzy values of migration [23]

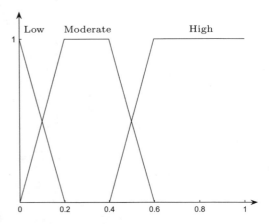

Fig. 10.17 Fuzzy values of fecundity [23]

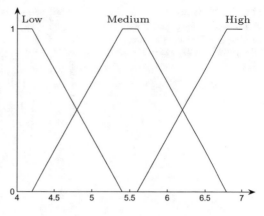

Fig. 10.18 Fuzzy values of survaival [23]

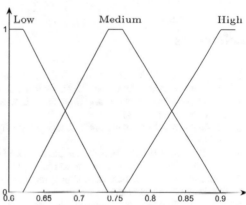

Fig. 10.19 Stability solution of the colonies for $N_{1,0} = 300$, $N_{2,0} = 700$, $E_{1,0} = 0.01$, and $E_{2,0} = 0.3$ [23]

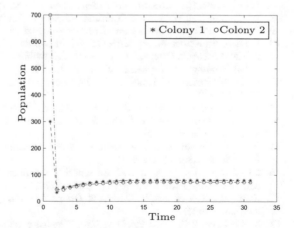

Fig. 10.20 Periodic
variations of the populations
for $N_{1,0} = 300$, $N_{2,0} = 400$,
$E_{1,0} = 1$, and $E_{2,0} = 0.9$
[23]

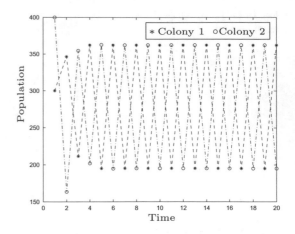

References

1. K.B. Athreya, S. Karlin, On branching processes with random environments: I: extinction probabilities. Ann. Math. Stat. **42**(5), 1499–1520 (1971)
2. R. McCredie May, *Stability and Complexity in Model Ecosystems*, vol. 6 (Princeton University Press, Princeton, 1973)
3. M. Turelli, Stochastic community theory: a partially guided tour. Biomathematics **17**, 321–339 (1986)
4. L.C. Barros, M.B.F. Leite, R.C. Bassanezi, The SI epidemiological models with a fuzzy transmission parameter. Int. J. Comput. Math. Appl. **45**, 1619–1628 (2003)
5. R.C. Bassanezi, L.C. Barros, A simple model of life expectancy with subjective parameters. Kybernets **7**, 91–98 (1995)
6. L. Arnold, *Random Dynamical Systems*, 2nd edn. (Springer, Berlin, 2003)
7. W.O. Bussab, P.A. Morettin, *Estatística básica*, 5th edn. (Editora Saraiva, São Paulo, 2002)
8. R.G. Bartle, *The Elements of Real Analysis* (Wiley, New York, 1964)
9. W. Rudin, *Principles of Mathematical Analysis* (McGraw-Hill Book Co., Tokyo, 1953)
10. L. Edelstein-Keshet, *Mathematical Models in Biology* (McGraw-Hill, México, 1988)
11. E. Massad, N.R.S. Ortega, L.C. Barros, C.J. Struchiner, *Fuzzy Logic in Action: Applications in Epidemiology and Beyond* (Springer, Berlin, 2008)
12. K. Sadegh-Zadeh, Fundamentals of clinical methodology: 3. nosology. Artif. Intell. Med. **17**, 87–108 (1999)
13. T.M. Apostol, *Calculus*, vol. 2, 2nd edn. (Editorial Reverté, Mexico, 1975)
14. H.L. Guidorizzi, *Um curso de cálculo*, vol. 1, 5th edn. (Livros Técnicos e Científicos Editora S. A, Rio de Janeiro, 2001)
15. B. James, *Probabilidade: um curso de nível intermediário*, Instituto de Matemática Pura e Aplicada, Rio de Janeiro (1981)
16. L.C. Barros, R.Z. Oliveira, R.C. Bassanezi, The influence of heterogeneity in the control of deseases. Front. Artif. intell. Appl. **85**, 88–95 (2002)
17. E. Massad, R. Menezes, P. Silveira, N. Ortega, *Métodos quantitativos em medicina* (Manole, São Paulo, 2004)
18. M.B.F. Leite, R.C. Bassanezi, H.M. Yang, The basic reproduction ratio for a model of directly transmitted infections considering the virus charge and the immunological response, IMA. J. Math. Appl. Med. Biol. **17**, 15–31 (2000)
19. L.C. Barros, R.Z. Oliveira, R.C. Bassanezi, M.B.F. Leite, A desease evolution model with uncertain parameters, in *Proceedings of Joint 9th IFSA World Congress and 20th NAFIPS International Conference (Vancouver, Canada), IFSA, NAFIPS* pp. 1626–1630 (2001)

20. R.M. Jafelice, *Um estudo da dinâmica de transferência de soropositivos para aidéticos via modelagem fuzzy*, Tese de Doutorado, FEEC-UNICAMP, Campinas (2003)
21. R.M. Jafelice, L.C. Barros, R.C. Bassanezi, F. Gomide, Fuzzy modeling in symptomatic HIV virus infected population. Bull. Math. Biol. **66**, 1597–1620 (2004)
22. R.M. Anderson, G.F. Medley, R.M. May, A.M. Johnson, A preliminaire study of the transmission dynamics of the human immunodeficiency virus (HIV), the causitive agent of AIDS. IMA J. Math. Med. Biol. **3**, 229–263 (1986)
23. M.J.P. Castanho, K.F. Magnago, R.C. Bassanezi, W. Godoy, Fuzzy subset approach in coupled population dynamics of blowflies. Biol. Res. **39**(2), 341–352 (2006)
24. W.A.C. Godoy, *Dinâmica determinística e estocástica em populações de dípteros califorídeos: acoplamento por migração, extinção local e global*, Tese de livre docência, UNESP, Botucatu (2002)
25. T. Prout, F. McChesney, Competition among immatures affects their adult fertility: population dynamics. Am. Nat. **126**, 521–558 (1985)
26. J. Roughgarden, *Primer on Ecological Theory* (Prentice-Hall, Upper Saddle River, 1998)
27. K.F. Magnago, *Abordagem fuzzy em modelos populacionais discretos*, Tese de Doutorado, IMECC-UNICAMP, Campinas (2005)

Chapter 11
End Notes

"If you obey all the rules you miss all the fun".

(Katharine Hepburn)

Abstract This chapter presents the concept of joint possibility distribution from the point of view of fuzzy number membership. The concept of completely correlated fuzzy numbers is presented. Next, an interactive fuzzy number subtraction operator is discussed. Finally, two bio-mathematical models are studied using these concepts. The first models the risk of getting dengue fever and second is an epidemiological SI-model with completely correlated initial conditions.

This last chapter is a collection of various fun topics. So, if Katherine Hepburn is correct, we are not following all rules. However, we are following fuzzy rule. Let us start by presenting some more advanced topics associated with fuzzy number arithmetic. Then we will present biomathematical models that use some of these concepts, specifically, the concepts of t-norm, Takagi-Sugeno inference method, and interactivity between fuzzy numbers.

The models that we will present here do not properly fit in either demographic or environmental uncertainty as developed in Chaps. 9 and 10. So we opted to present them into new chapter. In the first model we use the concepts of t-norm to represent the interactivity between the involved individuals, but the equations are deterministic. In the second model we employ the Takagi-Sugeno inference method in order to obtain a partial differential equation that represent the evolution of an epidemic system in time and space. Finally, in the third model we use a fuzzy differential equation whose the variables are given by completely correlated fuzzy numbers.

Our first section starts with subtraction of fuzzy numbers of special type, interactive fuzzy numbers. The reason we start with subtraction is that subtraction is where additive inverses and change (derivatives) begin. The reason we start with interactivity is that it is not always the case that the entities modeled by fuzzy numbers are non-interactive.

© Springer-Verlag Berlin Heidelberg 2017

L.C. de Barros et al., *A First Course in Fuzzy Logic, Fuzzy Dynamical Systems, and Biomathematics*, Studies in Fuzziness and Soft Computing 347, DOI 10.1007/978-3-662-53324-6_11

11.1   Subtration of Interactive Fuzzy Numbers

Intuitively, for the arithmetic presented in Chap. 2 there exists some type of independence (or non-interactive) between the α-levels of the two fuzzy numbers involved,
since all elements of both intervals contribute to the result of operation in question.
Such a fact is corroborated by the minimum t-norm in the united extension and
Zadeh's extension for fuzzy numbers. However, it is possible to define an arithmetic
for fuzzy numbers that resembles the arithmetic for random variables by means of
joint distributions.

The standard difference between two fuzzy numbers based on the difference
between intervals (see Proposition 2.5) and takes into account all the possible com-
binations between two elements, one at each α-level. Consequently, the result is
always greater (in diameter) than any of the sets involved in the operation. In fact,
the width of the result of subtracting of two intervals is the sum of the widths of these
two intervals. Thus, the difference between two non-crisp fuzzy numbers is always
a non-crisp number and subtracting a non-crisp number from itself is never zero.

Using the Hukuhara Difference (2.9), the result of subtracting a non-crisp number
A from itself ($A \ominus_H A$) is, in fact, non-zero. However, for this case, a necessary condition for the subtraction between two different fuzzy numbers A and B to exist is
that the first term must have a bigger diameter than the second one. A proposed rem-
edy to some of the issues involving interval subtraction is the Generalized Hukuhara
difference, which also satisfies $A -_{gH} A = 0$ [1, 2] and is defined for a bigger class
of fuzzy numbers than the Hukuhara difference. An extension of the generalized
Hukuhara difference is the generalized difference [1, 3], which has the same results
of the generalized Hukuhara operator (when it exists), but is defined for a larger class
of fuzzy numbers. Another possibility is CIA (Constraint Interval Arithmetic) [4].
In this case, the diameter of the difference between two fuzzy numbers using CIA is
often smaller than using standard difference.

All differences mentioned above make use of the interval arithmetic on α-levels.
Extensions to fuzzy numbers are computed via Negoita and Ralescu's Representation
Theorem (Theorem 1.4) over the resulting α-levels.

Another way to subtract is similar to the arithmetic for random variables, that is,
the subtractions between fuzzy numbers are obtained using the joint possibility (or
membership) distribution between the involved fuzzy numbers [5]. The comparison
between the results obtained from the two approaches (interval-valued and joint
possibility distribution) is made via a kind of Nguyen extension theorem [5].

The following concepts are from possibility theory and will be used to define the
interactive difference between fuzzy numbers [5]. Some these concepts have been
presented in Chap. 4.

Definition 11.1 Let A and B be fuzzy numbers and $J \in \mathcal{F}_C(\mathbb{R}^2)$, the class of fuzzy
normal subsets of $\mathbb{R}^2$. Then J is a joint possibility distribution of A and B if

$$\max_{y \in \mathbb{R}} \varphi_J(x, y) = \varphi_A(x) \quad \text{and} \quad \max_{x \in \mathbb{R}} \varphi_J(x, y) = \varphi_B(y).$$

Moreover, φ_A and φ_B are called marginal distributions of J.

If the joint possibility distribution is given by a t-norm $\triangle$, then

$$\varphi_J(x, y) = (\varphi_A(x)\triangle\varphi_B(y)).$$

When $\triangle = \min$, A and B are called non-interactive fuzzy numbers. The results of this section may be considered as a generalization of Zadeh's extension for fuzzy arithmetic which is a particular case of what is presented when the t-norm is the minimum norm. The next definition describes a joint possibility distribution which is not given by means of t-norm.

Definition 11.2 Two fuzzy numbers A and B are said to be completely correlated if there are $q, r \in \mathbb{R}$, with $q \neq 0$, such that their joint possibility distribution C is defined by

$$\begin{aligned}
\varphi_C(x, y) &= \varphi_A(x)\mathcal{X}_{\{qx+r=y\}}(x, y) \\
&= \varphi_B(y)\mathcal{X}_{\{qx+r=y\}}(x, y)
\end{aligned} \tag{11.1}$$

where

$$\mathcal{X}_{\{qx+r=y\}}(x, y) = \begin{cases} 1 & \text{if } qx + r = y \\ 0 & \text{if } qx + r \neq y \end{cases}$$

is the membership function on the real line $\{(x, y) \in \mathbb{R}^2 : qx + r = y\}$.

We have, in this case:

$$[C]^\alpha = \{(x, qx + r) \in \mathbb{R}^2 : x = (1 - s)a_1^\alpha + sa_2^\alpha, s \in [0, 1]\}$$

where $[A]^\alpha = [a_1^\alpha, a_2^\alpha]; [B]^\alpha = q[A]^\alpha + r$, for any $\alpha \in [0, 1]$. Moreover, if as $q \neq 0$,

$$\varphi_B(x) = \varphi_A\left(\frac{x - r}{q}\right), \forall x \in \mathbb{R}.$$

It is important to observe that some pairs of fuzzy numbers cannot be completely correlated. For example, a triangular fuzzy number can not be completely correlated with a trapezoidal fuzzy number. Recently, we presented a family of parametrized joint possibility distributions which extend the properties of completely fuzzy number [6, 7].

In Definition 11.2, if q is positive (negative), the fuzzy numbers A and B are said to be completely positively (negatively) correlated. If $[B]^\alpha = q[A]^\alpha + r$, the correlated addition of A and B is the fuzzy number $A + B$ with α-cuts

$$[A + B]^\alpha = (q + 1)[A]^\alpha + r. \tag{11.2}$$

We will formulate the extension principle in what follows for the joint possibility distribution of fuzzy numbers [5].

Definition 11.3 Let J be a joint possibility distribution with marginal possibility distributions φ_A and φ_B, and let $f : \mathbb{R}^2 \longrightarrow \mathbb{R}$ be a function. Then the extension f_J of f by J at pair (A, B) is the fuzzy set $f_J(A, B)$ whose membership function is given by

$$\varphi_{f_J(A,B)}(z) = \begin{cases} \sup_{z=f(x,y)} \varphi_J(x, y) & \text{if } f^{-1}(z) \neq \emptyset \\ 0 & \text{if } f^{-1}(z) = \emptyset \end{cases}$$

where $f^{-1}(z) = \{(x, y) : f(x, y) = z\}$.

The next result can be viewed as a generalization of Nguyen's theorem [8].

Theorem 11.1 ([5]) *Let $A, B \in \mathcal{F}(\mathbb{R})$ be completely correlated fuzzy numbers, C its joint possibility distribution and $f : \mathbb{R}^2 \longrightarrow \mathbb{R}$ a continuous function. Then,*

$$[f_C(A, B)]^\alpha = f([C]^\alpha), \forall \alpha \in [0, 1].$$

11.1.1   Difference Between Fuzzy Numbers

Next we present different ways, as found in literature, to obtain the difference between fuzzy numbers.

Difference Via Interval Analytic Theory

Initially we present the fuzzy differences arising from the interval analysis theory.

Definition 11.4 (*Standard difference*) Let A, B be fuzzy numbers with α-levels given by $[a_1^\alpha, a_2^\alpha]$ and $[b_1^\alpha, b_2^\alpha]$, respectively. The α-levels of the standard difference, $A - B$, are defined by

$$[A - B]^\alpha = [a_1^\alpha - b_2^\alpha, a_2^\alpha - b_1^\alpha].$$

This standard difference can also be called Minkowski difference and it coincides to the one introduced in Proposition 2.5.

Lodwick [4, 9] proposed constraint interval arithmetic (CIA) and in particular subtraction is defined as follows.

Definition 11.5 (*CIA*) The subtraction between two fuzzy numbers A and B is defined level-wise by

$$[A -_{\text{CIA}} B]^\alpha = \{[(1 - \lambda_A)a_1^\alpha + \lambda_A a_2^\alpha] - [(1 - \lambda_B)b_1^\alpha + \lambda_B b_2^\alpha], \\ 0 \leq \lambda_A \leq 1, 0 \leq \lambda_B \leq 1\}.$$

Remark 11.2 Using CIA, we have

$$[A -_{\text{CIA}} A]^\alpha =$$

$$\{[(1 - \lambda_A)a_1^\alpha + \lambda_A a_2^\alpha] - [(1 - \lambda_A)a_1^\alpha + \lambda_A a_2^\alpha]\} = \{0\}$$

where $0 \le \lambda_A \le 1$. Therefore, $A -_{\text{CIA}} A = \{0\}$.

Definition 11.6 Given two fuzzy numbers A, B the Hukuhara difference (H-difference) $A \ominus_H B = C$ is the fuzzy number C such that $A = B + C$, if it exists.

Note that the above definition was presented in Chap. 2 (see Definition 2.9).

Definition 11.7 ([1, 2]) Given two fuzzy numbers A, B the generalized Hukuhara difference (gH-difference) $A \ominus_{gH} B$ is the fuzzy number C (if it exists) such that in this case we write $A \ominus_{gH} B = C$.

$$\begin{cases} (i) \quad A = B + C \quad \text{or} \\ (ii) \ B = A - C. \end{cases}$$

Definition 11.8 ([1, 3]) Given two fuzzy numbers A, B the generalized difference (g-difference) $A \ominus_g B = C$ is the fuzzy number C with α-levels

$$[A \ominus_g B]^\alpha = \text{cl} \bigcup_{\beta \ge \alpha} ([A]^\beta \ominus_{gH} [B]^\beta), \forall \alpha \in [0, 1],$$

where the gH-difference $(\ominus_{gH})$ is related to the intervals $[A]^\beta$ and $[B]^\beta$.

Bede and Stefanini [1, 3] proposed the generalized difference between fuzzy numbers as a difference that always exists and results in a fuzzy number. But for this, as observed in [10], a convexification is required in order that the difference is always a fuzzy number. For each of the differences presented in this subsection, $A - B$ is a fuzzy number according to Theorem 1.4.

Differences Via Joint Possibility Distribution

Differences via joint possibility distribution are obtained with the help of Definition 11.3. Note that this form of dealing with fuzzy numbers is inspired by the arithmetic of random variables, which considers the joint probability distribution.

Definition 11.9 Suppose A and B are two fuzzy numbers. Let $f : \mathbb{R}^2 \to \mathbb{R}$ be defined by $f(x, y) = x - y$, that is, the subtraction operator for real numbers. The difference using the joint distribution J is the fuzzy number $A -_J B$, whose membership function is defined by

$$\varphi_{(A-_J B)}(z) = \sup_{(x,y) \in f^{-1}(z)} \varphi_J(x, y), \tag{11.3}$$

where $f^{-1}(z) = \{(x, y) : f(x, y) = x - y = z\}$.

Next the difference using the joint possibility distribution is given via t-norms.

Definition 11.10 (Differences via the t-norm) Let A, B be fuzzy numbers and $f(x, y) = x - y$ the subtraction operator, then the extension sup $-T$ of the fuzzy number $A -_\triangle B$ is obtained by the following membership function

$$\varphi_{A -_\triangle B}(z) = \sup_{(x,y) \in f^{-1}(z)} (\varphi_A(x) \triangle \varphi_B(y)), \ z \in \mathbb{R}.$$

where $f^{-1}(z) = \{(x, y) : f(x, y) = x - y = z\}$.

Note that Definition 2.9 (c) arises when $\triangle$ is the minimum t-norm. Moreover, the difference using joint possibility distributions may not necessarily be given by a t-norm.

Definition 11.11 ([5]) The subtraction of two completely correlated fuzzy numbers A and B is defined by

$$\varphi_{A -_c B}(z) = \sup_{(x,y) \in f^{-1}(z)} \varphi_C(x, y).$$

That is, $\varphi_{A -_c B}(z) = \sup\limits_{z = x - y} \varphi_B(y) \mathcal{X}_{\{qx + r = y\}}(x, y)$.

From Theorem 11.1, [5], we have that, for all $\alpha \in [0, 1]$,

$$[A -_c B]^\alpha = (q - 1)[B]^\alpha + r.$$

Remark 11.3 The sum of two completely correlated fuzzy numbers A and B is the fuzzy number $A +_c B$ which α-levels are given by

$$[A +_c B]^\alpha = (q + 1)[B]^\alpha + r.$$

Definition 11.12 Let C be a joint possibility distribution with marginal possibility distributions A and B, and let $f : \mathbb{R}^2 \longrightarrow \mathbb{R}^2$ be a function. If A and B are completely correlated fuzzy numbers, then the extension of f applied to (A, B) is the fuzzy set $f_c(A, B)$ whose membership function is defined by

$$\varphi_{f_C(A,B)}(u, v) = \begin{cases} \sup\limits_{(x,y) \in f^{-1}(u,v)} \varphi_c(x, y), & \text{if } f^{-1}(u, v) \neq \emptyset \\ \\ 0 & , \text{ if } f^{-1}(u, v) = \emptyset, \end{cases}$$

where $f^{-1}(u, v) = \{(x, y) : f(x, y) = (u, v)\}$.

The next theorem will be used to study the solution of an epidemiological model (SI) where S and I is considered completely correlated.

Theorem 11.4 *Let $A, B \in \mathcal{F}(\mathbb{R})$ be completely correlated fuzzy numbers, let C be their joint possibility distribution, and let $f : \mathbb{R}^2 \longrightarrow \mathbb{R}^2$ be a continuous function. Then,*

$$[f_c(A, B)]^\alpha = f([C]^\alpha).$$

The proof of the Theorem 11.4 is found in [11]. We end this section by recalling that the interactive difference can be used to define derivative for autocorrelated fuzzy process (see [12, 13]).

11.2 Prey-Predator

The study presented in this section is based on [14, 15]. The classical models of interaction between species of prey-predator type uses the hypothesis that the predation rates are related to the probability of encounters between a predator and a prey. A typical case is in the Lotka-Volterra model below, already seen in Sect. 9.3,

$$\begin{cases} \frac{dx}{dt} = ax - bxy \\ \frac{dy}{dt} = -cy + dxy \end{cases}, \tag{11.4}$$

where x and y are, respectively, the number (or density) of prey and predators, $a > 0$ is the growth rate of prey, $c > 0$ is the mortality rate of predators, $b > 0$ is the proportion of successful attacks of the predators and $d > 0$ is the biomass conversion rate of the prey to predators.

This model supposes that both of species are uniformly distributed in the habitat and this is implicit in the terms bxy and dxy which are proportional to the probability of the number of encounters between prey and predators. In other words, we can say that the rate of encounters is derived from the "mass action law" that in the context of physicochemical establishes that the rates of molecular collisions of two chemicals and is proportional to the product of their concentrations [16].

On the other hand, we know that if the habitat where the prey and predators are living together is small, that is the area in which the two populations exist is small, the predation happens immediately, because there are enough prey. Therefore it is possible that if the number of prey is bigger than the number of predators, the predation rate is proportional to just the number of predators. Now, if the number of predators is bigger than the prey, then the predation rate is given by the number of prey. So, in both cases the predation rate is proportional to the minimum between the populations of prey and predators [17, 18]. These observations translate into various t-norms operations, more specifically, other t-norms besides the product t-norm which is commonly used in models to represent the interaction between species. The more detailed analysis of this situation is found in Sect. 9.3.

11.2.1   Prey-Predator with the Minimum t-Norm

These observations and those found in [17] lead us to consider the predation rate
as proportional to the minimum between the populations of prey and predators. To
model this situation, we change the t-norm of the product to the minimum $t - norm$
to represent the interaction between species. Thus, we have the following model
[14, 15]:

$$\begin{cases} \frac{dx}{dt} = ax - b(x \wedge y) \\ \frac{dy}{dt} = -cy + d(x \wedge y) \end{cases}, \tag{11.5}$$

where a, b, c and d are the same as in (11.4).

The phase plane of the model (11.5) can be seen in the Fig. 11.1. From (11.5)
it is possible to see that the only equilibrium point is the trivial one $(0, 0)$. But the
qualitative aspect of phase plane of (11.5) is very different to that of the one in
Sect. 9.3.

11.2.2   Prey-Predator with the Hamacher t-Norm

The Hamacher t-norm (see Chap. 4), given by

$$\nabla_H (x, y) = \frac{xy}{p + (1 - p)(x + y - xy)}, \quad p \geq 0 \tag{11.6}$$

and it can replace the product t-norm in the prey-predator model (11.4). The parameter p can be tunned in order to fit the specific character of the population under
consideration. The various t-norms are obtained by a parameter p where the product
t-norm occurs for $p = 1$. Thus, we have the following model

Fig. 11.1 Phase plane of the
model (11.5) where
$a = 0.08, b = 0.09,$
$c = 0.075$ and $d = 0.07$

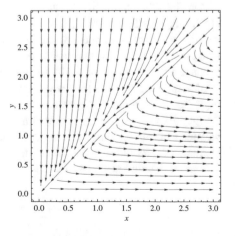

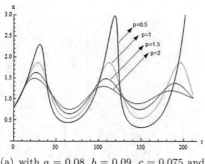

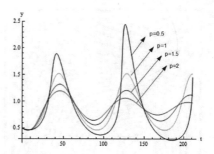

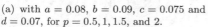

(a) with $a = 0.08$, $b = 0.09$, $c = 0.075$ and $d = 0.07$, for $p = 0.5, 1, 1.5$, and 2.

(b) with $a = 0.08$, $b = 0.09$, $c = 0.075$ and $d = 0.07$, for $p = 0.5, 1, 1.5$, and 2.

Fig. 11.2 Solution x and y for time t

$$\begin{cases} \frac{dx}{dt} = ax - \frac{bxy}{p+(1-p)(x+y-xy)} \\ \frac{dy}{dt} = -cy + \frac{dxy}{p+(1-p)(x+y-xy)} \end{cases}, \tag{11.7}$$

where a, b, c and d are the same as in (11.4). Figure 11.2a, b illustrate solutions of model (11.7) for some values of p.

It is interesting to note that the peaks of the solutions in Fig. 11.2a, b increase as p gets bigger. In cases where $p > 1$, the solutions go together to an equilibrium point, which differs from the classical case ($p = 1$), where there exists a periodic curve [15, 16].

Figures 11.3a up to 11.4b show the phase plane of the solutions of the model (11.7) for values of $p = 0.5, 1.0, 1.5, 2.0$. It is possible to observe that for $0 \le p < 1$ we

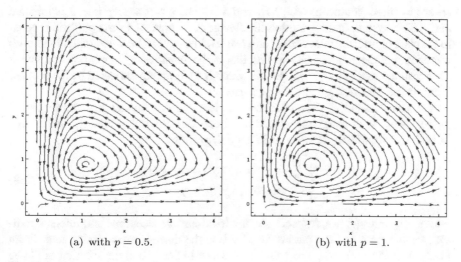

(a) with $p = 0.5$.

(b) with $p = 1$.

Fig. 11.3 Phase plane of the solution with parameters like Fig. 11.2a

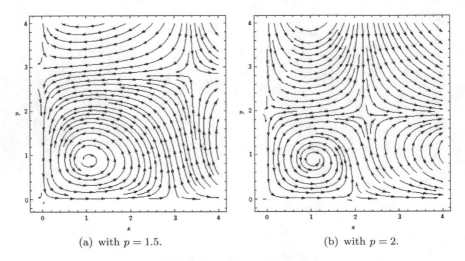

(a) with $p = 1.5$.   (b) with $p = 2$.

Fig. 11.4 Phase plane of the solution with parameters like Fig. 11.2a

have repelling equilibrium points, for $p = 1$ we have closed orbits around the equilibrium point and for $p > 1$ we have attractors equilibrium points and saddle points. Therefore, the choice of the parameter p will determine the stability of the system equilibrium (11.7).

11.3 Epidemiological Model

The more common epidemiological models that describe the dynamics of diseases spread by direct contact are SI, SIS and SIR where S is susceptible, I is infected and R is recovered. In these models the change of the state of a susceptible individual to the class of infected ones occurs as a result of the contact between individuals with infectious pathogens and healthy ones, that is, the transmission rate is proportional to the encounter rate of those individuals which is traditionally modeled by the product between the densities (quantities) [16, 19].

We have studied in Sect. 10.2 the simplest classical model that describes the dynamics of the diseases transmitted by direct contact without vital dynamics, that is, without birth/death. This is the SI model, given by

$$\begin{cases} \frac{dx}{dt} = -\beta xy; \quad x(0) = x_0 > 0 \\ \frac{dy}{dt} = \beta xy; \quad y(0) = y_0 > 0, \end{cases} \tag{11.8}$$

where $x(t)$ and $y(t)$ are, respectively, the fractions of susceptible and infected individuals at time t and the parameter $\beta > 0$ is the disease transmission rate. From (11.8) we have $x(t) + y(t) = 1$ and, as we saw in Sect. 10.2, the solution of (11.8) is given by

$$y(t) = \frac{y_0 e^{\beta t}}{x_0 + y_0 e^{\beta t}} \quad \text{and} \quad x(t) = 1 - y(t) = \frac{x_0}{x_0 + y_0 e^{\beta t}}. \tag{11.9}$$

In some epidemiological SI models, an individual who is infected can not recover. A typical case of this model is HIV, where the virus attacks the immune system which is responsible for protecting the body against diseases. For more details the reader might want to see [20].

One of the first models developed for populations of individuals that already have HIV is due to Anderson et al. [21]. The Anderson model studies the transfer between the individuals that are asymptomatic to the symptomatic ones, that is, it is not a direct transmission model [22]. This model is given by

$$\begin{cases} \dfrac{dx}{dt} = -\lambda x; \quad x(0) = x_0 > 0 \\ \dfrac{dy}{dt} = \lambda x; \quad y(0) = y_0 > 0, \end{cases} \tag{11.10}$$

where λ is the transfer rate from the asymptomatic to symptomatic phase (AIDS), $x(t)$ and $y(t)$ are, respectively, the fractions of infected individuals who did not develop AIDS and the others who did develop the disease. According to the model above we have the constraint

$$x(t) + y(t) = 1, \qquad \forall t \geq 0.$$

The solution of (11.10) is given by

$$x(t) = x_0 e^{-\lambda t} \quad \text{and} \quad y(t) = 1 - x_0 e^{-\lambda t}. \tag{11.11}$$

In (11.10) the dynamics of the disease is not modeled by the product operation. Since all individuals are already infected, the transmission does not depend on the encounter between them. Epidemiological modelers frequently discuss how to handle these types of models in which infections are not always transmitted by are interaction between a product-like accumulation of two populations (infected and susceptible).

Apparently the models (11.8) and (11.10) are not linked. However we will see that this is not one hundred percent true when different t-norms are used instead of the product.

11.3.1 SI Model with Minimum t-Norm

We base this section on [17, 23] where the model we have chosen uses the minimum t-norm, instead of product operation. This is because, when the susceptive population is small, its variation rate is proportional to susceptive population. On the other hand, the variation rate of infected population is proportional to this population when it is small. Thus, in both cases, the variation rate is proportional to the minimum between susceptive and infected population.

The model is given by the following differential equations [14, 15],

$$\begin{cases} \frac{dx}{dt} = -\lambda(x \wedge y) \\ \frac{dy}{dt} = \lambda(x \wedge y) \end{cases}. \tag{11.12}$$

The solution of (11.12) is given by

$$x(t) = \begin{cases} 1 - y_0 e^{\lambda t} & \text{if } t \leq \bar{t} \\ 0.5 e^{-\lambda(t-\bar{t})} & \text{if } t > \bar{t} \end{cases} \tag{11.13}$$

and

$$y(t) = \begin{cases} y_0 e^{\lambda t} & \text{if } t \leq \bar{t} \\ 1 - 0.5 e^{-\lambda(t-\bar{t})} & \text{if } t > \bar{t} \end{cases}, \tag{11.14}$$

where $\bar{t} = \frac{1}{\lambda} \ln \frac{0.5}{y_0}$. The model (11.10) coincides with (11.12) when the individuals of population interact and the majority is already symptomatic, that is, $(x \wedge y) = x$.

Illustrations of the solutions (11.13) and (11.14) can be seen in Fig. 11.5a and b, respectively. It is possible to verify the similarity between the curves that represent the proportion of infected individuals in this section to those in Sect. 10.2.

11.3.2 SI Model with Hamacher t-Norm

We will next use the t-norm of Hamacher, which is given by

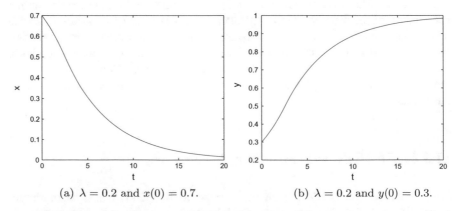

(a) $\lambda = 0.2$ and $x(0) = 0.7$. (b) $\lambda = 0.2$ and $y(0) = 0.3$.

Fig. 11.5 Proportion of susceptible and infected individuals versus time

$$\nabla_H (x, y) = \frac{xy}{p + (1 - p)(x + y - xy)},\tag{11.15}$$

to model the interaction between the individuals. Thus, we have

$$\begin{cases} \frac{dx}{dt} = \frac{-\lambda xy}{p+(1-p)(x+y-xy)} \\ \frac{dy}{dt} = \frac{\lambda xy}{p+(1-p)(x+y-xy)} \end{cases}.\tag{11.16}$$

Since $x + y = 1$, that is, there is no vital dynamics, we have

$$\nabla_H(x, 1 - x) = \frac{x(1 - x)}{p + (1 - p)(1 - x(1 - x))}.$$

The implicit solution of (11.16) for the susceptible is given by

$$c_1 + \lambda t = (1 - p)x(t) - \ln(1 - x(t)) + \ln x(t)$$

while the infected ones follows from the equation

$$(p - 1 - c_1) + \lambda t = (p - 1)y(t) - \ln(1 - y(t)) + \ln y(t).$$

We next do a comparative study of the models (11.8) and (11.16). Let us suppose that in (11.16) the interaction is proportional to the product (xy). Thus, in (11.16) we can interpret $\beta = \frac{\lambda}{p+(1-p)(x+y-xy)}$ as the transfer rate from susceptible to infected class of individuals. In this case, the rate $\beta = \beta(x, y)$ depends on both concentrations of x and y. Therefore, the number of susceptible individuals is provided by (11.16) and is inferior to the one that is provided by (11.8) for $p < 1$, and superior for $p > 1$. The illustration of the solutions for some values of p can be seen in Fig. 11.6a and b.

We finish this section by observing that all model presented here are in fact classical ones, in the sense that both are differential equation and their solutions are deterministic.

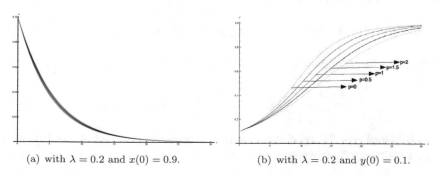

(a) with $\lambda = 0.2$ and $x(0) = 0.9$.   (b) with $\lambda = 0.2$ and $y(0) = 0.1$.

Fig. 11.6 Number of susceptible **a** and infected **b** versus time of the model (11.16)

11.4   Takagi–Sugeno Method to Study the Risk of Dengue

This section discusses concepts related to the formulation of models of Takagi–Sugeno and an application will be presented for the analysis of the risk of dengue[1] in the southern region of Campinas. The city of Campinas, located in southeast region of Brazil in the state of São Paulo, experienced the largest epidemic of dengue in 2007, with 1089.4 registered cases per 100, 000 inhabitants. High rates of incidence of dengue have been reported in the south region of the city, leading researchers from the Faculty of Medical Sciences of the University of Campinas to initiate a study on the phenomenon and its possible causes [24, 25].

11.4.1   Takagi–Sugeno Model

Chapter 5 developed the theory of fuzzy inference processes of the Takagi–Sugeno-Kang type where the consequent of each rule is explicitly given by a function of the input values of this rule. Currently, researchers are using this idea to construct fuzzy rules whose consequences are differential equations, applied to different problems [26–28].

The formulation of Takagi–Sugeno model for the risk of dengue in the southern region of Campinas, that will be presented, is based on references [24, 25]. The following is a summary of the main concepts used by these authors.

Consider the nonlinear partial differential equation (PDE) problem,

$$\frac{\partial y(x, t)}{\partial t} = \kappa(y(x, t)) \frac{\partial^2 y(x, t)}{\partial x^2} + f(y(x, t)) + g(x)u(t) \tag{11.17}$$

for $0 \leq x \leq L$, $t > 0$ where $y(x, t)$ is the displacement, $\kappa(y(x, t)) \geq 0$ and $f(x, t)$ are nonlinear functions satisfying $\kappa(0) = 0$ and $f(0, 0) = 0$, $u(t)$ is the distribution of the control force and $g(x)$ is an influence function. The initial and boundary conditions are given by

$$y(0, t) = y(L, t) = 0, \quad y_x(0, t) = y_x(L, t) = 0 \text{ and } y(x, 0) = y_0(x) \tag{11.18}$$

In the fuzzy formulation of systems (11.17)–(11.18) we will set $u(t) = 0$, i.e.,

$$\frac{\partial y(x, t)}{\partial t} = \kappa(y(x, t)) \frac{\partial^2 y(x, t)}{\partial x^2} + f(y(x, t)). \tag{11.19}$$

A model of type Takagi–Sugeno is used to approximate equation (11.19) and it has the following fuzzy rules:

---

[1]Dengue is a mosquito borne disease that causes fever and in some cases death.

$$\text{Rule } i : \text{If } y(x,t) \text{ is } F_i, \text{ then}$$

$$\frac{\partial y(x,t)}{\partial t} = \kappa_i \frac{\partial^2 y(x,t)}{\partial x^2} + a_i y(x,t) \qquad (11.20)$$

where F_i are fuzzy sets, $\kappa_i \geq 0$, a_i are known constants for $i = 1, 2, \ldots, M$; and M is the number of rules.

Fuzzy rule i means that if the input variable $y(x,t)$ is locally represented by the fuzzy set F_i, then the non-linear partial differential equation (11.19) can be represented by the linear equation (11.20). The process of fuzzy inference is done as follows

$$\frac{\partial y(x,t)}{\partial t} = \sum_{i=1}^{M} \varphi_i(y(x,t)) \left[\kappa_i \frac{\partial^2 y(x,t)}{\partial x^2} + a_i y(x,t) \right], \qquad (11.21)$$

where

$$\varphi_i(y(x,t)) = \varphi_{F_i}(y(x,t)) / (\sum_{k=1}^{M} \varphi_{F_k}(y(x,t)))$$

is the membership degree of $y(x,t)$ belonging to F_i. The denominator of $\varphi_i(y(x,t))$ is only for normalization so that the total sum is

$$\sum_{k=1}^{M} \varphi_i(y(x,t))) = 1.$$

11.4.2 Dengue Risk Model

This section develops a model of the risk of dengue epidemic from the point of view spacial temporal dynamics for the southeast part of the city of Campinas, Brazil. With the collaboration of the Laboratory for Spacial Analysis of Epidemiological Data (epiGeo) researchers of University of Campinas [29], we obtained data that generated the initial risk map of dengue in the region studied as shown in Fig. 11.7.

The mesh adopted corresponds to a 40×40 grid which covers approximately $20\,\text{km} \times 20\,\text{km}$ of the region. Note that higher risks are associated with warm colors, that is, with reddish hues.

The researchers of epiGeo determined, from the initial data that gave rise to the map, the relative risk. The relative risk is given as the quotient between the probabilities of the exposed individual and of the control (not exposed individual) [25]. For example, if the risk is 2, then at that geographic location, the individuals have twice the risk of contracting the dengue disease than individuals not exposed to risk factors. From Fig. 11.7, the risk of dengue was classified as *Low*, *Medium* and *High* and membership functions were constructed as illustrated in Fig. 11.8.

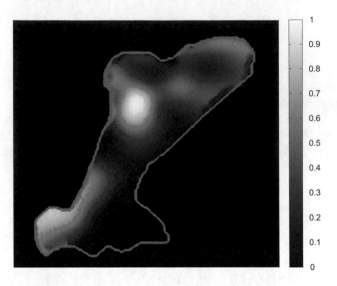

Fig. 11.7 Map of dengue risk developed by the epiGeo [25]

Fig. 11.8 Membership
functions for the risk of
dengue [25]

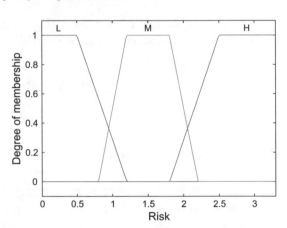

Let $r(x, y, t)$ be the risk of dengue. The fuzzy rules that were developed, using
the ideas presented by [26], were the following.

Rule 1 : If $r(x, y, t)$ is Low (L), then
$$\frac{\partial r(x, y, t)}{\partial t} = \kappa_B \left[\frac{\partial^2 r(x, y, t)}{\partial x^2} + \frac{\partial^2 r(x, y, t)}{\partial y^2} \right] + a_B r(x, y, t).$$

Rule 2 : If $r(x, y, t)$ is Medium (M), then

$$\frac{\partial r(x, y, t)}{\partial t} = \kappa_M \left[\frac{\partial^2 r(x, y, t)}{\partial x^2} + \frac{\partial^2 r(x, y, t)}{\partial y^2} \right] + a_M r(x, y, t).$$

Rule 3 : If $r(x, y, t)$ is High (H), then

$$\frac{\partial r(x, y, t)}{\partial t} = \kappa_A \left[\frac{\partial^2 r(x, y, t)}{\partial x^2} + \frac{\partial^2 r(x, y, t)}{\partial y^2} \right] + a_A r(x, y, t).$$

In this case ($M = 3$), and from (11.21) we have

$$\frac{\partial r(x, y, t)}{\partial t} = \sum_{i=1}^{M} \varphi_i(r(x, y, t)) \left[\kappa_i \left(\frac{\partial^2 r(x, y, t)}{\partial x^2} + \frac{\partial^2 r(x, y, t)}{\partial y^2} \right) + a_i r(x, t) \right].$$

(11.22)

The parameters κ_i in (11.22) represent the spatial distribution of risk for the given domain, that is, the associated geographical region.

A system based on fuzzy rules was constructed to find κ_i taking into account environmental factors that influence the dynamics of *Aedes aegypti* and the affect they have on the dispersion of risk. From this point of view, one might consider the dynamics of *Aedes aegypti* as environment fuzziness (see Chaps. 9 and 10). The input variables that affect the dynamics of *Aedes aegypti* are *rainfall, human inhabitants* and *mosquito breeding containers*. The membership functions adopted for the input variables can be found in [24, 25]. The membership functions constructed for the output variable κ_i are shown in Fig. 11.9. A stochastic model was constructed to determine the amount of rain, taking into account historical records provided by the Agronomic Institute of Campinas.

References [24, 25] contain the details of the procedures used to calculate the parameters a_i and the numerical methods to implement the equations.

Fig. 11.9 Membership functions for κ_i [25]

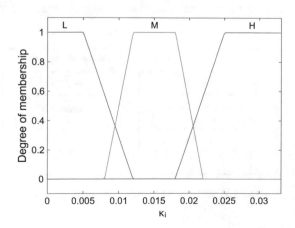

11.4.3 Simulations

We used MATLAB to implement computationally the PDE given in (11.22) and we coupled the MATLAB toolkit for stochastic systems and fuzzy logic to determine the parameters followed by their numerical methods solvers. The interested reader can find a detailed development in [24, 25].

The spatial discretization we chose was WENO-5 (weighted essentially non-oscillatory schemes) for the non-smooth regions of the map and CFDS-4 (centered finite difference scheme of fourth order) for the smooth regions of the map. The time discretization used Runge–Kutta TVD (Total Variation Diminishing). Figure 11.10 shows a representative scheme of our coupling.

Case 1

Simulations of the evolution of dengue risk over time were implemented for the months of December, January and February, corresponding to summer in the region. Figure 11.11 shows the results obtained.

These results show, in general, that there was a spread of the disease risk over the region. It is observed that there was a higher risk (red) of dengue that occurred in our simulation during the three months. We conclude that, for the summer months, the estimated values for the parameters κ_i and a_i in this simulation favored the spread of the risk of dengue in the southern region of Campinas.

Public health officials usually adopt measures to combat the *Aedes aegypti* mosquito breeding to decrease the incidence of dengue. So, the next simulation assumes a reduction of potential mosquito breeding sites available in the region and this is used in the fuzzy rules for κ_i, to see whether or not the model/simulation obtained a decreased risk of dengue.

The fuzzy rules were developed according to [26] and it was assumed $u(t) = 0$ in (11.17). The measure of control, which was the reduction of mosquito breeding sites, was inserted into the parameter estimation procedure κ_i through the system based on fuzzy rules. For a more comprehensive study, one could try to obtain a function $u(.)$ that takes into account other possible disease controls.

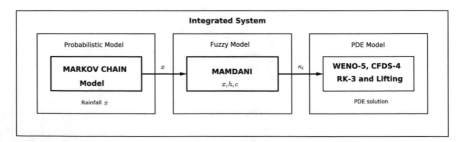

Fig. 11.10 Representative scheme of the coupling mathematical tools

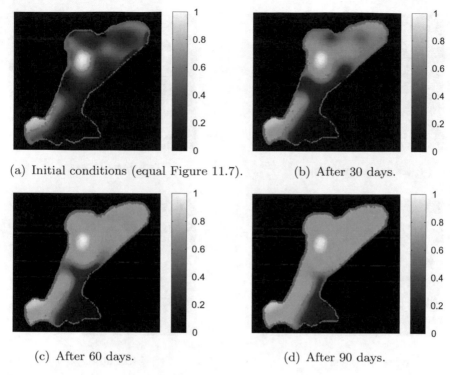

(a) Initial conditions (equal Figure 11.7).　　　(b) After 30 days.

(c) After 60 days.　　　　　　(d) After 90 days.

Fig. 11.11 Evolution of the risk of dengue [25]

Case 2

Suppose we have a reduction of 80 % in the number of mosquito breeding sites for *Aedes aegypti* in the region. Starting from the given initial conditions, we have the results illustrated in Fig. 11.12.

The figures show that after the first 30 days, there was reduction in the risk of dengue in virtually the entire region considered, indicating that a relatively important measure is to invest in a large reduction of sites available for the breeding of the dengue vector. However note that after 60 and 90 days, in the vicinity of the red regions, there was a growth and the spread of risk. This indicates that a public health policy needs to be one of continuing reduction of mosquito breeding sites.

11.4.4 Final Considerations

This section proposed a Takagi–Sugeno model to assess the risk of dengue in the southern region of Campinas. Preliminary studies regarding the risk of dengue in this region were conducted by researchers at EpiGeo Laboratory of the University

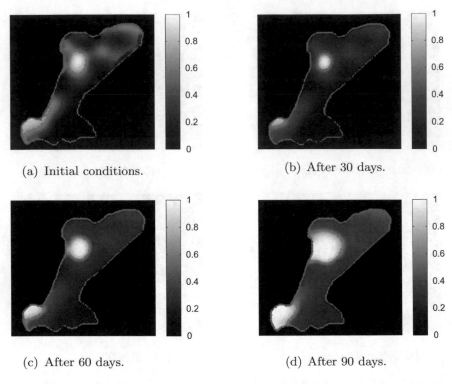

(a) Initial conditions.

(b) After 30 days.

(c) After 60 days.

(d) After 90 days.

Fig. 11.12 Evolution of the dengue risk [25]

of Campinas. Such information was the starting point for the proposed model. The model was comprised of rules where the consequences are PDEs. The inference combines such rules and the resulting equations are solved numerically by means of methods developed in [24].

We observe from the situation, that an effective measure to reduce the risk of dengue is to aggressively reduce the potential mosquito's, *Aedes aegypti*, breeding sites. For a more comprehensive study, one could try to obtain a function $u(t)$ that takes into account various possible disease controls such as genetically modified mosquitoes, house screens, and/or mosquito eating animals such as bats and swallows (birds).

11.5 The SI-model with Completely Correlated Initial Conditions

This section presents the SI epidemiological model by considering uncertain parameters modeled by completely correlated fuzzy numbers. More specifically we will analyze the model, via the extension principle that will account for the correlation among the variables. The initial conditions are given by interactive fuzzy numbers [11].

The SI-model, as we have already seen, is described by the system of differential equations

$$\begin{cases} \dfrac{dS}{dt} = -\beta SI, \quad S(0) = S_0 \\[2mm] \dfrac{dI}{dt} = \beta SI, \quad I(0) = I_0 > 0, \end{cases} \tag{11.23}$$

where $S(t)$ and $I(t)$ are, respectively, the fractions of susceptible and infected individuals at the time t. The parameter β is a positive constant representing the rate of contact of the disease.

Suppose that there is no variation in the total number of the population, that is, consider the model without vital dynamics,

$$S(t) + I(t) = 1, \qquad \forall t \geq 0. \tag{11.24}$$

Thus, we get for each $t \geq 0$, the deterministic solution of problem (11.23) given by

$$L_t(S_0, I_0) = \left(\frac{S_0}{S_0 + I_0 e^{\beta t}}, \frac{I_0 e^{\beta t}}{S_0 + I_0 e^{\beta t}} \right). \tag{11.25}$$

Now, consider system (11.23) where the initial conditions are uncertain and modeled by fuzzy numbers. Since $S_0 + I_0 = 1$, we are dealing with completely correlated fuzzy numbers where $r = 1$ and $q = -1$ which we explain next. According to Definition 11.2, $S_0 + I_0 = 1$ means that the joint possibility distribution C of S_0 and I_0 is such that

$$\varphi_C(s_0, i_0) = \varphi_{S_0}(s_0)\mathcal{X}_{\{s_0+i_0=1\}}(s_0, i_0) = \varphi_{I_0}(i_0)\mathcal{X}_{\{s_0+i_0=1\}}(s_0, i_0). \tag{11.26}$$

In this case, for each $\alpha \in [0, 1]$, we have

$$\varphi_{I_0}(i_0) = \varphi_{S_0}(1 - i_0), \quad [I_0]^\alpha = [a_1^\alpha, a_2^\alpha], \quad [S_0]^\alpha = (-1)[I_0]^\alpha + 1$$

and

$$[C]^\alpha = \{(1 - i_0, i_0) \in \mathbb{R}^2 : i_0 = (1 - \gamma)a_1^\alpha + \gamma a_2^\alpha, \gamma \in [0, 1]\}. \tag{11.27}$$

Thus, $S_0 + I_0 = 1$ implies $q = -1$ and $r = 1$.

Taking into consideration (11.27), and remembering the notions found in Sect. 8.1.3, Eq. (11.23) becomes

$$\begin{cases} \left(\dfrac{dS}{dt}, \dfrac{dI}{dt} \right) = \left(-\beta SI, \beta SI \right) \\[2mm] (S_0, I_0) \quad \in \quad C \end{cases}. \tag{11.28}$$

Solution of the Fuzzy SI-model Via Differential Inclusion

The solution to the Eq. (11.28) via fuzzy differential inclusion requires that we apply the method described in Sect. 8.1.3 of Chap. 8, so that the solution of the problem (11.28), using differential inclusion, is obtained from the solution of the auxiliary problem

$$
\begin{cases}
(\frac{dS}{dt}, \frac{dI}{dt}) = (-\beta SI, \beta SI) \\[2mm]
(S_0, I_0) \in \quad [C]^\alpha,
\end{cases}
\tag{11.29}
$$

where $[C]^\alpha$ is given by Eq. (11.27). The attainable sets of the problem (11.29) are given by

$$
\begin{aligned}
\mathcal{A}_t([C]^\alpha) &= \left\{ x(t, S_0, I_0) : x(., S_0, I_0) \text{ is solution of (11.29)} \right\} \\
&= \left\{ x(t, S_0, I_0) : x'(t, S_0, I_0) = (-\beta SI, \beta SI), \ (S_0, I_0) \in [C]^\alpha \right\} \\
&= \left\{ \left(\frac{s_0}{s_0 + i_0 e^{\beta t}}, \frac{i_0 e^{\beta t}}{s_0 + i_0 e^{\beta t}} \right) : (s_0, i_0) \in [C]^\alpha \right\} \\
&= \left\{ \left(\frac{1 - i_0}{(1 - i_0) + i_0 e^{\beta t}}, \frac{i_0 e^{\beta t}}{(1 - i_0) + i_0 e^{\beta t}} \right) : \right. \\
&\qquad\qquad \left. i_0 = (1 - \gamma) a_1^\alpha + \gamma a_2^\alpha, \gamma \in [0, 1] \right\}.
\end{aligned}
$$

Solution of the Fuzzy SI-model Via Extension Principle

We will study the fuzzy SI-model given by (11.28) using as a tool the extension principle via Definition 11.12 in (11.25). According to Theorem 11.4, the α-levels of the solution obtained by the extension principle of the problem (11.28) are given by the expression

$$
[(L_t)_C(S_0, I_0)]^\alpha = L_t([C]^\alpha).
$$

Therefore, the α-levels of the solution of the problem (11.28) are

$$
\begin{aligned}
[(L_t)_C(S_0, I_0)]^\alpha &= L_t([C]^\alpha) \\
&= \left\{ L_t(s_0, i_0) : (s_0, i_0) \in [C]^\alpha \right\} \\
&= \left\{ L_t(1 - i_0, i_0) : i_0 = (1 - \gamma) a_1^\alpha + \gamma a_2^\alpha, \gamma \in [0, 1] \right\} \\
&= \left\{ \left(\frac{1 - i_0}{(1 - i_0) + i_0 e^{\beta t}}, \frac{i_0 e^{\beta t}}{(1 - i_0) + i_0 e^{\beta t}} \right) : \right. \\
&\qquad\qquad \left. i_0 = (1 - \gamma) a_1^\alpha + \gamma a_2^\alpha, \gamma \in [0, 1] \right\}.
\end{aligned}
$$

That is, as predicted by Theorem 3.2 in [11], for every $t \geq 0$, the sets $(L_t)_C(S_0, I_0)$ and $\mathcal{A}_t(C)$ are identical.

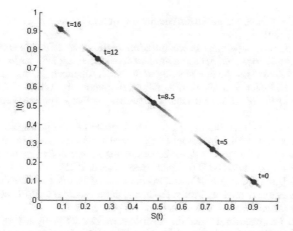

Fig. 11.13 Fuzzy solution to the problem (11.28) in the phase-portrait. The *dots* correspond to the deterministic solution for different values of time t. The initial conditions are the completely correlated triangular fuzzy numbers $I_0 = (0.05; 0.08; 0.11)$ and $S_0 = (0.89; 0.92; 0.95)$, with $S_0 + I_0 = 1$, and the contact rate is $\beta = 0.3$. Darker regions (for each $t \geq 0$) mean greater possibility (membership) of the number of susceptible and infected to the solution of the problem. The deterministic solution has membership degree equal to 1 in the fuzzy solution [11, 30]

Figure 11.13 represents the solution to the problem (11.28) employing the completely correlated triangular fuzzy numbers $I_0 = (0.05; 0.08; 0.11)$ and $S_0 = (0.89; 0.92; 0.95)$ as initial conditions, with $S_0 + I_0 = 1$ (according to Formula (11.3)) and contact rate $\beta = 0.3$. Note that the fact that the fuzzy numbers are completely correlated forces the solution to problem (11.28) to be a curve contained within the line $S + I = 1$, for each $t \geq 0$.

We conclude this study by commenting that the solutions $S(t)$ and $I(t)$, of a general epidemiological model are trajectories out of line $x + y = 1$ (see [16]). The deterministic solution of problem (11.23), belong to line $x + y = 1$ because we admit the correlation $S(t) + I(t) = 1$ for each $t \geq 0$. If bise this we admit that $S(t)$ and $I(t)$ are fuzzy numbers, then due $S(t) + I(t) = 1$, we have fuzzy numbers negatively completely correlated.

Acknowledgments The authors would like to acknowledge and thank the partial support received from CNPq.

References

1. L. Stefanini, A generalization of hukuhara difference and division for interval and fuzzy arithmetic. Fuzzy Sets Syst. **161**(11), 1564–1584 (2010)
2. L. Stefanini, B. Bede, Generalized hukuhara differentiability of interval-valued functions and interval differential equations. Nonlinear Anal. Theory, Methods Appl **71**(3–4), 1311–1328 (2009)

3. B. Bede, L. Stefanini, Generalized differentiability of fuzzy-valued functions. Fuzzy Sets Syst. **230**, 119–141 (2013)
4. W.A. Lodwick, E.A. Untiedt, *A comparison of interval analysis using constraint interval arithmetic and fuzzy interval analysis using gradual numbers*, Fuzzy Information Processing Society, 2008. NAFIPS 2008. Annual Meeting of the North American (2008), pp. 1–6
5. C. Carlsson, R. Fuller, P. Majlender, Additions of completely correlated fuzzy numbers, in *Proceedings of the IEEE International Conference on Fuzzy Systems, 2004* vol. 1 (2004), pp. 535–539
6. E. Esmi, G. Barroso, L.C. Barros, P. Sussner, A family of joint possibility distributions for adding interactive fuzzy numbers inspired by biomathematical models, in *2015 Conference of the International Fuzzy Systems Association and the European Society for Fuzzy Logic and Technology (IFSA-EUSFLAT-15)* (Atlantis Press, France, 2015)
7. P. Sussner, E. Esmi, L.C. Barros, Controlling the width of the sum of interactive fuzzy numbers with applications to fuzzy initial value problems, in *Proceedings in IEEE World Congress on Computational Intelligence* (2016). (accepted for publication)
8. H.T. Nguyen, On conditional possibility distributions. Fuzzy Sets Syst. **1**(4), 299–309 (1978)
9. W.A. Lodwick, Constrained interval arithmetic, Technical report (Denver, Colorado, 1999)
10. L.T. Gomes, L.C. Barros, A note on the generalized difference and the generalized differentiability. Fuzzy Sets Syst. **280**, 142–145 (2015)
11. V.M. Cabral, L.C. Barros, Fuzzy differential equation with completely correlated parameters. Fuzzy Sets Syst. **265**, 86–98 (2015)
12. L.C. Barros, F.S. Pedro, Fuzzy differential equations with interactive derivative, in *Fuzzy Sets and Systems* (2016). (accepted for publication)
13. E. Esmi, F.S. Pedro, L.C. Barros, W.A. Lodwick, *Fréchet derivative for linearly correlated fuzzy function* (2016). (submitted for publication)
14. F.S. Pedro, *Modelos matemáticos para dinâmica de doenças de transmissão direta e de presa-predador considerando parâmetros interativos e t-normas* (Dissertação de Mestrado, IMECC-UNICAMP, Campinas, 2013)
15. F.S. Pedro, L.C. Barros, The use of t-norms in mathematical models of epidemics, in *2013 IEEE International Conference on Fuzzy Systems (FUZZ)* (2013), pp. 1–4
16. L. Edelstein-Keshet, *Mathematical Models in Biology* (McGraw-Hill, México, 1988)
17. V. Kreinovich, O. Fuentes, *High-concentration Chemical Computing Techniques for Solving Hard-to-solve Problems, and their Relation to Numerical Optimization, Neural Computing, Reasoning Under Uncertainty, and Freedom of Choice* (Wiley-VCH Verlag GmbH and Co. KGaA, 2012), pp. 209–235
18. O. Kosheleva, V. Kreinovich, L.C. Barros, Chemical kinetics in situations intermediate between usual and high concentrations: fuzzy-motivated derivation of the formulas, in *Proceedings of the 2016 World Conference on Soft Computing* (Berkeley, California, 2016)
19. L.C. Barros, M.B.F. Leite, R.C. Bassanezi, The SI epidemiological models with a fuzzy transmission parameter. Int. J. Comput. Math. Appl. **45**, 1619–1628 (2003)
20. R.M. Jafelice, L.C. Barros, R.C. Bassanezi, F. Gomide, Fuzzy modeling in symptomatic HIV virus infected population. Bull. Math. Biol. **66**, 1597–1620 (2004)
21. R.M. Anderson, G.F. Medley, R.M. May, A.M. Johnson, A preliminaire study of the transmission dynamics of the human immunodeficiency virus (HIV), the causitive agent of AIDS. IMA J. Math. Med. Biol. **3**, 229–263 (1986)
22. J. Murray, *Mathematical Biology* (Springer, USA, 1990)
23. J.M. Baetens, B.D. Baets, Incorporating fuzziness in spatial susceptible-infected epidemic models, in *Proceedings of IFSA-EUSFLAT Conference on Cd-rom* (Lisbon, 2009)
24. G.P. Silveira, *Métodos numéricos integrados à lógica fuzzy e método estocástico para solução de edp's: uma aplicação à dengue*, Phd thesis, IMECC–UNICAMP, Campinas (2011). (in portuguese)
25. G.P. Silveira, L.C. Barros, Analysis of the dengue risk in a model of the kind takagi-sugeno. Fuzzy Sets Syst. **277**, 122–137 (2015)

26. B.S. Chen, Y.T. Chang, Fuzzy state-space modeling and robust observer-based control design for nonlinear partial differential systems. IEEE Trans. Fuzzy Syst. **17**(5), 1025–1043 (2009)
27. J.-W. Wang, H.-N. Wu, H.-X. Li, Distributed fuzzy control design of nonlinear hyperbolic pde systems with application to nonisothermal plug-flow reactor. IEEE Trans. Fuzzy Syst. **19**(3), 514–526 (2011)
28. H.-N. Wu, H.-X. Li, H_∞ fuzzy observer-based control for a class of nonlinear distributed parameter systems with control constraints. IEEE Trans. Fuzzy Syst. **16**(2), 502–516 (2008)
29. R. Cordeiro, M. Donalisio, V. Andrade, A. Mafra, L. Nucci, J. Brown, C. Stephan, *Spatial Distribution of the Risk of Dengue Fever in Southeast Brazil, 2006–2007*, vol. 11(1) (BMC Public Health, (2011), p. 355
30. V.M. Cabral, L.C. Barros, The SI epidemiological model withinteractive fuzzy parameters, in *2012 Annual meeting of the North American Fuzzy Information Processing Society (NAFIPS)* (IEEE, New York, 2012), pp. 1–4

Index

© Springer-Verlag Berlin Heidelberg 2017
L.C. de Barros et al., *A First Course in Fuzzy Logic, Fuzzy Dynamical Systems, and Biomathematics*, Studies in Fuzziness and Soft Computing 347, DOI 10.1007/978-3-662-53324-6

Printed in the United States
By Bookmasters